Dengue Fever in a One Health Perspective

Edited by Márcia Aparecida Sperança

Published in London, United Kingdom

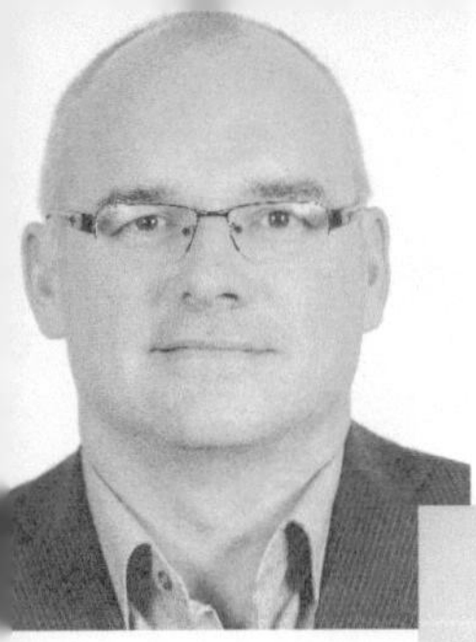
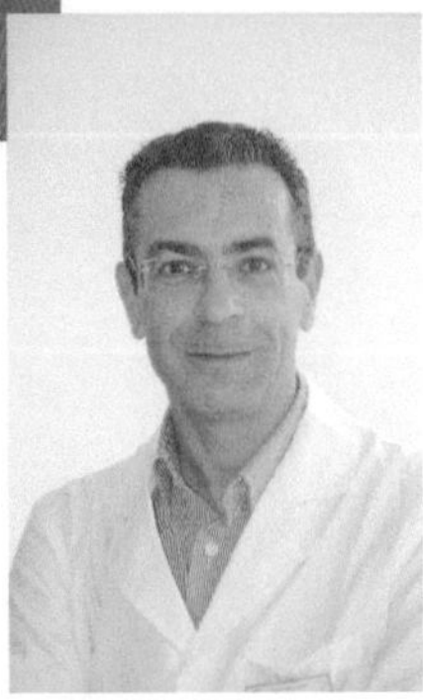
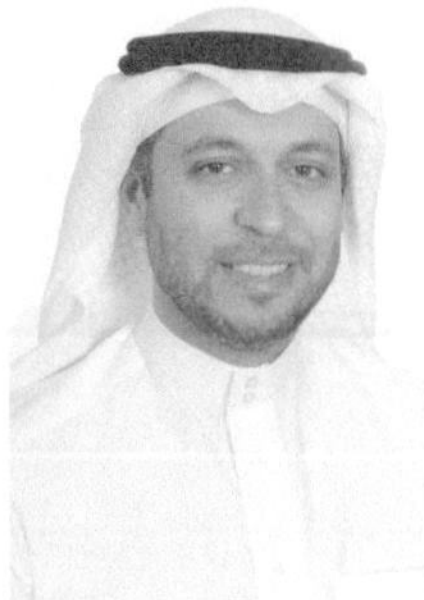
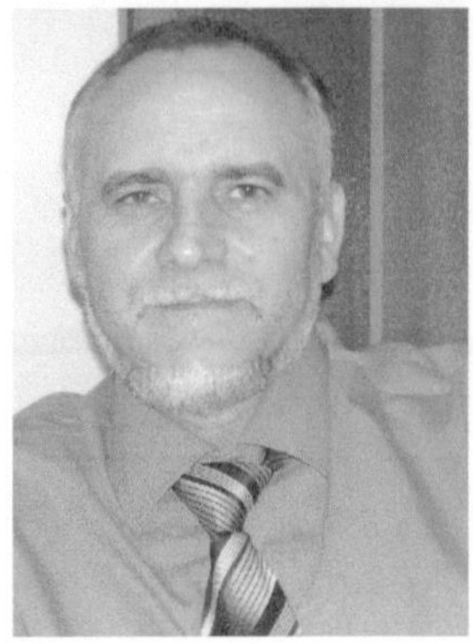
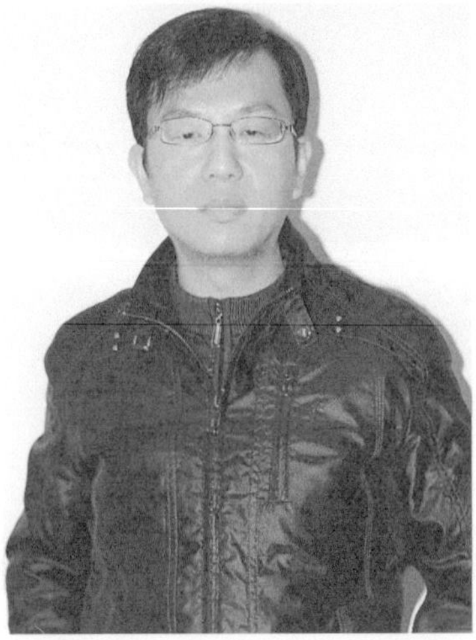
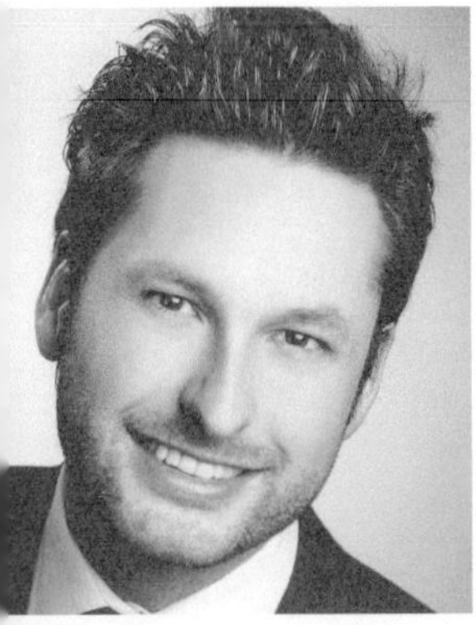
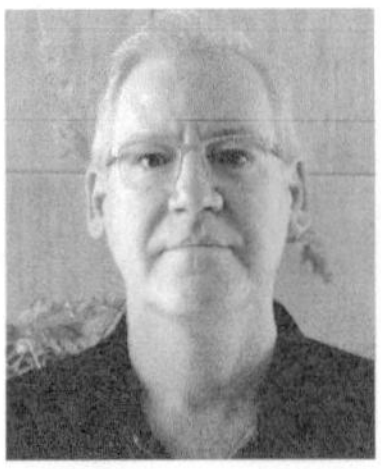

IntechOpen

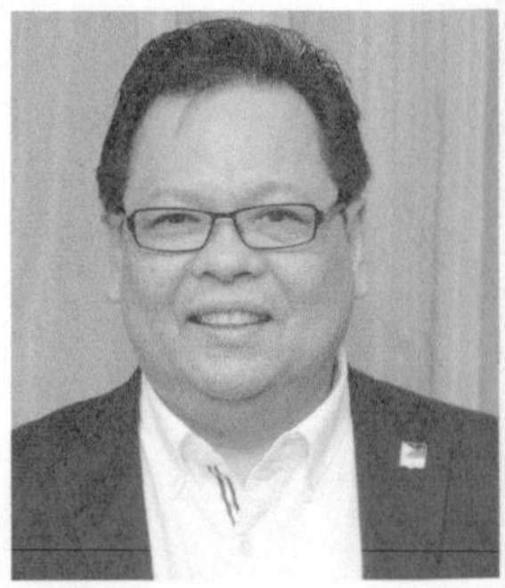
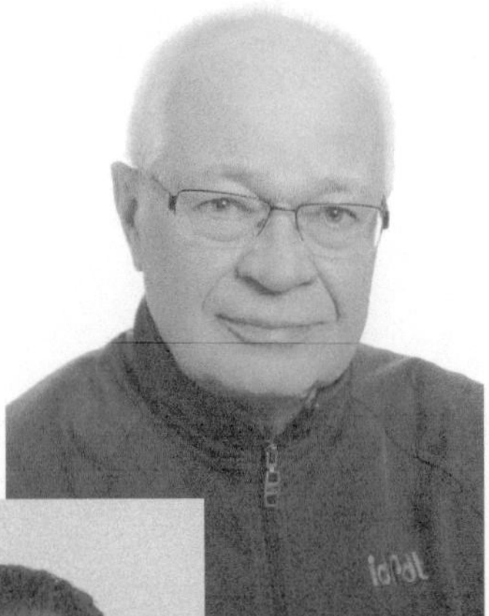
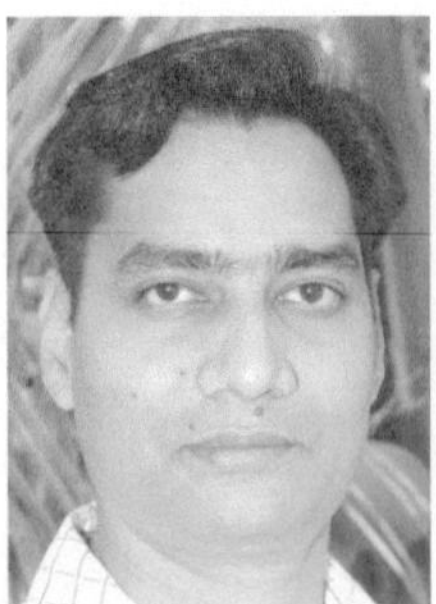
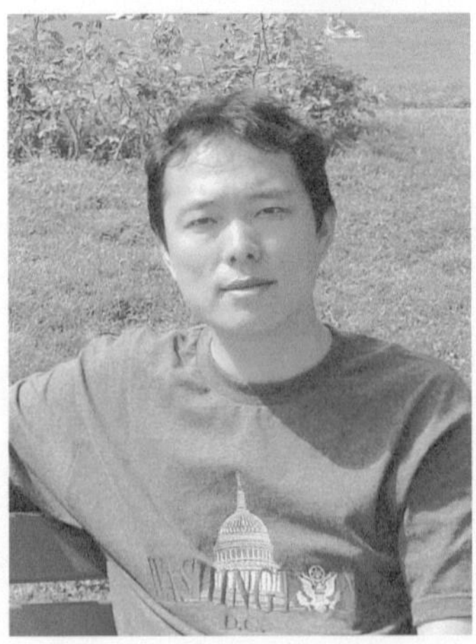
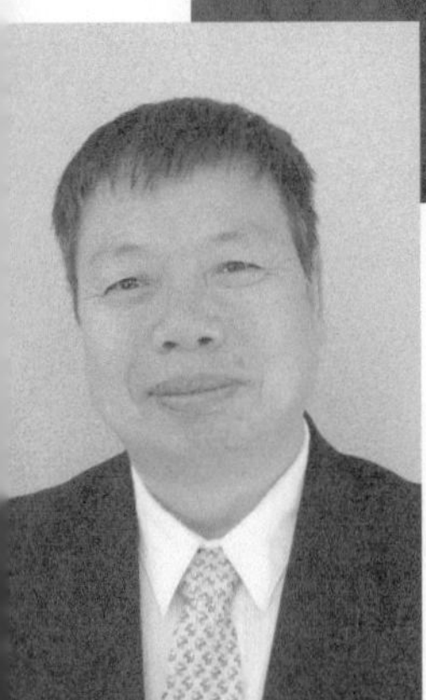
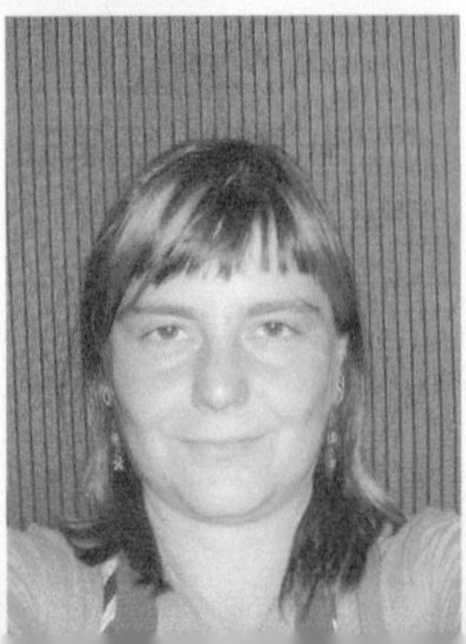

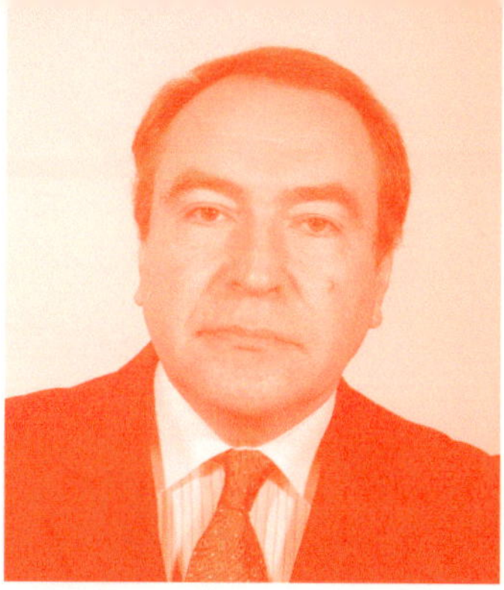
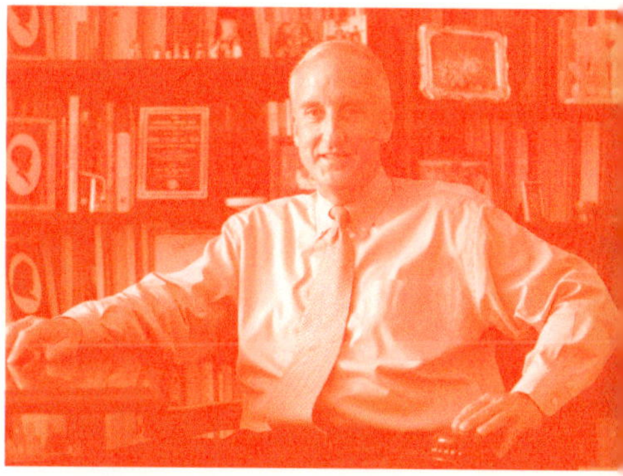
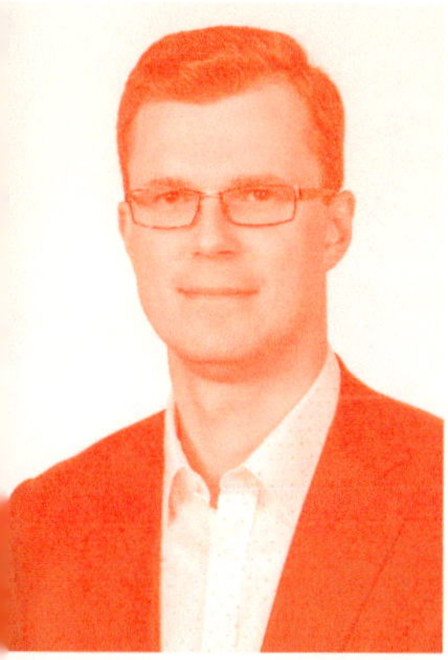
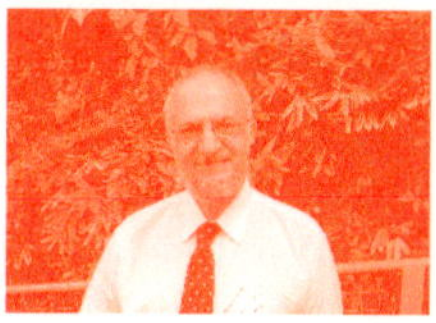
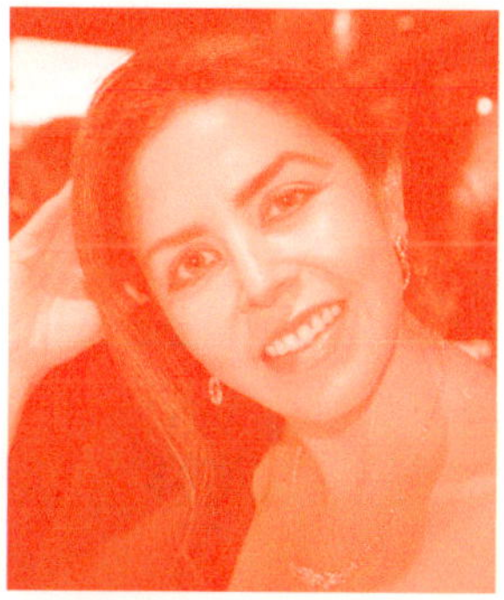

Supporting open minds since 2005

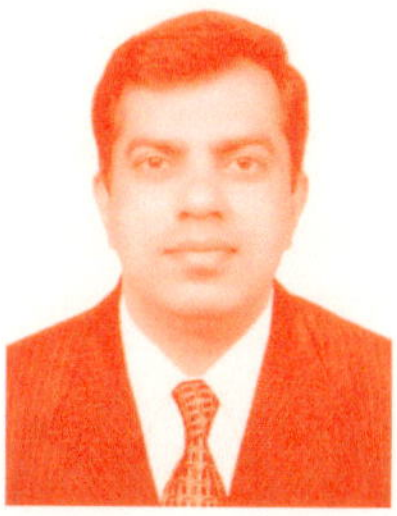
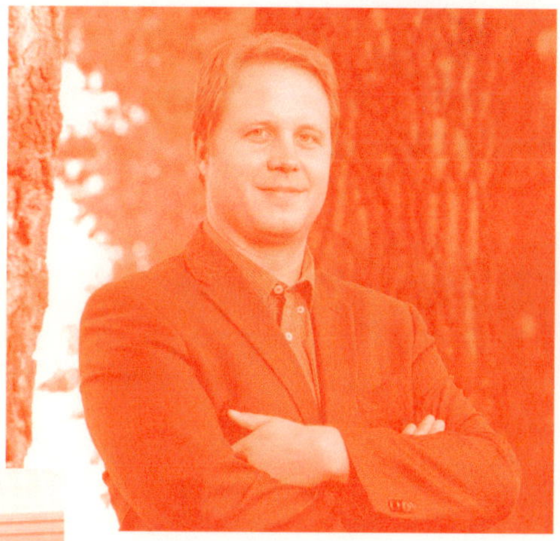
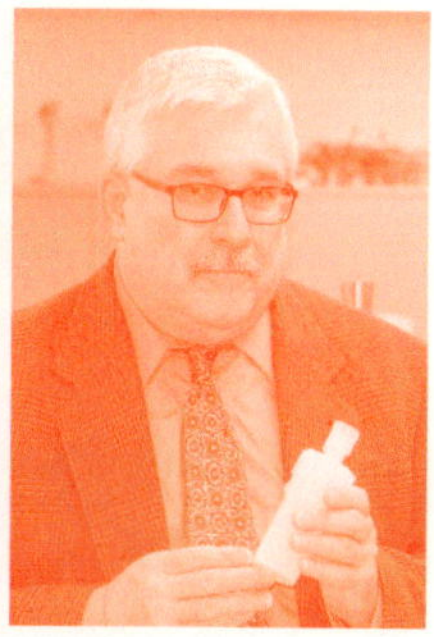
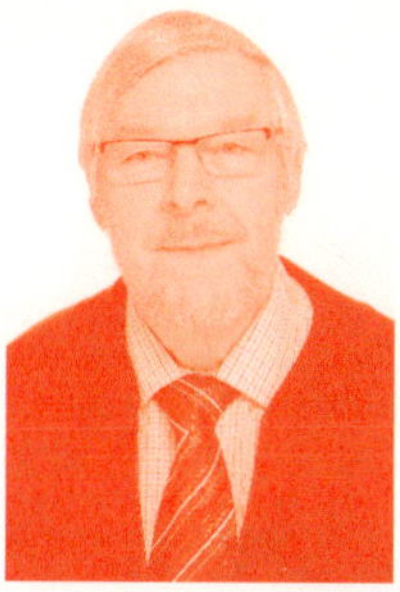
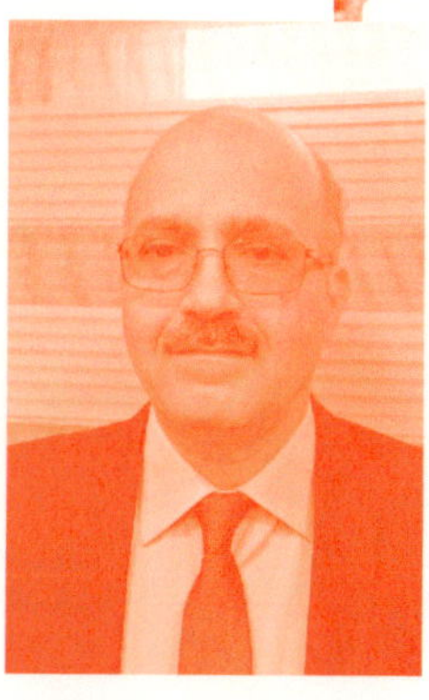
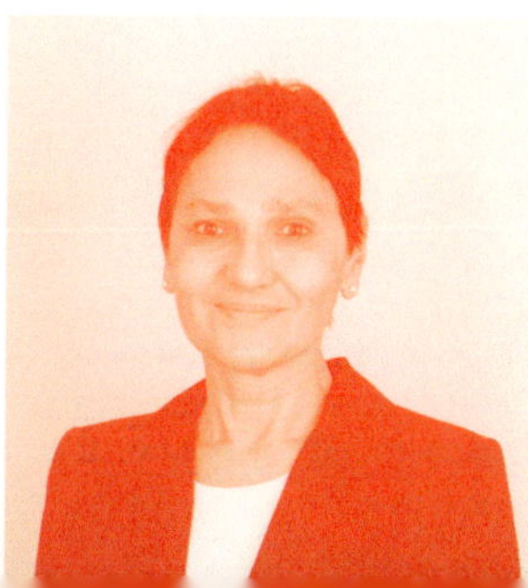
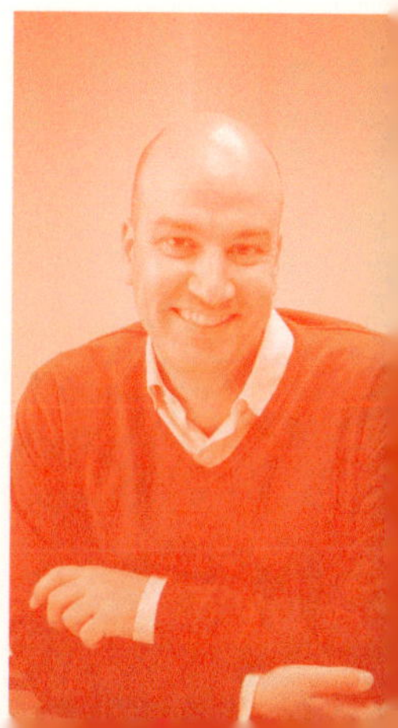

Dengue Fever in a One Health Perspective
http://dx.doi.org/10.5772/intechopen.87409
Edited by Márcia Aparecida Sperança

Part of IntechOpen Book Series: Infectious Diseases, Volume 7
Book Series Editor: Shailendra K. Saxena

Contributors
Samir Casseb, Karla Melo, Juan Samuel Sulca Herencia, Cristian Díaz-Vélez, Jorge Luis Fernández-Mogollon, John Alexis Cabrera-Enríquez, Stalin Tello Vera, Oscar Medrano-Velásquez, Elmer Córdova-Calle, Balasubramanian Arul, Ramalingam Kothai, Henry Puerta-Guardo, Eva Harris, Scott B. Biering, Norma Pavia Ruz, Gonzalo Vazquez-Prokopec, Pablo Manrique-Saide, Guadalupe Ayora-Talavera, Márcia Aparecida Sperança, Juliana Sá Teles De Oliveira Molina, Andreia Moreira Dos Santos Carmo, Gabriel Lopes Pereira, Leticia Abrantes Andrade, Felipe Trovalim Jordão, Rodrigo Buzinaro Suzuki, Luana Prado Rolim De Oliveira, Aline Diniz Cabral, Isaura Beatriz Borges Silva, Renato Kaylan Alves De Oliveira França, Jacyelle Medeiros Silva, Andrea Queiroz Maranhão, Carlos Roberto Prudencio

First published in London, United Kingdom, 2020 by IntechOpen
IntechOpen is the global imprint of INTECHOPEN LIMITED, registered in England and Wales, registration number: 11086078, 5 Princes Gate Court, London, SW7 2QJ, United Kingdom
Printed in Croatia

British Library Cataloguing-in-Publication Data
A catalogue record for this book is available from the British Library

Additional hard and PDF copies can be obtained from orders@intechopen.com

Dengue Fever in a One Health Perspective
Edited by Márcia Aparecida Sperança
p. cm.
Print ISBN 978-1-78985-202-8
Online ISBN 978-1-78985-649-1
eBook (PDF) ISBN 978-1-78985-650-7
ISSN 2631-6188

For EU product safety concerns:
IN TECH d.o.o., Prolaz Marije Krucifikse Kozulić 3, 51000 Rijeka, Croatia, info@intechopen.com or visit our website at intechopen.com.

IntechOpen Book Series

Infectious Diseases

Volume 7

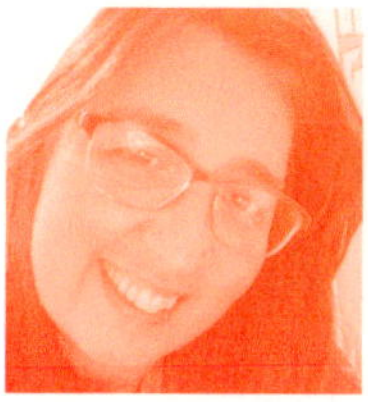

Márcia Aparecida Sperança is Associate Professor at the Center for Natural and Human Sciences of Universidade Federal do ABC (UFABC, São Bernardo do Campo, São Paulo, Brazil). After obtaining a PhD in Biology of Parasite–Host Interaction from the Parasitology Department of the Biomedical Institute of University of São Paulo (Brazil), Dr. Sperança worked as an assistant professor and researcher at Marilia Medical School (Marilia, São Paulo, Brazil). Her scientific experience is in diagnosis, molecular biology, and molecular epidemiology of different infectious agents including arboviruses, the bacteria *Helicobacter pylori*, malaria parasites, and trypanosomatids. Presently, Dr. Sperança is the head of the Laboratory of Pathogenic Agents at UFABC, an institution with multi and interdisciplinary academic proposals, which are characteristics of her investigation field.

Editor of Volume 7:
Márcia Aparecida Sperança
Universidade Federal do ABC - Center for Natural and Human Sciences,
São Paulo, Brazil

Book Series Editor:
Shailendra K. Saxena
King George's Medical University

Scope of the Series

The series will give a most comprehensive overview of recent trends in various infectious diseases (as per the most recent Baltimore classification), as well as general concepts of infections, immunopathology, diagnosis, treatment, epidemiology and etiology to current clinical recommendations in management of infectious diseases, highlighting the ongoing issues, recent advances, with future directions in diagnostic approaches and therapeutic strategies. This book series will focus on various aspects and properties of infectious diseases whose deep understanding is very important for safeguarding human race from more loss of resources and economies due to pathogens.

Contents

Preface

The One Health approach from the World Health Organization has emerged to translate the interrelationships between human, animal, and environmental health. Anthropogenic movements result in modifications of the wild natural habitat, such as the destruction of forest areas, the introduction of domestic animals, and the improvisation of sanitation conditions. Climate changes can affect and modulate pathogen epidemics by providing conditions for the proliferation of arthropod vectors of infectious diseases. In this scenario, dengue fever is the most important arthropod-borne disease worldwide.

The dengue virus (DENV) occurs in four different serotypes and is transmitted by mosquitoes from the genus *Aedes*, principally *Ae. aegypti* and *Ae. Albopictus*. The first section of the book contains chapters on general aspects of virus biology, epidemiology, transmission routes, natural history, and vector biology. Chapters 1 and 2 describe for the first time the role of *Aedes* species in the transmission cycle of DENV in different global regions, and Chapter 3 examines the role of environmental changes associated to proliferation of *Aedes* vectors.

The pathophysiologic characteristics of diseases caused by DENV infection is a result of the complex interaction of different virus serotypes and genotypes with the immune system of the human host. Chapters 4 and 5 in the second section of the book cover humoral and cellular immune responses associated to immunopathology caused by DENV infection. Knowledge of immune response to DENV is of major importance to development of a secure vaccine.

In the third section of the book, three different chapters describe how molecular biology tools can help in the establishment of new strategies for the study and management of epidemics caused by dengue viruses. Chapter 6 focuses on miRNA studies to investigate DENV replication, vector proliferation, and infection, bringing new possibilities to vector control strategies. Chapter 7 present an excellent review on phage display technologies and discusses its use in DENV diagnosis and drug therapy. Chapter 8 describes a simple method to extract RNA from single specimen of mosquitoes, contributing to new possibilities to explore arthropod vector biology.

This book contributes to the knowledge of different aspects of DENV biological interactions in the perspective of the One Health concept, inspiring a broad public, including undergraduate and post-graduate students, researchers from different knowledge areas, and health professionals, to reflect on global recurrent emergent and reemergent arthropod-borne diseases. I am grateful to all authors for their contributions and to IntechOpen for the opportunity to participate as editor of this book on an important global life-threatening disease.

Márcia Aparecida Sperança, PhD
Universidade Federal do ABC - Center for Natural and Human Sciences,
São Paulo, Brazil

Section 1

Biological and Environmental Aspects

Chapter 1

Dengue Fever: An Overview

Ramalingam Kothai and Balasubramanian Arul

Abstract

Dengue fever is a disease caused by a family of viruses transmitted by mosquitoes. Dengue virus (DENV), a member of the *Flaviviridae* family, causes the most widespread mosquito-borne viral infection in humans around the world today. Dengue can affect anyone but tends to be more severe in people with compromised immune systems. Dengue hemorrhagic fever is a more severe form of a viral illness. Symptoms include headache, fever, rash, and evidence of bleeding (hemorrhage) in the body. This form of dengue fever can be life-threatening and can progress to the most severe form of the illness, dengue shock syndrome. This chapter reviews the etiology, epidemiology, diagnosis, pathophysiology, transmissions, manifestations, diagnosis, treatment, and prevention of dengue.

Keywords: dengue, etiology, epidemiology, pathophysiology

1. Introduction

Dengue fever is a mosquito-borne viral infection which has a sudden onset that follows symptoms such as headache, nausea, weakness, intense muscle and joint pain, swelling of lymph nodes (lymphadenopathy), and rashes on the skin. Many symptoms of dengue fever include gingivitis, sharp pain in the eyes, and swollen palms and soles.

Dengue can affect any person but appears to be more serious in immunocompromised people. Because it is caused by one of the five dengue virus serotypes, it is possible to have dengue fever multiple times. Nonetheless, a dengue attack provides lifelong immunity to the specific viral serotype to which the patient has been exposed. This disease may also be called "breakbone fever" or "dandy fever."

This dengue fever may become more serious and then named as dengue hemorrhagic fever and dengue shock syndrome. Dengue hemorrhagic fever is a more severe form in which hemorrhages occurs in the body. It is a life-threatening condition, and it may progress to the most critical form called dengue shock syndrome [1].

2. Etiology

Dengue virus (DENV) is a single-stranded, positive-sense RNA virus in the *Flaviviridae* family and the *Flavivirus* genus. When viewed under the transmission electron micrograph, the virions appear as a bunch of black spots. Yellow fever virus, West Nile virus, St. Louis encephalitis virus, Japanese encephalitis virus, tick-borne encephalitis virus, Kyasanur Forest disease virus, and Omsk hemorrhagic fever virus belong to this family, and majority of them is transmitted by arthropods (mosquitoes or ticks) [2].

Approximately 11,000 nucleotide bases were present in the dengue genome, which codes for a single polyprotein. It is made up of three structural protein molecules (C, prM, and E) that constitute the virus particle and seven nonstructural proteins (NS1, NS2a, NS2b, NS3, NS4a, NS4b, and NS5) which are required for viral replication [3, 4]. The five strains of the virus (DENV-1, DENV-2, DENV-3, DENV-4, and DENV-5) are referred to as serotypes because they vary in serum reactivity (antigenicity) [5].

The main cause of dengue fever is an infected mosquito bite [6], and besides it, it may be accidentally acquired after vertical transmission, especially in near-term pregnant women through the placenta [7], infected blood products [8], through organ transplantation [9], and even after needle stick injury [10].

3. Epidemiology

Awareness about the terrestrial spread and impact of dengue is relevant for assessing its relation to worldwide morbidity and mortality and knowing how to utilize the available resources for controlling the dengue globally.

Only nine countries had suffered major epidemics of dengue, before 1970. Currently it is common in most of the regions of the WHO. The Americas, South East Asia, and Western Pacific areas are the most severely affected, with Asia responsible for around 70% of the global disease burden. Throughout the recent decades, the prevalence of dengue has significantly elevated around the globe. The vast majority of cases are asymptomatic or mild and self-managed, and therefore the actual number of dengue cases is underreported. Many cases are also misdiagnosed as other febrile disorders [11].

One report indicates 390 million dengue virus infections per year, of which 96 million occur clinically (with any disease severity). The report on dengue prevalence reports that 3.9 billion people are at risk of infection with dengue viruses. Despite the risk of infection in 128 countries, 70% of the real burden is from Asia [12].

The number of dengue cases recorded to WHO has risen ~6 fold, from <0.5 million in 2010 to more than 3.34 million in 2016. The year 2016 was marked by massive dengue outbreaks worldwide. A major reduction in the number of dengue cases in the Americas was reported in 2017, from 2,177,171 cases in 2016 to 584,263 cases in 2017. It reflects a drop of 73%. Following a drop in the number of cases in 2017–2018, a sharp increase in cases is reported in 2019. Cases have increased in Australia, Cambodia, China, Lao PDR, Malaysia, the Philippines, Singapore, and Vietnam. An estimated 500,000 people with severe dengue require hospitalization every year, and an estimated 2.5% of cases are fatal each year. Nevertheless, several countries have lowered the case fatality rate to less than 1%, and internationally, there has been a decline in case of fatality between 2010 and 2016, with a significant improvement in case management through country-level capacity building. The only continent that has not witnessed dengue transmission is Antarctica.

The global burden of dengue is formidable and is a growing challenge for public health officials and policymakers. Success in addressing this growing global threat depends, in part, on strengthening the evidence base on which planning control decisions and their impact are assessed. It is hoped that this assessment of the distribution and burden of contemporary dengue risk will help to advance this objective.

4. Pathophysiology

The pathophysiology of DENV and the immune response of the host are not fully understood. Primary manifestations of disease include capillary leak syndrome (plasma leakage due to DHF-specific endothelial cell dysfunction), thrombocytopenia (seen in all types of DENV infection, but extreme in DHF), hemorrhagic tendencies, and leukopenia. It is known that the major viral envelope (E) of glycoprotein in the virus helps to bind the host cells, followed by viral replication [13] . Data suggest that monocytes are the primary target [14]. Infected monocytes induce the production of interferon-a (IFN-a) and IFN-b [15]. Envelope (E), precursor membrane protein (pre-M), and nonstructural protein 1 (NS1) are the major DENV proteins targeted by antibodies as part of the host immune response. Studies have shown that DENV-specific CD4+ and CD8+ T lymphocytes attack infected cells and release IFN-g, tumor necrosis factor-a (TNF-a), and lymphotoxin. Primary infection induces a lifetime immunity of the individual to that particular serotype, but not to secondary infection by another serotype.

Bite of *Aedes Aegypti*

↓

The virus penetrates to the skin

↓

The virus infects and replicates inside the Langerhans cell [immunity of the skin]

↓

Langerhans cells release interferons [to limit the spread of infections]

↓

Infected Langerhans cells go to the lymphatic system to make the immune system alert

↓

Then goes to circulation

↓

Results in viremia—high levels of virus in the bloodstream

↓

Activation of immune response—increases lymphocyte

↓

Decreases neutrophils and white blood cells

↓

Release of pyrogen causes fever and increased blood pressure in vessels—causes rashes

↓

Dengue

5. Transmission

Dengue virus is the most common mosquito-borne infection in humans all over the world. It belongs to the family *Flaviviridae*, which contains more than 70 viruses [16], in which DENV is transmitted by the *Aedes aegypti* and *Aedes albopictus* mosquitoes [17].

Dengue virus is spread primarily by *Aedes* mosquitoes, in particular *Aedes aegypti*. These mosquitoes usually live between 35°N and 35°S below an altitude of 1000 m (3300 feet) [5]. They usually bite especially in the early morning and in the evening. Certain *Aedes* disease-borne species include *Aedes albopictus*, *Aedes scutellaris*, and *Aedes polynesiensis*. Human beings are the primary hosts of this virus, arousing even nonhuman primates. An infection may be obtained through a single bite. A female mosquito that consumes an infected person's blood (within a febrile, viremic span of 2 to 12 days) becomes infected with the virus in its intestine. The virus then spread into other tissues, including the salivary glands of the mosquito, approximately after a period of 8–10 days and is subsequently released into its saliva. When it bites the other person, the virus is transmitted through its saliva to that person. The virus does not cause any harm to the mosquito [18]. *Aedes aegypti* is a main concern as it prefers to lay its eggs in containers of freshwater and stay close to humans. Infected blood products and organ donation can also cause dengue [8, 9, 19]. Even in countries like Singapore, the incidence is approximately 1.6 to 6 in 10,000 transfusions [20]. The vertical transmission (from mother to child) during pregnancy or at birth is also documented [8]. Other person-to-person forms of transmission have also been reported, but are very rare [21]. Dengue's genetic variants are regionally specific, indicating that the creation of new territories is relatively rare, despite the fact that dengue has appeared in new regions in recent decades [22].

5.1 The virus

DENV is a small single-stranded RNA virus consisting of five different serotypes (DENV-1 to DENV-5). The virus particle is spherical in shape with a diameter of 50 nm. The genome is divided into three structural proteins (capsid C prM, membrane precursor M protein, and envelope E) and seven nonstructural proteins (NS) by the host and viral proteases.

Within each serotype, distinct genotypes or lineages (viruses closely related in nucleotide sequence) have been identified, demonstrating the substantial genetic variability in dengue serotypes. However, purifying selection continues to be a dominant theme in the evolution of dengue viruses, so only viruses that are "fit" for both humans and vectors are retained. Between these, severe secondary dengue infections are often associated with "European" genotypes DENV-2 and DENV-3 [23–25]. The human hosts have established intra-host viral diversity (quasi-species).

5.2 The vectors

Different dengue virus serotypes are transmitted to humans through the bites of infected *Aedes* mosquitoes, mainly *Aedes aegypti*. This mosquito is a tropical and subtropical species widely distributed around the world, mostly between 35°N and 35°S latitudes. Such geographical limits correspond roughly to the 10°C winter isotherm. *Aedes aegypti* was located as far north as 45°N, but in warmer months, these invasions took place, and the mosquitoes did not survive the winter months. *Aedes aegypti* is also relatively uncommon over 1000 m, due to lower temperatures. The embryonic stages are found in water-filled settings, mostly in artificial containers that are closely linked to human dwellings, and often inside. Research suggests that mostly female *Aedes aegypti* may spend their lives in or around the homes where the adults emerge. It means people are spreading the virus quickly within and between populations, rather than mosquitoes. *Aedes albopictus*, *Aedes polynesiensis*, and several species of *Aedes scutellaris* were also attributed to outbreaks of the dengue [26]. Each of these species has a specific ecological, behavioral, and geographical distribution. *Aedes albopictus* has spread from Asia to Africa, Americas, and Europe in recent decades, aided particular by international trade in used tires, where eggs are deposited as they contain rainwater. Eggs can remain viable for many months, in the absence of water.

5.3 The host

After an incubation period of 4–10 days, infection with any of the four virus serotypes can cause a wide range of illnesses, although most infections are asymptomatic or subclinical. Primary infection is thought to cause long-term defensive immunity to serotype infections [27]. Around 2–3 months of primary infection, but without long-term cross-protective immunity, individuals suffering from infection are protected from clinical illness with a specific serotype.

Personal risk factors influence the severity of the disease and also include secondary infections (bronchial asthma, sickle cell anemia, and diabetes mellitus), age, race, and potentially chronic diseases. In particular, young children may be less able to compensate for capillary leakage than adults and are thus at a higher risk of dengue shock [5].

Seroepidemiological reports conducted in Cuba and Thailand strongly support the position of secondary heterotypic infection as a risk factor for severe dengue, although there is little evidence of serious primary infection cases [28–31]. Also, the time interval between infections and the specific viral infection sequence may be significant. For example, a higher fatality rate was observed in Cuba when DEN2 infection followed DEN-1 infection at an interval of 20 years compared to 4 years. Severe dengue is also commonly seen in infants born to dengue-infected mothers. Antibody-dependent enhancement (ADE) of the infection has been hypothesized [32] as a mechanism to explain severe dengue in the course of secondary infection and in infants with primary infections. In this model, non-neutralizing, cross-reactive antibodies produced during primary infection or acquired passively at birth bind to epitopes on the surface of the heterologous infective virus and promote the entry of the virus into Fc-bearing cells. The increased number of infected cells is expected to result in increased viral load and robust host immune response activation including inflammatory cytokines and mediators, some of which may contribute to capillary leakage. Cross-reactive memory T cells are also rapidly triggered during secondary infection, proliferate, release cytokines, and die of apoptosis in a manner that usually correlates with overall disease severity. Host genetic determinants may have an effect on the clinical outcome of infection [33], although most studies have not been able to address this problem adequately. Studies in the American region indicate that the levels of extreme dengue in individuals of African descent are lower than in other ethnic groups [34].

Recent data suggest that endothelial cell activation could mediate plasma leakage [35, 36]. Plasma leakage is believed to be associated with functional effects on endothelial cells, rather than harmful ones. Endothelial cell dysfunction may also be associated with the activation of infected monocytes and T cells, the complement system, and the production of mediators, monokines, cytokines, and soluble receptors.

Thrombocytopenia may be associated with alterations in megacaryocytopoiesis due to human hematopoietic cell infection and impaired progenitor cell growth, resulting in platelet dysfunction (activation and aggregation of platelets), increased destruction, or consumption (peripheral sequestration and consumption). Hemorrhage may result from thrombocytopenia and related platelet dysfunction or intravascular coagulation. In short, a transient and reversible imbalance of inflammatory mediators, cytokine, and chemokine occurs during severe dengue times, probably due to high early viral loads, leading to vascular endothelial cell dysfunction, hemocoagulation disorders, and then plasma leakage, shock, and bleeding.

6. Manifestations

One of three clinical forms can be used in humans, such as dengue fever (DF), dengue hemorrhagic fever (DHF), and dengue shock syndrome (DSS).

Approximately one-half of the DENV infections are asymptomatic, and some are undifferentiated (in which the patient develops fever and mild symptoms, but the source of the infection is not diagnosed as DENV). The three clinical forms of the disease vary in the severity of their symptoms, with the influenza-like DF being the least severe and the DSS being the most severe. In most cases, mild febrile DF is not fatal; however, infections that develop into DHF or DSS may be life-threatening and cause death in many cases. Patients with DHF and DSS were found to have virus titers 100- to 1000-fold higher than those with DF from the initial stage of infection [37]. Overall, DENV infection has been found to be more severe in children than adults [38].

Based on the outcome of several studies, the WHO has developed a new dengue classification. It differentiates dengue cases into cases with or without warning signs and serious cases of dengue.

Usually, signs begin to appear after an incubation period of 3–10 days [39]. The severity of clinical presentations ranges from mild symptoms to extreme life-threatening symptoms for dengue hemorrhagic fever and dengue shock syndrome [40]. Predicting the progression of mild signs to severe DHF/DSS remains a challenge due to unspecific clinical presentation and incomplete understanding of disease pathophysiology and its underlying molecular mechanisms.

The early signs of the disease are nonspecific. According to WHO, DF is characterized by febrile episodes (≥40°C for 2–7 days) often associated with rash, nausea, vomiting, and headache. Even though the disease affects all ages of people from infant to adulthood [41], epidemiological data showed that children tend to control this disease better than adults [42]. The severity of the above symptoms and the emergence of other symptoms, such as abdominal pain, mucosal bleeding, and lethargy and restlessness, can be seen after 3–7 days. Laboratory examination of mild dengue fever cases usually reveals elevated leukocyte counts and a small increase in hepatic aminotransferase activity. The emergence of these symptoms is a warning sign of disease progression to severe form (DHF/DSS) if therapeutic action is not undertaken. At this level, clinical intervention and continuous surveillance are necessary to prevent vascular leakage, especially in the endemic region.

Extreme dengue infection can be due to any of the four recognized DENV 1–4 serotypes. The likelihood of developing DHF/DSS is high in patients who have had dengue infection with heterogeneous serotype [43] in the past, with approximately 5–10% of patients developing extreme DHF/DSS that can be fatal unless treated promptly [44].

This type evolves at a late stage of DF, where patients will experience a defervescent process characterized by a sudden drop in body temperature. This phase is also characterized by severe bleeding, especially from the gastrointestinal tract (black, tarry stool) and thrombocytopenia (<50,000/mm^3), which may affect up to 50% of DHF cases [45]. Ironically, there was a negative correlation between the frequency of DHF and the number of platelets in the blood. The exact mechanism of this association is yet to be identified. Decreased platelet counts and loss of function contribute to vascular fragility, increasing the risk of hemorrhage and plasma leakage59. It has been proposed that DENV replicates rapidly in platelets during the acute phase of infection, as this is very important to the survival and dissemination of the virus [46]. The existence of other signs such as retro-orbital pain, maculopapular rash, petechiae, or nose or gum bleeding may help to make a definitive diagnosis of DF [47]. Subsistence in systolic pressure and hypotension can result in profound shock, known as dengue shock syndrome. Long-term DSS duration can predispose to additional complications such as severe bleeding, diffuse intravascular coagulopathy (DIC), respiratory failure, multiorgan failure, and infrequently encephalopathy leading to death [48, 49]. It was estimated that DHF-related case fatality could exceed 15% of all cases, but proper medical treatment and symptomatic management could minimize the mortality rate to less than 1%.

Signs and symptoms depending on the stage of the disease reflect the dengue fever. People with dengue virus normally become asymptomatic (80%) or have mild symptoms such as uncomplicated fever [50, 51]. 5 % of the people have more severe illness and, in a small proportion of cases (<1%), are life-threatening and cause death despite care. The incubation period (time between exposure and onset of symptoms) ranges from 3 to 14 days, but most of the time is 4 to 7 days. Children are more likely to have atypical symptoms, often with common cold or gastroenteritis (vomiting and diarrhea)-like symptoms [52].

The characteristic symptoms of dengue are sudden fever, headache (typically behind the eyes), muscle and joint pain, and rash. The course of infection is divided into three phases: febrile, serious, and recovery. The febrile phase includes high fever, possibly over 40°C (104°F) and is associated with severe pain and headache; this period usually lasts 2–7 days. Vomiting and rash will be there along with flushed skin. In some cases, the illness is progressing to a serious stage as the fever clears. This process is characterized by major, diffuse plasma leakage usually lasting 1–2 days. Organ dysfunction and severe bleeding, usually from the gastrointestinal tract, may also occur [53]. Shock (dengue shock syndrome) and hemorrhage (dengue hemorrhagic fever) occur in less than 5% of all dengue cases. This serious phase is more common among children and young adults. The recovery phase is followed by the resorption of the leaked fluid into the bloodstream over a duration of 2–3 days. The change is often startling and can be followed by serious pruritus and bradycardia. The rash can occur, with either a maculopapular or a vasculitic appearance accompanied by desquamation. A fluid-overloaded condition can occur during this stage, in rare cases.

Dengue also affects a variety of other body systems, either in isolation or along with typical dengue symptoms. Decreased sensitivity occurs in 0.5–6% of severe cases, due to encephalitis or, indirectly, to compromised vital organs (e.g., hepatic encephalopathy). Other neurological disorders similar to dengue, such as transverse myelitis and Guillain-Barré syndrome, have been identified. Myocarditis and acute liver failure are among the most rare complications.

7. Diagnosis

Signs and symptoms of dengue fever are similar to some other illnesses, such as typhoid fever or malaria, which can sometimes hinder the likelihood of a timely and correct diagnosis. It may be diagnosed by the patient's signs and symptoms, patient's medical history, and testing blood samples (preliminary by platelet count, followed by ELISA, HI assay, and RT-PCR).

The early and precise diagnosis of dengue infection in the laboratory is of paramount importance for disease control. It was estimated that the number of cases of dengue misdiagnosed could reach a record of 50% of all cases, mainly due to a wide disparity in dengue signs and symptoms that conflict with symptoms of other viral infections, particularly for people living in or traveling to endemic areas of tropical infectious diseases. Until the antiviral vaccine is available, early and accurate diagnosis relies heavily on the prevention of serious cases and the reduction of the disease's economic burden. To date, two screening methods have been employed for early diagnosis of the disease. The first is a direct approach for the acute dengue disease phase which is focused on an antigen detection of genomic RNA from viremic patient's blood samples. The second is an indirect approach that relies on serological tests to detect dengue-related immunoglobulins by Mac-ELISA for the capture of real IgM or indirect ELISA for the capture of antiDEN IgGs.

Dengue diagnosis is usually performed clinically on the basis of recorded symptoms and physical examination, especially in endemic areas. However, early dengue fever can be difficult to differentiate from other viral infections. Tourniquet testing, which is particularly useful in environments where laboratory tests are not available, includes applying a blood pressure cuff, inflating it to the midpoint between diastolic and systolic pressure for 5 minutes, and then counting any petechial hemorrhages that occur. The higher number of petechiae makes dengue diagnosis more likely; the lower limit for diagnosis is variably specified as 10–20 petechiae per 2.5 cm^2 [54].

8. Treatment

There are no particular antiviral medicines for dengue, but it is necessary to maintain a proper fluid balance [55]. Treatment is dependent on the severity of the symptoms. Those who can drink and pass urine have no warning signs can be treated with daily follow-up and oral rehydration therapy at home. Those who have serious health problems, who have warning signs, or who are unable to handle daily follow-up should be admitted to the hospital for treatment. For areas with access to an intensive care unit, treatment should be given for those with extreme dengue fever. Intravenous hydration usually takes 1 or 2 days, if necessary. Fluid administration dose is titrated to 0.5–1 mL/kg per hour of urinary output, stabilizing vital signs, and normalizing hematocrit. The volume of fluid that is provided should be the smallest to achieve such markers. Bearing in mind the risk of infection, invasive medical procedures such as nasogastric intubation, intramuscular injections, and arterial punctures should be avoided. Paracetamol (acetaminophen) is used for fever and nausea, and it is important to avoid nonsteroidal anti-inflammatory drugs such as ibuprofen and acetylsalicylic acid as they may increase the risk of bleeding. For patients with compromised vital signs faced with declining hematocrit, blood transfusion should begin early, rather than waiting for the concentration of hemoglobin to decline to some predetermined "cause of transfusion" level. It is advised to deliver red blood cells or whole blood; platelets and fresh, frozen plasma are not typically recommended. Intravenous fluids are removed during the recovery phase to avoid fluid overload. When fluid overload occurs and vital signs are stable, stopping the administration of fluid can be all that is required to remove excess fluid. If the individual is outside the critical phase, a diuretic loop, such as furosemide, may be used to remove excess fluid from circulation.

9. Prevention

In December 2015, after decades of research and clinical progress, the first dengue vaccine (CYD-TDV or Dengvaxia®, by Sanofi Pasteur) was authorized [56]. Now regulatory authorities have approved it in ~20 countries.

CYD-TDV was found to be effective and safe in clinical trials in people who had past infections with the dengue virus (seropositive individuals). It does, however, bring an increased risk of severe dengue in those who undergo their first normal dengue infection after vaccination (those who were seronegative at vaccination time). It was confirmed in November 2017 by the results of an additional retrospective study analysis which determines the serostatus at the time of vaccination.

Pre-vaccination screening is the recommended strategy for countries which consider vaccination as part of their dengue control program. With this approach only individuals under evidence of past dengue infection would be vaccinated (based on an antibody test or confirmed dengue infection in the past by a verified laboratory).

Decisions on implementing a pre-vaccination screening strategy would require careful country-level evaluation, including consideration of the sensitivity and specificity of the available tests and local priorities, dengue epidemiology, country-specific hospitalization levels, and availability of both CYD-TDV and screening tests [57].

But prevention depends on the monitoring and safety of the bite of the mosquito that transmits it. The primary tool used to monitor *Aedes aegypti* is by destroying its habitats, which include standing water in urban areas (e.g., abandoned tires, ponds, irrigation ditches, and open barrels). If habitat destruction is not possible, the application of insecticides or biological control agents to standing water is another option. Reducing open water collection is the preferred and simplest method of control. Generalized spraying is often done with organophosphate or pyrethroid insecticides but is not considered successful. People can avoid mosquito bites by wearing clothes that completely cover the skin, wearing a repellent scarf, or staying in air-conditioned, screened, or nested areas. However, these approaches do not seem to be sufficiently effective, as the frequency of outbreaks in certain areas appears to be increasing, probably because urbanization is increasing the habitat of *Aedes* mosquitoes; however, the range of diseases appears to be expanding, possibly due to climate change.

10. Conclusion

Dengue fever is a terrible disease and a growing public health problem. A rapid increase in unplanned urbanization leads to more mosquito breeding sites, hence a greater number of people are exposed to *Aedes Aegypti* mosquitoes bite. These include semi-urban and slum areas where household water storage is normal and where solid waste disposal facilities are inadequate. The urgent need for a vaccine to minimize morbidity and mortality due to this disease has been recognized in a cost-effective manner in recent years.

Conflict of interest

The authors have none to declare.

Author details

Ramalingam Kothai* and Balasubramanian Arul
Department of Pharmacology, Vinayaka Mission's College of Pharmacy, Vinayaka Mission's Research Foundation (Deemed to be University), Salem, Tamil Nadu, India

*Address all correspondence to: kothaiarul@yahoo.co.in

References

[1] Cunha JP. Dengue fever [Internet]. MedicineNet. 2017. Available from: https://www.medicinenet.com/dengue_fever/article.htm [Accessed: 02 January 2020]

[2] Gould EA, Solomon T. Pathogenic flaviviruses. The Lancet (London, England). 2008;**371**(9611):500-509. DOI: 10.1016/S0140-6736(08)60238-X

[3] Rodenhuis-Zybert IA, Wilschut J, Smit JM. Dengue virus life cycle: Viral and host factors modulating infectivity. Cellular and Molecular Life Sciences. 2010;**67**(16):2773-2786. DOI: 10.1007/s00018-010-0357-z

[4] Guzman MG, Halstead SB, Artsob H, Buchy P, Farrar J, Gubler DJ, et al. Dengue: A continuing global threat. Nature Reviews. Microbiology. 2010;**8**(12 Suppl):S7-S16. DOI: 10.1038/nrmicro2460

[5] WHO. Epidemiology, burden of disease and transmission. In: Dengue: Guidelines for Diagnosis, Treatment, Prevention and Control. Geneva: World Health Organization; 2009. pp. 3-25

[6] Pozzetto B, Memmi M, Garraud O. Is transfusion-transmitted dengue fever a potential public health threat? World Journal of Virology [Internet]. 2015;**4**(2):113-123. DOI: 10.5501/wjv.v4.i2.113

[7] Pouliot SH, Xiong X, Harville E, Paz-Soldan V, Tomashek KM, Breart G, et al. Maternal dengue and pregnancy outcomes: A systematic review. Obstetrical & Gynecological Survey. 2010;**65**(2):107-118. DOI: 10.1097/OGX.0b013e3181cb8fbc

[8] Teo D, Ng LC, Lam S. Is dengue a threat to the blood supply? Transfusion Medicine [Internet]. 2009;**19**(2):66-77. DOI: 10.1097/OGX.0b013e3181cb8fbc

[9] Tan FL-S, Loh DLSK, Prabhakaran K, Tambyah PA, Yap H-K. Dengue haemorrhagic fever after living donor renal transplantation. Nephrology, Dialysis, Transplantation. 2005;**20**(2):447-448. DOI: 10.1097/OGX.0b013e3181cb8fbc

[10] Chen LH, Wilson ME. Nosocomial dengue by mucocutaneous transmission. In: Emerging Infectious Diseases. 2005;**11**(5):775. DOI: 10.3201/eid1105.040934

[11] Waggoner JJ, Gresh L, Vargas MJ, Ballesteros G, Tellez Y, Soda KJ, et al. Viremia and clinical presentation in Nicaraguan patients infected with Zika virus, chikungunya virus, and dengue virus. Clinical Infectious Diseases. 2016;**63**(12):1584-1590. DOI: 10.1093/cid/ciw589

[12] Bhatt S, Gething PW, Brady OJ, Messina JP, Farlow AW, Moyes CL, et al. The global distribution and burden of dengue. Nature. 2013;**496**(7446):504-507. DOI: 10.1093/cid/ciw589

[13] Anderson R, King AD, Innis BL. Correlation of E protein binding with cell susceptibility to dengue 4 virus infection. The Journal of General Virology. 1992;**73**(Pt 8):2155-2159. DOI: 10.1099/0022-1317-73-8-2155

[14] Scott RM, Nisalak A, Cheamudon U, Seridhoranakul S, Nimmannitya S. Isolation of dengue viruses from peripheral blood leukocytes of patients with hemorrhagic fever. The Journal of Infectious Diseases. 1980;**141**(1):1-6. DOI: 10.1093/infdis/141.1.1

[15] Kurane I, Ennis FA. Production of interferon alpha by dengue virus-infected human monocytes. The Journal of General Virology. 1988;**69**(Pt 2):445-449. DOI: 10.1099/0022-1317-69-2-445

[16] Kuno G, Chang GJ, Tsuchiya KR, Karabatsos N, Cropp CB. Phylogeny of the genus *Flavivirus*. Journal of Virology [Internet]. 1998;**72**(1):73-83. DOI: 10.1099/0022-1317-69-2-445

[17] Surasombatpattana P, Hamel R, Patramool S, Luplertlop N, Thomas F, Despres P, et al. Dengue virus replication in infected human keratinocytes leads to activation of antiviral innate immune responses. Infection, Genetics and Evolution. 2011;**11**(7):1664-1673. DOI: 10.1016/j.meegid.2011.06.009

[18] Tomashek KM. Dengue fever. In: CDC Health Information for International Travel 2012: The Yellow Book. USA: Oxford University Press; 2011

[19] Wilder-Smith A, Chen LH, Massad E, Wilson ME. Threat of dengue to blood safety in dengue-endemic countries. Emerging Infectious Diseases. 2009;**15**(1):8-11. DOI: 10.3201/eid1501.071097

[20] Stramer SL, Hollinger FB, Katz LM, Kleinman S, Metzel PS, Gregory KR, et al. Emerging infectious disease agents and their potential threat to transfusion safety. Transfusion. 2009;**49**(Suppl 2):1S-29S. DOI: 10.1111/j.1537-2995.2009.02279.x

[21] Wiwanitkit V. Unusual mode of transmission of dengue. Journal of Infection in Developing Countries. 2009;**4**(1):51-54. DOI: 10.3855/jidc.145

[22] Chen LH, Wilson ME. Dengue and chikungunya infections in travelers. Current Opinion in Infectious Diseases. 2010;**23**(5):438-444. DOI: 10.1097/QCO.0b013e32833c1d16

[23] Simmons CP, Farrar JJ, van Vinh CN, Wills B. Dengue. The New England Journal of Medicine [Internet]. 2012;**366**(15):1423-1432. DOI: 10.1056/NEJMra1110265

[24] Leitmeyer KC, Vaughn DW, Watts DM, Salas R, Villalobos I, de Chacon, et al. Dengue virus structural differences that correlate with pathogenesis. Journal of Virology. 1999;**73**(6):4738-4747

[25] Lanciotti RS, Lewis JG, Gubler DJ, Trent DW. Molecular evolution and epidemiology of dengue-3 viruses. The Journal of General Virology. 1994;**75**(Pt 1):65-75. DOI: 10.1099/0022-1317-75-1-65

[26] Bhattacharya MK, Maitra S, Ganguly A, Bhattacharya A, Sinha A. Dengue: A growing menace—A snapshot of recent facts, figures & remedies. International Journal of Biomedical Science [Internet]. 2013;**9**(2):61-67

[27] Messer WB, Gubler DJ, Harris E, Sivananthan K, de Silva AM. Emergence and global spread of a dengue serotype 3, subtype III virus. Emerging Infectious Diseases. 2003;**9**(7):800-809. DOI: 10.3201/eid0907.030038

[28] Halstead SB. Etiologies of the experimental dengues of Siler and Simmons. The American Journal of Tropical Medicine and Hygiene. 1974;**23**(5):974-982. DOI: 10.4269/ajtmh.1974.23.974

[29] Halstead SB, Nimmannitya S, Cohen SN. Observations related to pathogenesis of dengue hemorrhagic fever. IV. Relation of disease severity to antibody response and virus recovered. The Yale Journal of Biology and Medicine. 1970;**42**(5):311-328

[30] Sangkawibha N, Rojanasuphot S, Ahandrik S, Viriyapongse S, Jatanasen S, Salitul V, et al. Risk factors in dengue shock syndrome: A prospective epidemiologic study in Rayong, Thailand. I. The 1980 outbreak. American Journal of Epidemiology. 1984;**120**(5):653-669. DOI: 10.1093/oxfordjournals.aje.a113932

[31] Guzman MG, Kouri G, Valdes L, Bravo J, Alvarez M, Vazques S, et al. Epidemiologic studies on dengue in Santiago de Cuba, 1997. American Journal of Epidemiology. 2000;**152**(9):793-799; discussion 804. DOI: 10.1093/aje/152.9.793

[32] Halstead SB. Antibody, macrophages, dengue virus infection, shock, and hemorrhage: A pathogenetic cascade. Reviews of Infectious Diseases. 1989;**11**(Suppl 4):S830-S839. DOI: 10.1093/clinids/11.supplement_4.s830

[33] Halstead SB, Heinz FX, Barrett ADT, Roehrig JT. Dengue virus: molecular basis of cell entry and pathogenesis, 25-27 June 2003, Vienna, Austria. Vaccine. 2005;**23**:849-856. DOI: 10.1016/j.vaccine.2004.03.069

[34] Kouri GP, Guzman MG, Bravo JR, Triana C. Dengue haemorrhagic fever/dengue shock syndrome: Lessons from the Cuban epidemic, 1981. Bulletin of the World Health Organization. 1989;**67**(4):375-380

[35] de la C Sierra B, Kouri G, Guzman MG. Race: A risk factor for dengue hemorrhagic fever. Archives of Virology. 2007;**152**(3):533-542. DOI: 10.1007/s00705-006-0869-x

[36] Avirutnan P, Malasit P, Seliger B, Bhakdi S, Husmann M. Dengue virus infection of human endothelial cells leads to chemokine production, complement activation, and apoptosis. Journal of Immunology. 1998;**161**(11):6338-6346

[37] Cardier JE, Marino E, Romano E, Taylor P, Liprandi F, Bosch N, et al. Proinflammatory factors present in sera from patients with acute dengue infection induce activation and apoptosis of human microvascular endothelial cells: Possible role of TNF-alpha in endothelial cell damage in dengue. Cytokine. 2005;**30**(6):359-365. DOI: 10.1016/j.cyto.2005.01.021

[38] Vaughn DW, Green S, Kalayanarooj S, Innis BL, Nimmannitya S, Suntayakorn S, et al. Dengue viremia titer, antibody response pattern, and virus serotype correlate with disease severity. The Journal of Infectious Diseases. 2000;**181**(1):2-9. DOI: 10.1086/315215

[39] Hammond SN, Balmaseda A, Perez L, Tellez Y, Saborio SI, Mercado JC, et al. Differences in dengue severity in infants, children, and adults in a 3-year hospital-based study in Nicaragua. The American Journal of Tropical Medicine and Hygiene. 2005;**73**(6):1063-1070

[40] Chan M, Johansson MA. The incubation periods of Dengue viruses. PLoS One [Internet]. 2012;**7**(11):e50972. DOI: 10.1371/journal.pone.0050972

[41] Guha-Sapir D, Schimmer B. Dengue fever: New paradigms for a changing epidemiology. Emerging Themes in Epidemiology [Internet]. 2005;**2**(1):1. DOI: 10.1186/1742-7622-2-1

[42] Khan NA, Azhar EI, El-Fiky S, Madani HH, Abuljadial MA, Ashshi AM, et al. Clinical profile and outcome of hospitalized patients during first outbreak of dengue in Makkah, Saudi Arabia. Acta Tropica. 2008;**105**(1):39-44. DOI: 10.1016/j.actatropica.2007.09.005

[43] Ooi E-E, Goh K-T, Gubler DJ. Dengue prevention and 35 years of vector control in Singapore. Emerging Infectious Diseases. 2006;**12**(6):887-893. DOI: 10.3201/10.3201/eid1206.051210

[44] Low JGH, Ooi E-E, Tolfvenstam T, Leo Y-S, Hibberd ML, Ng L-C, et al. Early dengue infection and outcome study (EDEN)—Study design and preliminary findings. Annals of the Academy of Medicine, Singapore. 2006;**35**(11):783-789

[45] Wichmann O, Jelinek T. Dengue in travelers: A review. Journal of Travel Medicine. 2004;**11**(3):161-170. DOI: 10.2310/7060.2004.18503

[46] Schexneider KI, Reedy EA. Thrombocytopenia in dengue fever. Current Hematology Reports. 2005;**4**(2):145-148

[47] Martina BEE, Koraka P, Osterhaus ADME. Dengue virus pathogenesis: An integrated view. Clinical Microbiology Reviews. 2009;**22**(4):564-581. DOI: 10.1128/CMR.00035-09

[48] Noisakran S, Chokephaibulkit K, Songprakhon P, Onlamoon N, Hsiao H-M, Villinger F, et al. A re-evaluation of the mechanisms leading to dengue hemorrhagic fever. Annals of the New York Academy of Sciences. 2009;**1171**(Suppl 1):E24-E35. DOI: 10.1111/j.1749-6632.2009.05050.x

[49] Marques N, Gan VC, Leo Y-S. Dengue myocarditis in Singapore: Two case reports. Infection. 2013;**41**(3):709-714. DOI: 10.1007/s15010-012-0392-9

[50] Misra UK, Kalita J, Syam UK, Dhole TN. Neurological manifestations of dengue virus infection. Journal of the Neurological Sciences. 2006;**244**(1-2):117-122. DOI: 10.1016/j.jns.2006.01.011

[51] Whitehorn J, Farrar J. Dengue. British Medical Bulletin. 2010;**95**: 161-173. DOI: 10.1093/bmb/ldq019

[52] Reiter P. Yellow fever and dengue: A threat to Europe? Euro Surveillance: Bulletin Europeen Sur les Maladies Transmissibles = European Communicable Disease Bulletin. 2010;**15**(10):19509

[53] Varatharaj A. Encephalitis in the clinical spectrum of dengue infection. Neurology India. 2010;**58**(4):585-591. DOI: 10.4103/0028-3886.68655

[54] Ranjit S, Kissoon N. Dengue hemorrhagic fever and shock syndromes. Pediatric Critical Care Medicine. 2011;**12**(1):90-100. DOI: 10.1097/PCC.0b013e3181e911a7

[55] Ramalingam K, Varghese CS, Elias C, Mathew GM, Balasubramanian A, Nadu T. A retrospective study on the effect of Vitamin C in the management of dengue fever in three different states of India. International Journal of Research in Pharmaceutical Sciences. 2019;**10**(4):2670-2673. DOI: 10.26452/ijrps.v10i4.1525

[56] Vannice KS, Wilder-Smith A, Barrett ADT, Carrijo K, Cavaleri M, de Silva A, et al. Clinical development and regulatory points for consideration for second-generation live attenuated dengue vaccines. Vaccine [Internet]. 2018;**36**(24):3411-3417. DOI: 10.1016/j.vaccine.2018.02.062

[57] WHO. Dengue vaccine: WHO position paper, September 2018-Recommendations. Vaccine [Internet]. 2019;**37**(35):4848-4849. DOI: 10.1016/j.vaccine.2018.09.063

Chapter 2

Lessons Learned and Recent Advances in Dengue Research

Juan Samuel Sulca Herencia

Abstract

Dengue is the most important arbovirus, many research have contributed to the diagnosis, management, prevention and control of this disease, which will be described in this chapter, for example: the importance of serotypes and genotypes for the development of the disease, the relationship of the viral load between symptomatic and asymptomatic people, the influence of antibodies on the development of the disease, co-infections with microorganisms and chronic diseases, possible reservoirs, the diagnostic assays, cross-reactions in the diagnosis, the influence of climate change on the disease and the vector, mechanisms of transmission of the disease, new drugs and plant extracts with antiviral activity, the dengue vaccine, the results of immunizations, etc. This information gives a concrete idea of the advances and challenges against this disease.

Keywords: dengue, dengue virus, arbovirus, flavivirus, *Flaviviridae*

1. Introduction

Dengue is a single systematic and dynamic disease that includes severe and non-severe clinical manifestations [1]. It is caused by any of the four dengue virus serotypes and it is transmitted by *Aedes* mosquito bites, being the main vector *Aedes aegypti* [1]. Dengue can be maintained in an urban cycle which involves humans and it is a serious health problem worldwide [1]. For the past decades, this disease has been spread alarmingly due to different factors like climate change, migration of people, tourism, lack of access to basic services, etc. [1, 2]. Not only does it affect a large portion of the world's population but also it offers lessons in health sector, research and epidemiology which must be skilled to help in better understanding of the cycle of this disease, set out control strategies and lead the way to future investigations. Thus, in this chapter we are going to discuss some of the main lessons learnt throughout work experiences with this disease and we will learn new strategies designed for studies, assessment and control.

2. Dissemination of the disease in urban areas and transmission mechanisms

Dengue is the most important and common arbovirus in more than 100 countries [1]. This disease is caused by one of the four serotypes of dengue virus (DENV), more than one dengue serotype can be found in many geographical areas (phenomenon called hyperendemicity) [1]. Outbreaks of this disease have been reported in America, Africa, Mid-west, Asia and the Pacific islands [2]. Nearly 3 billion people (40% of world population) are at risk in areas where dengue occurs, and about 70% of the population at risk are in South East Asia and Western Pacific region [2]. About 400 million people are infected with dengue annually, of which 100 million people are sick and 22,000 die of severe dengue [3]. A virus, a vector and a sensitive population must be in the same geographic area for a dengue onset outbreak [1]. Travelers contribute to dengue dissemination to non-endemic areas but they may also serve as sentinels for warning dissemination. Some studies indicate that dengue represents about 2% of the diseases from travelers returning to from endemic areas [4]. Based on GeoSentinel, a data-collection network between 1997 and 2006, dengue was imported from South-east Asia (51%), South Central Asia (17%), Latin America (15%), the Caribbean (9%), parts of Africa (5%) and Oceania (2%) [4]. The number of febrile travelers returning from the tropics and sub-tropical areas being diagnosed with dengue has increased from 2% in the 1990s to 16% by 2005 [4]. A study of paedriatic travelers in 19 countries reported dengue and typhoid fever as the most often febrile diseases in children returning from tropical regions and sub-Saharan Africa [4]. *Aedes aegypti* vector can be disseminated relatively easy in urban areas because of its strong anthropophilic habits, its biological features like egg resistance to desiccation, its permanence within and not away from the urban centers, and the search for water with low load of organic matter for its oviposition making its arrival in rural areas, where the temperature enables its replication, relatively simple; transform cemeteries, tire repair shop, bus terminals, etc. in critical points of infestation where the vector surveillance must be carried out [5]. The virus can reach new areas where cases of symptomatic and asymptomatic persons or cases of people's incubation period of the disease have not been reported. Around three-quarters of dengue infections presented each year are clinically inapparent, the asymptomatic ones were considered dead-end hosts because they do not produce high enough viremia to infect mosquitoes [6]. Some studies provide evidence that despite a low level of viremia, dengue asymptomatic persons were capable of transmitting the disease to mosquitoes and potentially enabling a high virus transmission. Since it has no symptoms, they could continue in their day-to-day work and be exposed to mosquito bites [6]. The virus can also be spread through infected mosquitoes so that once the mosquito is infected and the extrinsic incubation period is passed, it can be a lifelong carrier of the virus which is about 2 weeks or a month. The interruption of dengue transmission was possible in the 60s and at the beginning of the 70s as a result of an *Aedes aegypti* eradication. The lack of surveillance and vector control followed outbreaks in the Caribbean, Central America and South America [1]. From this experience, it is considered that vector control and epidemiological services detecting and studying dengue cases have to work together and maintain a constant vigilance [1]. The monitoring service should be capable of making the difference between a seasonal and/or temporary increase and increases in the number of cases resulting from a dengue outbreak so that tools of epidemiology as the endemic channel are highly important. If the number of cases reported is higher in two standard deviations above the endemic channel in monthly or weekly notifications, a warning of dengue is produced [1, 7]. However, the lack of notifications continues to be one of the most significant problems in order to prevent and control this disease in many countries as well as in the western Pacific region [1]. The Geographic Information Systems (GIS) allows the analysis of this information on the geographical reference basis in space and time. This type of systems is important for vector-borne disease surveillance and vector control strategy planning [8]. DENV can be transmitted to humans through the bite of female mosquitoes of the *Aedes aegypti*. Other dengue transmission mechanism is the perinatal transmission and it occurs when a mother is infected near the childbirth so that the infection can be transmitted through microtransfusion when a placental abruption occurs or during delivery when the mother's blood gets in contact with the newborn's mucosal. Dengue in pregnancy is related to premature delivery, fetal distress in labour, intrauterine death and miscarriages. DENV can also be transmitted through breast milk or exposure to blood, organs or infected tissues like bone marrow [9]. In a study carried out at the Brazilian blood center from February to June in 2012, donors tested positive for DENV-3 and DENV-4 were found and 42 units of PCR tested positive were transfused in 35 recipients. Of these findings, 16 units testing positive were transfused in 16 sensitive recipients in which 5 possible cases transmitted by transfusion (TT) were found, 1 case was considered as a possible TT, and 10 of them were not transmitted. However, no significant differences were found between symptoms and mortality in cases and controls [10].

3. Dengue virus serotypes and genotypes and its relation to clinical cases

The evolution of molecular biology and phylogenetic analysis has enabled molecular epidemiology studies binding DENV-phylogenetic analysis which was found in different geographic areas within a certain period of time and clinical and epidemiological data in order to establish a relation to genotypes and lineages which are found with other circulating strains as well as to identify the origin and the transmission route, the severity of the disease, etc. There are four related DENV serotypes but antigenically different DENV-1, DENV-2, DENV-3, DENV-4 and each of them generates an immune response to the infection. The nucleotide sequences show 63–68% homology within the DENV group in comparison with 44% between DENV and Yellow Fever virus (YFV), and 51% between DENV and West Nile virus (WNV), and it shares a minor homology at 80% at a level of amino acids [11]. Previous studies based on partial (prM/E), partial or complete E gene; or complete genomic sequences recognized distinct DENV genotypes [12] (**Table 1**).

The genotypes may present different lineages or clades. The genetic changes in the virus are caused by mutations or the introduction of a new variant from other region, thus genotyping of strain virus is used to identify the epidemic outbreak source and spread [12]. Some dengue genotypes are related to a higher virulence. DENV-2 and DENV-3 Asian genotypes are associated with severe infections [1]. In South East Asia, dengue hemorrhagic fever (DHF) and/or dengue shock syndrome (DSS) outbreaks are caused by DENV-2 southeast Asian genotype strain, meanwhile epidemics caused by DENV-2 in Latin America presents solely dengue fever (DF) in most cases. The DENV-2 genotypes circulating in the United States seem to be less virulent. Because of the introduction of the South East Asian genotype virulent, the number of cases of DHF and DSS in America has increased [1, 11].

It is thought that an infection with DENV serotype provides lifelong immunity against the same serotype infection and short-term protection against infection by a 2 or 3 month-heterologous serotype [1, 11]. Some studies contradict the hypothesis that has been accepted until now. In 2010–2011 a study in DENV-2 American/Asian genotype outbreak was conducted in Iquitos, Peru. It was carried out 15 years after the first DENV-2 American genotype in that region. The results on the study showed that protection against homologous DENV-2 may be incomplete [13]. In another study carried out in Peru, it was found that the antibodies of a primary infection against DENV-1 neutralized more efficiently in American DENV-2 than in Asian DENV-2. It is believed that this cross-protective immunity is not so strong to inhibit viremia but it may contribute to reduce DENV-2 infection

Dengue serotype	Genotype	Geographical distribution
DENV-1	I	Southeast Asia, China, The Middle East
	II	Thailand
	III (Sylvatic)	Malaysia
	IV	Countries of the Pacific Rim, the Western Pacific, islands and Australia
	V	The Americas, West Africa and Asia
DENV-2	Asian I	Thailand, Malaysia, Cambodia, Myanmar, Vietnam and Australia
	Asian II	China, Indonesia, The Philippines, Taiwan, Sri Lanka, India, Honduras and Mexico
	Southeast Asian/ American	Southeast Asia, Central and South America and the Caribbean
	Cosmopolitan	East and West Africa, the Middle East, the Indian subcontinent, Indian and Pacific Ocean Islands, Australia, Mexico
	American	Central and South America, the Caribbean and the Indian subcontinent and the Pacific Islands
	Sylvatic	West Africa and Southeast Asia
DENV-3	I	Southeast Asia, the Philippines and the South Pacific islands
	II	Continental Southeast Asia
	III	Asia, East Africa, the Americas
	IV	Puerto Rico and Tahiti
DENV-4	I	The Philippines, Thailand, Vietnam, Myanmar, Malaysia, Sri Lanka, India
	II	Southeast Asia (Indonesia, Malaysia, Singapore), China, islands of the Western Pacific Ocean, Australia, the Caribbean and the Americas
	III	Thailand
	IV	Malaysia

Table 1.
Dengue virus serotypes and genotypes and its geographical distribution.

symptomatology [14]. In 2013 evidences of a new dengue serotype appearance (DENV-5) that was identified in serum samples collected in 2007 during an epidemic in Malaysia were documented. Initially, it was thought that DENV-4 cases will circulate between primates and *Aedes nivalis* mosquitoes in the woods at South East Asia. However, it was shown that this virus was genetically different to DENV-4 from the rainforest and it had certain similarities to DENV-2 when the virus was isolated and after sequencing the whole genome, *rhesus macaques* were infected with four dengue serotypes. Once recovered from the infection, the monkeys were inoculated with DENV-5 which produced different antibodies. Moreover, it was observed that the infection with DENV-5 virus titer was four times higher than other serotypes. On the basis of this, it was concluded that DENV-5 will be a new serotype. It is thought that this new serotype may mainly circulate in non-human primates (NHP). This new serotype has only been found in the Woods of Sarawak [15]. However, there is a possibility that this new serotype may spread to human population becoming a public health concern. Thus, phylogenetics and epidemiological surveillance studies are required.

4. Factors that increase dengue severity, cases and co-infection classification

Most of dengue infections are subclinical or asymptomatic. Dengue epidemics were presented in Cuba in 1981 and 1987, and most cases of dengue shock and hemorrhagic dengue were mainly found in white population than in afro-descendants [16]. In studies carried out in Brazil and El Salvador, it was found that the African descent was a protective factor in dengue hemorrhagic manifestations [16]. In a dengue outbreak in Santiago de Cuba in 1997, it was found that hemorrhagic dengue cases were reported more frequently in patients aged between 15 and 39 years old. Additionally, they found a history of asthma in a 16.5% of the cases [17]. The WHO estimates that, by 2030, the diabetes mellitus will have been the 7th leading cause of death. A study carried out for evaluating the influence of diabetes mellitus and its relation to clinical manifestations of dengue, indicated higher risks of dengue symptoms potentially fatal within patients developing diabetes mellitus [18]. Other risk factors such as sickle-cell disease, uremia, allergies, hypertension, chronic renal failure may enable disease severity [1]. Regarding age, the lower compensation capacity of capillary plasma extravasation in children increases dengue shock risk. It has been observed that serious dengue cases were continuously presented in primary infections from breastfeeding babies whose mothers were developing immunity to some dengue serotype. The non-neutralizing antibodies produced by cross reaction during a primary infection or passively obtained from a mother to newborns are adhered to epitopes of dengue virus infections facilitating the entry of cells to Fc-receptors. This may contribute to a person's viral load increase resulting in strong immune response that includes inflammatory mediators [19]. Cytosines may enable plasma extravasation. In secondary infections, memory T-cells caused by previous reactions to dengue activate, replicate, produce cytosines and die of apoptosis. This can be correlated with disease severity [16]. The patient's background is important when ruling out other causes of this disease, for instance, other flavivirus presence like YFV, Saint Louis encephalitis virus (SLEV), Zika virus (ZIKV), WNV. Alphavirus like Chikungunya (CHIKV), Mayaro virus (MAYV), Venezuelan Equine Encephalitis virus (VEE), Bunyavirus like Oropouche virus (OROV), group C virus, Guaroa virus (GROV), Influenza virus, arenavirus, filovirus as well as other microorganisms can cause the disease with symptoms with similar symptoms such as malaria, Leptospirosis, typhoid fever, rickettsia diseases, etc. [1]. Dengue infections with different serotypes as well as the sequence of these infected patients may influence on the severity of the disease. In a study carried out in Singapore, between 2005 and 2011, febrile adult patients found in DENV-1 cases that were associated with dengue hemorrhagic fever (adjusted RR = 1.74) and severe dengue (adjusted RR = 2.1) were assessed, while DENV-2 had a low risk of dengue hemorrhagic fever (adjusted RR = 0.5) [20]. A special attention should be given to the clinical features of this disease in order to learn differences that lead to the identification of microorganisms causing the disease. It was found that there were no elevated hematocrit or shock cases in CHIKV infection as compared to dengue cases with high hematocrit in 40–69% of cases and shock in 10–39% of cases when comparing the clinical data and laboratory features within dengue infections and chikungunya [21]. The arthralgias were more frequent in CHIKV in 70–100% of cases as compared to at least 10% of dengue cases. The Zika infections may present Oedema in limbs as compared to dengue and chikungunya which is low or nil. The presence of this type of differences does not exclude atypical complications and presentations of the disease, thus the laboratory diagnosis plays a crucial role [22].

DENV, ZIKV and CHIKV are transmitted by *Aedes aegypti* vector. Therefore, the areas where the disease is spread may be the same leading potentially to co-infections. Co-infection cases within different dengue serotypes have been reported in various countries like Peru where isolation of DENV-1 and DENV-3 in the department of Madre de Dios was reported [23]. Although this type of findings, the connection between dengue co-infections and severity of the infection needs to be further examined. Reports of DENV and CHIKV co-infections have been exhibited since 1964 in Asia, Africa, the Caribbean, North America, South America. Dengue and malaria co-infections have been reported in various countries such as India, Pakistan, Indonesia, Japan, Malaysia, Brazil and many others; and even co-infections among dengue, malaria and chikungunya have been reported in South Africa and Asia. A systematic review to determine global prevalence and distribution of malaria, dengue and chikungunya coinfections reported evidence of coinfections within these agents in 42 countries. The most prevalent confection was malaria/dengue followed by dengue/chikungunya, Malaria/Chikungunya and Malaria/Dengue/Chikungunya [24]. Clinical presentations between dengue and malaria are alike so it can sometimes cause a co-infection misdiagnosis. Anemia is a major symptom of infections caused by malaria which are not presented in dengue cases but it is often in this type of co-infections. On the other hand, lowering of platelets and hemoglobin content, reduced aspartate aminotransferase levels and elevated alanine aminotransferase levels are also observed [25].

In 1970, dengue disease was classified as non-classical dengue fever, classical dengue fever, dengue hemorrhagic fever and dengue shock syndrome. Sometime after this, various studies reported lack of correlation between classification and disease severity [26]. This classification showed a high specificity in the identification of hemorrhagic dengue; however, its sensitivity was low when detecting severe dengue cases requiring medical care and/or hospitalization. Thus, the WHO proposed a new classification according to the level of clinical severity by dividing dengue disease in two categories, severe dengue and non-severe dengue in 2008 [1]. This classification makes possible to establish the management and improve notifications for a better epidemiological surveillance so that warning signs and early warning of severe cases requiring hospitalization are proposed [1]. Regarding a study conducted to compare both classifications, it was found that the sensitivity of the new classification to detect severe cases was 65%, and the old classification was 30%. The new classification had 72% of sensitivity to detect patients needing advanced medical services and the old classification only had 32%. Further studies alike indicate that the WHO classification in 2009 has brought benefits in epidemiology and clinical use, some others have proposed to include other variables on severe dengue categories in order to increase sensitivity in a case detection that may require advanced medical care [27].

5. Dengue vectors and mechanisms of infection

Dengue virus is mainly transmitted by *Aedes aegypti* and *Aedes albopictus* mosquitoes. *Aedes aegypti* is a tropical mosquito regarded as the most important disease transmission vector in urban areas, there are also other vector viruses like ZIKV and CHIKV. Dengue outbreaks have also been attributed to *Aedes albopictus*, *Aedes polynesiensis* and various species of complex *Aedes scutellaris* [1]. *Aedes aegypti* is a species with a strong predilection for human blood adapted to urban zones, especially in human dwellings; it is an efficient vector due to certain features like the egg-laying in a wide range of containers, the egg resistance to drying and the capacity of the female mosquito to bite in multiple occasions until they meet their need of blood. *Aedes albopictus* has adapted to temperate and tropical climates and it is a zoophilic and anthrophilic species and as well as *Aedes aegypti*, they both feed during the day [1]. Some laboratory studies have reported that *Aedes albopictus* can become infected and transmit other 22 arboviruses such as CHIKV, Eastern equine encephalitis virus (EEEV), Ross river virus (RRV), Western equine Encephalitis (WEE), YFV among others [28]. The vertical virus transmission (transovarial or transovum) of an infected female mosquito to its eggs and subsequent progeny provides a mechanism as the arbovirus may be maintained in nature during climate conditions such as cold periods in temperate and hot regions, and dry in tropical areas or during the lack of susceptible vertebrate host. Many flaviviruses like YFV, Japanese encephalitis virus (JEV), SLEV, WNV can be transmitted in a vertical manner in its natural vectors [29]. Such natural transmission for DENV has already been approved by *Aedes aegypti* and *Aedes albopictus*; however, it occurs in a smaller proportion in *Aedes aegypti*. Moreover, its potential for transmission and maintenance of disease in nature has not been established yet. The preference of *Aedes aegypti* for little organic matter in water or clean water when it comes to lay eggs provides information about the possible places that these mosquito larvae may be found. However, some studies reported that septic tanks have been identified as places where a high *Aedes aegypti* replication can occur [30]. A study in Brazil assessed rudimentary cesspits as possible *Aedes aegypti* breeding sites identifying immature and adult forms of *Aedes aegypti* in cesspits. The average number of insects found was similar to the one reported in common breeding habitats which confirmed the new place of breeding of this vector [30]. Thus, the identification of new *Aedes aegypti* breeding sites indicates a change in habits or an adaptation of the mosquito in its environment that also need to be considered in vector control strategies of *Aedes aegypti*. Climatic factors play a significant role in its biological cycle and displacement of dengue vector. In a study about the effect of temperature on mosquitoes, it was found that mosquitoes maintained at 20°C were less sensitive to the infection and died in less time which lessened the likelihood of midgut infection without affecting the extrinsic incubation period of DENV as compared to a constant 10°C temperature range [31].

6. Dengue virus jungle cycle and reverse zoonosis

DENV can circulate in jungle cycles where virus can remain in place using *non-human primates* (NHP) as reservoirs or viruses transmitted in an urban cycle can infect non-human primates ('spillback' or 'reverse zoonosis') [12]. The urban and jungle cycles are shown to exist in Asia and Africa, in countries such as Malaysia, Senegal, the Philippines where DENV would be identified by a virus isolation from species such as *Presbytis obscura*, *Erythrocebus patas,* and *Macaca fascicularis* respectively [32]. Studies conducted in South East Asia reported antibodies in non-human primates in Indonesia, the Philippines, Cambodia, Vietnam and Malaysia. DENV viral isolation or identification by RT-PCR in NHP has not been reported in Americas but wild caught patas monkeys (*Erythrocebus patas*) and rhesus macaques (*Macaca mulatta*) showing antibodies against DENV by PRNT were reported in a study carried out between 2010 and 2012 in Puerto Rico [32]. As no evidences of DENV jungle cycle in America were shown, it is believed that these results may represent a spillback infection and non-human primates would get the infection of urban cycles presented in the population. In Argentina 2020, antibodies against DENV-1 y DENV-3 in howler monkeys (*Alouatta caraya*) were found; and in Brazil between 2006 and 2014, low antibodies against DENV in free-living golden headed lion tamarins (*Leontopithecus chrysomelas*) were found [32]. These cases were also assumed to result from spillback infection. A study in Thailand in 2008–2009 identified 6 DENV positive-dogs by RT-PCR and/or viral isolation in urban areas,

2 were DENV-2 positive and 4 were DENV-3 positive in a rubber plantation area [33]. It is necessary to continue with this type of studies in these animals in order to develop a viremia high enough to infect mosquitoes. More than 200 viruses from 27 families, including *flaviviridae*, was isolated or detected in bats and several studies have shown DENV nucleic acids and/or antibodies present in Neotropical wildlife. A study in Costa Rica suggest that bats are infected accidentally by DENV because the RNA quantification in blood was low below the minimum infectious dose of mosquito that is needed to maintain the transmission cycle for the virus. Thus, they were considered as dead-end hosts for dengue virus [34].

7. Problems of dengue diagnosis

A series of multiple variant testing have been carried out for dengue diagnosis depending on a person's infection phase, these tests are conducted with different immunological targets for virus recognition, a part of its structure or a reaction in an infected person or an animal's body indicating an exposure to DENV [35] (**Table 2**).

In a dengue study, diagnostic tests display numerous problems which we will describe briefly. The presence of false positive as a result of contamination and different variants of RT-PCR such as endpoint PCR, nested PCR, real-time PCR as well as the use of different primers and enzymes lead to variations in levels of sensitivity and specificity. Some commercial test enables the identification of different microorganisms by utilizing RT-PCR, PCR tests and the detection of the product in about an hour. The RUO Film Array Global Fever Panel tests are utilized for the detection of 6 bacterias, 4 protozoans and 9 viruses like Chikungunya virus, Crimean-Congo hemorrhagic fever virus, Ebola virus, Lassa virus, Marburg virus, West Nile virus, Yellow fever virus, Zika virus and Dengue virus. Whole blood (EDTA) is used as a sample. The use of automation equipment can help to reduce contamination problems and deliver results in a short time as well as providing diagnosis for 19 pathogens. Regarding to improvements for this type of systems the equipment can only process one sample at a time, and the study is expensive. The rapid tests do not need sophisticated equipment or qualified staff, it is feasible in situ and they are inexpensive. Nonetheless, its sensitivity and specificity are not as higher as other techniques. Cell cultures are often used for dengue virus isolation. Many cell lines are used for virus isolation; however, their sensitivity can vary depending on the type of cell line, the clone, the system used for viral isolation and the sample type used for isolation [35, 36]. In order to isolate DENV, it is preferable to use C6/36 cell line obtained from *Aedes albopictus* mosquito salivary glands that is replicated at 28°C as

Diagnostic test	Immunological target
Polymerase chain reaction (PCR)	RNA detection
Rapid tests	NS1, IgM, IgG
Virus isolation	Virus
Immunofluorescence (IF)	Virus, IgM, IgG
Plaque assay (PA) and fluorescent focus assay (FFA)	Virus (titer)
Enzyme-linked immunosorbent assay (ELISAS)	NS1, IgM, IgG, IgA
Neutralization tests	Neutralizing antibodies (IgG)

Table 2.
Most commonly used diagnostic tests for diagnosing dengue.

it has higher sensitivity than Vero or BHK-21 (mammalian lines). Some researchers suggest using a variety of C6/36 HT which grows at 33°C. Such cell is considered to be more sensitive than the traditional C6/36, and it is recommended to use the shell vial or shell vial modified method instead of the traditional or standard isolated system in order to achieve better results. In the modified shell vial method, the cell culture is infected, centrifuged and incubated for 10–15 days, then positive cultures by indirect immunofluorescence are identified [35, 36]. Many laboratories do two or three passages from cell cultures following an assessment of virus presence conducted by IFI. This increases more the number of isolations but the cost of the testing goes up and the time needed to obtain the results raises. The quantification or viral load may be run by real time PCR utilizing a standard reference that in comparison with the sample allow us to assess the number of genetic material copies from the sample [35, 36]. When it is intended to quantify infecting viruses in biological samples for producing antigens or vaccines, is preferred to use PA in Vero or BHK-21 cells [35, 36]. One alternative for viral titration, depending on the study performed and especially when evaluating viral load in mosquitoes, is the use of FFA that is a mixture of plaque assay and immunofluorescence test and it allows the use of C6/36 cells containing higher sensitivity than the above-mentioned cells [35, 36]. IF and ELISAS tests are relatively low cost and they may occur commercially or may be designed. Many of their components as antibodies and antigens can be produced in the laboratory at lower costs but it is necessary a good quality control of production so that there can be variations in job titles of lots that may affect test results [35, 36]. Neutralization tests can be performed under different techniques such as PRNT, microneutralization, microneutralization-ELISA. These tests facilitate the high specificity type IgG neutralizing antibodies detection. However, the levels of sensitivity in relation to the cell line, the strain of virus and the technique used are due to cell cultures. Other problems have yet been overcome are DENV cross-reactions with other flavivirus and within the same serotypes in serological tests like ELISAS, IFI and even considered to be gold standard like neutralization test by plaque reduction (PRNT) exhibiting cross-reactions. Cross-reactivity between serotypes is frequent and it occurs particularly in epitope on NS protein for the conservation or in conserved epitopes on E glycoprotein and may vary according to homology between every DENV serotype and genotype. The use of specific monoclonal antibodies for every dengue serotype in the IFI tests improve greatly the specificity of the test as compared to the use of HMAF. The use of tests allows to detect multiple pathogens at the same time like CDC DENV-1-4 rRT-PCR multiplex detecting infecting dengue virus serotype and it was approved by FDA in 2013 [35, 37]. The CDC Trioplex rRT-PCR assay uses real-time (TaqMan®) RT-PCR assays for detection and differentiation of RNA from DENV, CHIKV and ZIKV in serum samples, whole blood (EDTA), cerebrospinal fluid. This also enables the RNA detection of ZIKV in urine and amniotic fluids. FDA has authorized the use of this test under an Emergency Use Authorization (EUA) [38].

8. Animal models for dengue

It is not yet found a suitable animal model expressing all characteristics for dengue disease [39]. Among the most common models used for research are mice showing drawbacks with low-level virus replication of clinical samples, and non-human primates showing a problem for not expressing the clinical disease in the same manner as humans [39]. The use of nursing mice used in intracranial inoculations with high viral load inducing neurological diseases and paralysis are still been used; however, its use continues more for the production of biological supplies. DENV can slightly replicate in mice A/J, BALB/c and C57BL/6. Mice A/J and BALB/c can die of paralysis [39, 40]. For animal studies, it is considered that an infection with DENV 10^4–10^6 PFU (plaque-forming units) concentrations imitate inoculum concentrations of a mosquito bite [39]. The mouse model is generally used initially to assess vaccines being the most suitable the immunocompetent mice but when it exhibits low viremia may result in the underestimation of the results. The use of nursing mice is a good way to assess possible candidate vaccines inducing neurovirulence. Although the NHP do not develop the disease, the antibody seroconversion produced is human-like [39, 40].

9. Antivirals for treating dengue

At the moment, there is no antiviral therapy for DENV treatment. It is believed that the compounds working as inhibitors of RNA-dependent RNA polymerase have shown low efficiency. Moreover, there is a possibility that viral epitopes of DENV may trigger an immune cell response, preceded by development of severe disease. Thus, these epitopes are examined as targets for antiviral productions and they are known as DENV entry inhibitors and can be used in combination with inhibitors of the virus replication in order to increase efficiency.

Inhibition of DENV attachment and entry into the host cell can inhibit immune activation.

Various compounds as peptide entry inhibitors, DN59 and 1OAN1 may inhibit the antibody-dependent enhancement (ADE) in vitro. The doxorubicin antibiotic SA-17 is structured similarly to tetracycline and it has an antiviral activity against DENV serotype 1, 2 and 3 in Vero and C6/36 cells interfering with viral entry by binding to the hydrophobic pocket of the E-protein without exhibiting virucidal activity. The glycosidase inhibitors are unpopular due to its toxicity and low specificity but may help understand E-protein glycosylation processes. The binding agents to carbohydrates occur only during the stage of virus adsorption to the host cell. Concanavalin and agglutinins of wheat germ can bind N-acetylglucosamine residues and the percentage of DENV-lytic plaques in BHK cells can be reduced. Plant lectins such as *Hippeastrum hybrid*, *Galanthus nivalis*, and *Urtica dioica* inhibit DENV-2 infection in Raji/DC-SIGN cells. The compounds of heparan sulfate are potential recipients for DENV. Dengue E protein domain III is responsible for the interaction of heparan sulfate, and it is believed to be in all DENV serotypes and to have epitopes that are recognized by neutralizing antibodies. The suramin is similar to heparan sulfate and persulfated glycosaminoglycan, they bind to a polyanion-binding site of DENV E protein by inhibiting infection. The sulfated polysaccharides extracted from red algae, carrageenans and DL-galactan presented antiviral activity against 4 serotypes of dengue; however, the antiviral activity of DENV-4 DENV-1 weakened in Vero cells and in human Hepatocytes [41, 42].

10. Dengue vaccine

In May 2019, the U.S. Food and Drug Administration (FDA) approved the use of Dengvaxia®, a vaccine against DENV that may be used in people aged from 9 to 45 years old [43]. This vaccine utilizes a live attenuated chimeric yellow fever/dengue virus based on a Yellow fever 17D vaccine virus backbone chimerized with prM and E proteins from DENV1–4 replacing the YF prM and E, and 3 doses are administered every 6 months. In phase III trials the overall protective efficacy was 56.7% and 60.8% in South East Asia and Latin America countries, respectively. In 2017, the vaccine manufacturer, Sanofi Pasteur, announced that some people getting the vaccine without having been previously infected by DENV may be at risk for developing severe dengue if the disease is acquired after immunization [43]. The vaccine candidates utilize strategies such as vaccines of Live-attenuated virus, Inactivated virus, Recombinant protein, DNA vaccine, Viral vector vaccine, Virus like particles and others. Two vaccine candidates (DENVax and TV003/TV005) are being tested in efficacy trials in both Asia and Latin America. DENVax is a tetravalent recombinant live-attenuated dengue vaccine licensed to Takeda. The live virus vaccine utilizes chimerization with DENV-2 PDK-53 as the backbone with DENV-2/-1, -2/-3, and -2/-4 chimeras are created by replacing the DENV-2 prM and E genes with the respective genes from the other DENV serotypes. Other vaccine candidate is TV003/TV00 with a whole attenuated virus for three of four serotypes (attenuated by deletion of 30 nucleotides from 3′ UTR of DENV-1, DENV-3, DENV-4, and a chimeric DENV-2/DENV-4) [44]. In spite of having already a vaccine available to prevent dengue, there is a need to further research in order to improve the vaccine for dengue or to produce a new vaccine which enables improvements in certain aspects, for example, a single dose that may immunize for extended periods of time even lifelong, the vaccine effectiveness no longer relying on previous exposure to flavivirus or DENV, the age of group to provide protection being the broadest possible including children under 9 years old, and its administration decreasing the chances of getting the most aggressive dengue disease at no point post vaccination.

11. Conclusions

Dengue is still a major public health concern worldwide. Several natural and social factors have contributed to the number of cases increased in recent decades. The efforts attained in the search of new antivirals and vaccines, and prevention and control strategies for this disease have not proved sufficient. However, the science and knowledge development acquired up to now provide us the tools we need to, and mark the way to follow, in order to achieve a control of this disease.

Conflict of interest

The authors declare no conflict of interest.

Disclaimer

The views expressed in this chapter are those of the author and do not necessarily reflect the official policy or position of the Department of the Navy, Department of Defense, nor the U.S. Government.

Copyright statement

Author details

Juan Samuel Sulca Herencia
U.S. Naval Medical Research Unit No. 6, Universidad Nacional Mayor de San Marcos, Lima, Peru

*Address all correspondence to: juan.sulca4@unmsm.edu.pe; juan.s.sulca.ln@mail.mil

References

[1] WHO. Dengue guías para el diagnóstico, tratamiento, prevención y control [Internet]. Ginebra: World Health Organization; 2009. Available from: http://www.who.int/iris/handle/10665/44504

[2] Brathwaite Dick O, San Martín J, del Diego J, Montoya R, Dayan G, Zambrano B. The history of dengue outbreaks in the Americas. The American Journal of Tropical Medicine and Hygiene. 2012;**87**(4):584-593

[3] Dengue |CDC [Internet]. Cdc.gov. 2020. Available from: https://www.cdc.gov/dengue/index.html

[4] Wilder-Smith A. Dengue infections in travellers. Paediatrics and International Child Health. 2012;**32**(sup1):28-32

[5] dos Reis I, Honório N, Codeço C, Magalhães M, Lourenço-de-Oliveira R, Barcellos C. Relevance of differentiating between residential and non-residential premises for surveillance and control of Aedes aegypti in Rio de Janeiro, Brazil. Acta Tropica. 2010;**114**(1):37-43

[6] Duong V, Lambrechts L, Paul R, Ly S, Lay R, Long K, et al. Asymptomatic humans transmit dengue virus to mosquitoes. Proceedings of the National Academy of Sciences. 2015;**112**(47):14688-14693

[7] Hernández M, Arboleda D, Arce S, Benavides A, Tejada P, Ramírez S, et al. Metodología para la elaboración de canales endémicos y tendencia de la notificación del dengue, Valle del Cauca, Colombia. Biomédica. 2016;**36**(2):98-107

[8] Zambrano L, Sierra M, Lara B, Rodríguez-Núñez I, Medina M, Lozada-Riascos C, et al. Estimating and mapping the incidence of dengue and chikungunya in Honduras during 2015 using geographic information systems (GIS). Journal of Infection and Public Health. 2017;**10**(4):446-456

[9] Table of Contents | 2020 Yellow Book | Travelers' Health | CDC [Internet]. Wwwnc.cdc.gov. 2020. Available from: https://wwwnc.cdc.gov/travel/yellowbook/2020/table-of-contents

[10] Sabino E, Loureiro P, Lopes M, Capuani L, McClure C, Chowdhury D, et al. Transfusion-transmitted dengue and associated clinical symptoms during the 2012 epidemic in Brazil. Journal of Infectious Diseases. 2015;**213**(5):694-702

[11] Kokara P. Dengue Virus Specific Immune Response: Implications for Laboratory Diagnosis and Vaccine Development [to Obtain the Degree of Doctor]. Rotterdam: Erasmus University; 2007

[12] Chen R, Vasilakis N. Dengue—Quo tu et quo vadis? Viruses. 2011;**3**(9):1562-1608

[13] Forshey B, Reiner R, Olkowski S, Morrison A, Espinoza A, Long K, et al. Incomplete protection against dengue virus type 2 Re-infection in Peru. PLOS Neglected Tropical Diseases. 2016;**10**(2):1-17

[14] Kochel TJ, Watts DM, Halstead SB, Hayes CG, Espinoza A, Felices V, et al. Effect of dengue-1 anti-bodies on American dengue-2 viral infection and dengue haemorrhagic fever. Lancet. 2002;**360**:310-312

[15] Mustafa M, Rasotgi V, Jain S, Gupta V. Discovery of fifth serotype of dengue virus (DENV-5): A new public health dilemma in dengue control. Medical Journal Armed Forces India. 2015;**71**(1):67-70

[16] Restrepo B, Ramírez R, Agudelo-Florez P, Avendaño E, Chacón J, Rojas W, et al. Características clínicas y niveles de citocinas en pacientes con dengue y su relación con la raza, Colombia. Revista Biomédica. 2010;**21**:137-147

[17] González Cortiñas M, Vidal González D, Cepero Cordero J, Lashley OM. Dengue hemorrágico. Estudio clínico de 200 pacientes. Revista Cubana de Medicina. 1999;**38**(1):13-18

[18] Htun N, Odermatt P, Eze I, Boillat-Blanco N, D'Acremont V, Probst-Hensch N. Is diabetes a risk factor for a severe clinical presentation of dengue?—Review and meta-analysis. PLOS Neglected Tropical Diseases. 2015;**9**(4):e0003741

[19] Sinhababu V, Sathananthan R, Malavige G. Perinatal transmission of dengue: A case report. BMC Research Notes. 2014;7(1):795

[20] Yung C, Lee K, Thein T, Tan L, Gan V, Wong J, et al. Dengue serotype-specific differences in clinical manifestation, laboratory parameters and risk of severe disease in adults, Singapore. The American Journal of Tropical Medicine and Hygiene. 2015;**92**(5):999-1005

[21] United States, National Center for Emerging and Zoonotic Infectious Diseases (CDC), Pan American Health Organization. Preparedness and Response for Chikungunya Virus: Introduction in the Americas. Washington D.C.: United States, National Center for Emerging and Zoonotic Infectious Diseases (CDC), Pan American Health Organization; 2011

[22] Beltrán-Silva S, Chacón-Hernández S, Moreno-Palacios E, Pereyra-Molina J. Clinical and differential diagnosis: Dengue, chikungunya and Zika. Revista Médica del Hospital General de México. 2018;**81**(3):146-153

[23] Sulca J, Guevara C, Halsey E, Ampuero J. Aislamiento de los serotipos 1 y 3 del virus dengue por shell vial modificado en un paciente coinfectado. Revista Peruana de Medicina Experimental y Salud Pública. 2014;**30**(2):354-355

[24] Salam N, Mustafa S, Hafiz A, Chaudhary AA, Deeba F, Parveen S. Global prevalence and distribution of coinfection of malaria, dengue and chikungunya: A systematic review. BMC Public Health. 2018;**18**(1):710. PMID: 29879935

[25] Selvaretnam A, Sahu P, Sahu M, Ambu S. A review of concurrent infections of malaria and dengue in Asia. Asian Pacific Journal of Tropical Biomedicine. 2016;**6**(7):633-638

[26] Horstick O, Jaenisch T, Martinez E, Kroeger A, See L, Farrar J, et al. Comparing the usefulness of the 1997 and 2009 WHO dengue case classification: A systematic literature review. The American Journal of Tropical Medicine and Hygiene. 2014;**91**(3):621-634

[27] Ajlan B, Alafif M, Alawi M, Akbar N, Aldigs E, Madani T. Assessment of the new World Health Organization's dengue classification for predicting severity of illness and level of healthcare required. PLOS Neglected Tropical Diseases. 2019;**13**(8):1-16

[28] Moore C. Aedes albopictus in the United States: Ten-year presence and public health implications. Emerging Infectious Diseases. 1997;**3**(3):329-334

[29] Thangamani S, Huang J, Hart C, Guzman H, Tesh R. Vertical transmission of Zika virus in Aedes aegypti mosquitoes. The American Journal of Tropical Medicine and Hygiene. 2016;**95**(5):1169-1173

[30] Gil L, Katsuragawa T, Lima A, Tada M, Ozaki L, Julião G. Rudimentary

cesspits as breeding sites for Aedes aegypti in urban areas of Northern Brazil. Revista Pan-Amazônica de Saúde. 2015;**6**(3):73-80

[31] Lambrechts L, Paaijmans K, Fansiri T, Carrington L, Kramer L, Thomas M, et al. Impact of daily temperature fluctuations on dengue virus transmission by Aedes aegypti. Proceedings of the National Academy of Sciences. 2011;**108**(18):7460-7465

[32] Valentine MJ, Murdock CC, Kelly PJ. Sylvatic cycles of arboviruses in non-human primates. Parasit Vectors. 2019;**12**:463. DOI: 10.1186/s13071-019-3732-0

[33] Thongyuan S, Kittayapong P. First evidence of dengue infection in domestic dogs living in different ecological settings in Thailand. PLoS One. 2017;**12**(8):e0180013. DOI: 10.1371/journal.pone.0180013

[34] Vicente-Santos A, Moreira-Soto A, Soto-Garita C, Chaverri LG, Chaves A, Drexler JF, et al. Neotropical bats that co-habit with humans function as dead-end hosts for dengue virus. PLoS Neglected Tropical Diseases. 2017;**11**(5):e0005537. DOI: 10.1371/journal.pntd.0005537

[35] Herencia JSS. Laboratory tests used in the diagnostic and research of dengue virus: Present and future, dengue fever—A resilient. In: Falcón-Lezama JA, Betancourt-Cravioto M, Tapia-Conyer R, editors. Threat in the Face of Innovation. Rijeka: IntechOpen; 2018. DOI: 10.5772/intechopen.80519. Available from: https://www.intechopen.com/books/dengue-fever-a-resilient-threat-in-the-face-of-innovation/laboratory-tests-used-in-the-diagnostic-and-research-of-dengue-virus-present-and-future

[36] Instituto de Medicina Tropical Pedro Kourí. Técnicas de laboratorio para el diagnóstico y la caracterización del virus dengue. La Habana: Instituto de Medicina Tropical Pedro Kourí; 2013. p. 128

[37] Centers for Disease Control and Prevention. Ensayo de RT-PCR en tiempo real para DENV-1-4 de los CDC. Puerto Rico: Centers for Disease Control and Prevention; 2013. p. 56

[38] Colombo T, Versiani A, Dutra K, Rubiato J, Galvão T, Negri Reis A, et al. Performance of CDC Trioplex qPCR during a dengue outbreak in Brazil. Journal of Clinical Virology. 2019;**121**:104208

[39] Zompi S, Harris E. Animal models of dengue virus infection. Viruses. 2012;**4**:62-82

[40] Na W, Yeom M, Choi I, Yook H, Song D. Animal models for dengue vaccine development and testing. Clinical and Experimental Vaccine Research. 2017;**6**(2):104-110

[41] Alen M, Schols D. Dengue virus entry as Target for antiviral therapy. Journal of Tropical Medicine. 2012;**2012**:1-13

[42] Low J, Ooi E, Vasudevan S. Current status of dengue therapeutics research and development. The Journal of Infectious Diseases. 2017;**215**(suppl_2):S96-S102

[43] Dengue Vaccine | Dengue | CDC [Internet]. Cdc.gov. 2020. Available from: https://www.cdc.gov/dengue/prevention/dengue-vaccine.html

[44] Prompetchara E, Ketloy C, Thomas SJ, Ruxrungtham K. Dengue vaccine: Global development update. Asian Pacific Journal of Allergy and Immunology. 2019. DOI: 10.12932/AP-100518-0309 [epub ahead of print]. Available from: http://apjai-journal.org/wp-content/uploads/2019/02/AP-100518-0309.pdf

Chapter 3

Situation of Dengue after the Phenomenon of the Coastal El Niño

Cristian Díaz-Vélez, Jorge Luis Fernández-Mogollón, John Alexis Cabrera-Enríquez, Stalin Tello-Vera, Oscar Medrano-Velásquez and Elmer Córdova-Calle

Abstract

Coastal El Niño is a weather phenomenon that is caused by abnormal warming (above 0.4°C) of the Pacific Ocean waters near the coasts of Ecuador and Peru, and it can even reach the central and southern Peruvian coast. As a result of the climatic phenomenon, the Aedes *aegypti* vector (which in turn is a vector of chikungunya and Zika fever) had been quickly installed in 448 districts of Peru, and emergency was declared in 10 regions, which reported 231,874 victims; 1,129,013 affected and 143 dead. It is necessary to know this, because the direct impact of the weather phenomena contributes to the dengue vector conditioning, facilitating its dissemination with ease. The geographical and climatic conditions of the cities most affected by the El Niño Costero phenomenon turned them into zones of epidemics; in these places, there is an important population growth, from urbanization to sectorization in young towns and urban slums, where in many there is no basic infrastructure and water supply is insufficient, which requires temporary water storage, as well as high temperatures, migratory movement, and beaches with influx of people, which make not only dengue proliferate but also other arbovirosis such as chikungunya.

Keywords: dengue, natural phenomenon, natural disaster, public health

1. Epidemiology of dengue and the coastal El Niño phenomenon in Peru and Ecuador

1.1 Epidemiological data

Coastal El Niño is a weather phenomenon that is caused by abnormal warming (above 0.4°C) of the Pacific Ocean waters near the coasts of Ecuador and Peru, and it can even reach the central and southern Peruvian coasts. As a result, it produces intense rains that, in turn, cause overflow of streams, floods, and allow the accumulation of stagnant waters, which forms the ideal scenario for the appearance of outbreaks of vector-borne diseases such as dengue (DENV), other arbovirosis, and zoonotics such as leptospirosis [1–4]. This phenomenon was presented more clearly in the summer of 2017; however, rains and floods have been reported for Peru even since December 2016 [5].

As a result of the climatic phenomenon, the *Aedes aegypti* vector (which in turn is a vector of chikungunya and Zika [ZIKV] fever) had been quickly installed in 448 districts of Peru, where more than 14 million people live, by July 2017 [6]. Thus, the Peruvian State in June 2017, declared emergency in 10 regions, which reported 231,874 victims; 1,129,013 affected and 143 dead. It is necessary to know this, because the direct impact of the weather phenomena contributes to the dengue vector conditioning, facilitating its dissemination with ease. Thus, the Peruvian Ministry of Health reported that at the end of 2017, the epidemiological surveillance system reported 76,093 cases of dengue (among probable and confirmed), marking an increase of up to three times more cases compared to 2016 (25,236 cases) (**Figure 1**) [7].

Among the most frequently reported forms were dengue without warning signs (88.6%), dengue with warning signs (11%), and severe dengue (0.3%). The cumulative national incidence for 2017 was 239.1 cases per 100,000 inhabitants and there were 93 deaths, of which 79 were confirmed cases and 14 were probable [8].

There was a marked increase in cases, in those places where there was a greater presence of rain and floods. Thus, for example, Piura concentrated 64% of dengue cases: this place being one of the most affected cities and even presented an overflow from its main river that crosses through the same city, the river Piura [9].

Do not forget that northern Peru is an endemic area due to climate, geography, and other factors that make it a vector-friendly ecosystem, being considered one of the countries with the greatest impact due to climate change [10].

1.2 Dengue and climate

Dengue transmission occurs through an insect vector, predominantly *Aedes aegytpi* but also *Aedes albopictus*. Environmental parameters, especially temperature and precipitation, affect the demography and behavior of these vectors, making dengue an obvious candidate to investigate the impact of climate on the disease. The incidence of dengue is very seasonal; this seasonality is the footprint of local meteorological variables, which also vary seasonally, and their impact on the demographics of mosquito vectors and transmission dynamics [11].

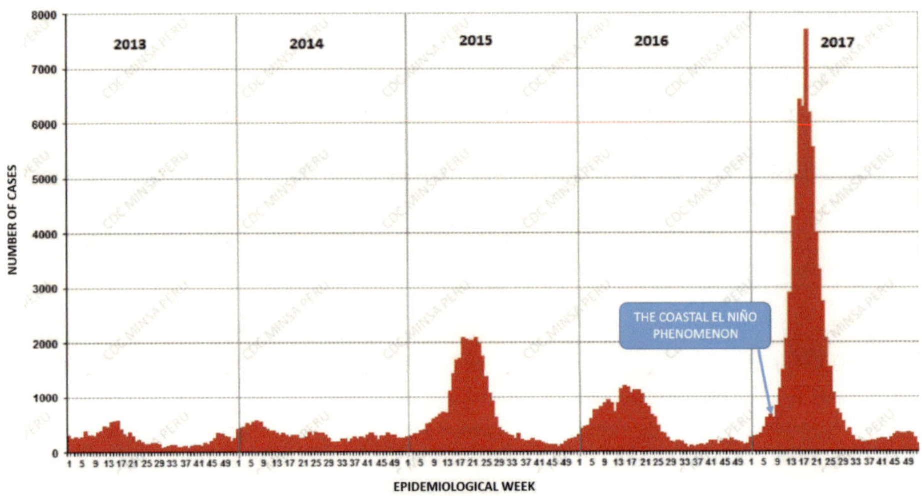

Figure 1.
Number of dengue cases, according to epidemiological weeks. Peru, 2013–2017. Taken from: Ministry of Health of Peru MINSA [12].

The geographical and climatic conditions of the cities most affected by the El Niño Costero phenomenon turned them into zones of epidemics; in these places, there is an important population growth, from urbanization to sectorization in young towns, urban slums, where in many there is no basic infrastructure and water supply is insufficient, which requires temporary water storage, as well as high temperatures, migratory movement, and beaches with influx of people, which make not only dengue proliferate but also other arbovirosis such as chikungunya [13].

1.3 Epidemiology of other metaxenic diseases

The propagation of the vector for decades is conditioned by the climatic changes. For example, in May 2004, heat waves and droughts were observed in the coastal areas of Kenya, toward Lamu and Mombasa, two large coastal cities. That period was also the beginning of a large chikungunya outbreak in these two cities (with reported attack rates of 75%) before its spread to the Indian Ocean [14]. Entomologists have explained how and why droughts can be associated with increases in diseases transmitted by *Aedes*, such as chikungunya, dengue, Zika, and yellow fever [15, 16]. During droughts, due to water scarcity, people store a greater amount of water outside or inside the home for longer periods of time, providing shelters to mosquito eggs and larvae [13].

In Peru, the consequence of this weather phenomenon allowed the dissemination of the *Aedes* vector and consequently led to the increase in cases of emerging diseases, such as Zika and chikungunya (**Figure 2**). Thus, from 2016 to 2018, 1113 gestating women entered the surveillance system for Zika, of which 61% were notified in 2017. Of the total number of pregnant women notified, 31% had laboratory confirmation for Zika virus through molecular tests like polymerase chain reaction-reverse transcription (RT-PCR) [7].

1.4 Dengue and coinfections

The fluvial precipitations that the phenomenon of the coastal El Niño brought with it during 2017 triggered the collapse of the sewerage system, generating floods and the exposure of wastewater, which together with the rains gave an adequate

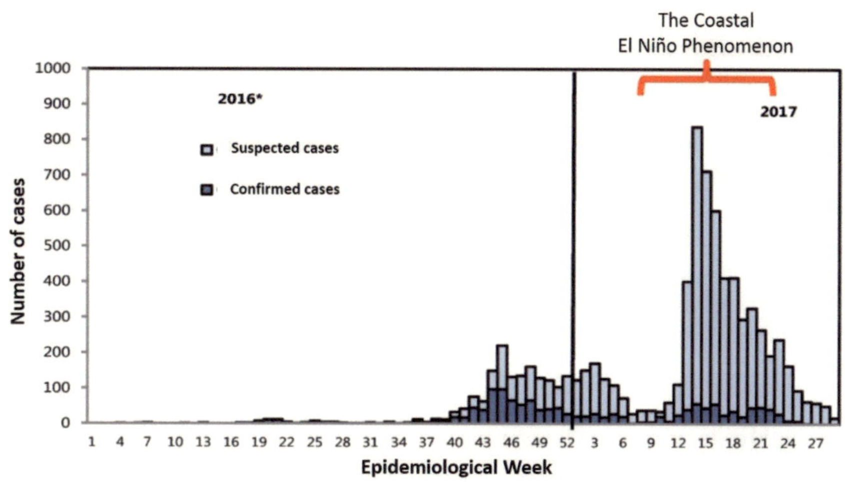

Figure 2.
Distribution of indigenous cases of Zika by onset of symptoms. Peru 2016–2017. Taken from: Ministry of Health of Peru MINSA [17].

environment for the transmission of leptospirosis in urban areas of the Lambayeque region. It was even possible to demonstrate that during this period, laboratory findings compatible with dengue and leptospirosis were reported simultaneously. While it is true that many of the immunoglobulin can remain for years in the patient and do not necessarily require an acute infection, the similarity of clinical symptoms between dengue and leptospirosis makes both pathologies confusing to health personnel, even more so during the appearance of a weather phenomenon where there is an outbreak [18].

1.5 Dengue and seasonality

Dengue in Ecuador fluctuates with a very similar seasonality. The season is an important determinant of infectious disease rates, including mosquito-propagated arboviruses, such as dengue, chikungunya, and Zika. Seasonal disease patterns are driven by a combination of climatic or environmental factors, such as temperature or rainfall, and trends in human behavior time, such as school year schedules, vacations, and weekend patterns. These factors affect both disease rates and medical care-seeking behavior. The seasonality of dengue fever has been studied in the context of climatic factors. Thus, between 2009 and 2016, a predictive model of dengue detection was studied using data from the same patients in rural areas in Ecuador. Thus, compared to the average of every day, cases were more likely to be diagnosed on Tuesdays (relative risk [RR]: 1.26; 95% confidence interval [CI]: 1.05–1.51) and Thursdays (RR: 1.25; 95% CI: 1.02–1.53), and were less likely to be diagnosed on Saturdays (RR: 0.81; 95% CI: 0.65–1.01) and Sundays (RR: 0.74; 95% CI: 0.58–0.95). The holidays were not significant predictors of dengue diagnoses, except for an increase in diagnoses the day after Christmas (RR: 2.77; 95% CI: 1.46–5.24) [19].

From the political sphere, the coastal El Niño phenomenon caused the Ministry of Health and the Ministry of Defense of Ecuador to take into account the declaration of emergency for the Peruvian city of Piura, issued by the Ministry of Health of that country. This is because that city is close to the border of Ecuador, and the trade between the two countries is very high, which makes it necessary to work in a multisectoral way to eradicate the vector [20].

1.6 Impact on the epidemiological surveillance system

It is very necessary to maintain entomological surveillance, especially in those cities where the phenomenon left vector presence. Migration and population increase, in addition to raising awareness and educating the population about the risk factors of dengue occurrence, should always be taken into account to avoid a disease that was installed in the Americas decades ago, precisely because of migration from other areas. The consequences of climate change must be learned as it not only destroys our habitat but directly interferes with our health [21]. Health authorities have the responsibility to plan strategies and evaluate their impact progressively. Many times it is not enough to plan, but to change strategies to avoid having the same results.

2. Clinical behavior of dengue

2.1 Definitions

Classically, the disease presents with an incubation period of 3–14 days; after that a febrile phase (1–4 days); viremia, the critical phase from 4 to 7 days; and a recovery phase from day 7 onward [22]. This disease course depends on the virus serotype and whether or not the individual has previously had a dengue infection. In this spectrum of disease, one can have:

- Dengue without warning signs: Person with a fever of 7 or less days, with at least two of the following symptoms such as eye pain, myalgia, headache, arthralgia, low back pain, rash, and nausea [23, 24].

- Dengue with warning signs: Person with a probable case of dengue with one or more of the clinical signs such as severe abdominal pain, dyspnea, serous effusion, persistent vomiting, hypothermia, mucosal bleeding, altered mental status, increased hematocrit, and hepatomegaly [23, 24].

- Severe dengue: A probable case with or without warning signs presenting one of the following signs such as signs of hypovolemic shock, severe bleeding, respiratory distress syndrome due to plasma extravasation, and severe organ involvement (encephalitis, hepatitis, and myocarditis) [25].

2.2 Signs and symptoms

It is known that the cross-immunity of dengue serotypes is limited, which increases the possibility of reinfections and with them more florid clinical pictures [25, 26].

Previous studies observed the outbreaks from 2010 onward, observing that dengue cases occurred in a greater proportion due to DENV-2, the most frequent clinical symptom being retro-ocular pain, myalgias associated with a 7-day fever [27]. Also, it was observed that in dengue cases, many of them were reinfections and DENV-2 continued to prevail, which was one of the worst at presenting cross-immunity (**Figure 3**).

A study conducted in the north coast of Peru found that, among the referred symptoms, 82% reported fever, being less than half quantified (values from 37to 41°C), followed by headache (75.6%), arthralgias (69.7%), myalgias (62.4%), retroocular pain (55.5%), lumbar pain (44.7%), and only 24.4% presenting rash. The presence of platelet decrease (78.4%) was the most frequent among cases with alarm signs [28] (**Figure 4**).

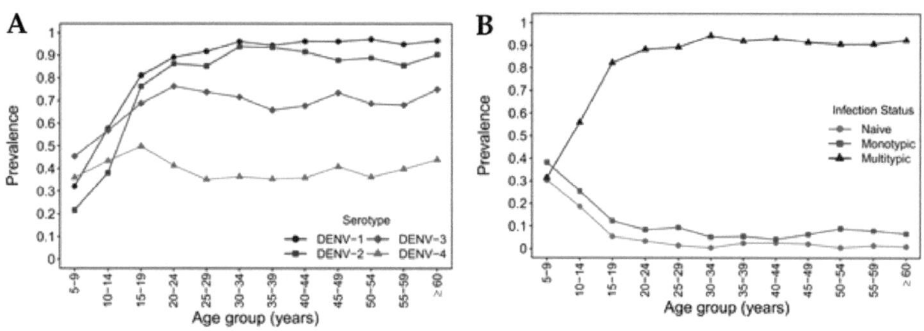

Figure 3.
Age distribution of DENV-neutralizing antibodies in 2010. Samples were collected between March and June 2010, approximately 6 months prior to a large dengue epidemic largely caused by American/Asian genotype DENV-2. Panel A: Age distribution of serotype-specific DENV-neutralizing antibodies. Panel B: Age distribution of number of prior DENV infections. Naive indicates absence of detectable DENV-neutralizing antibodies against any serotype, monotypic indicates DENV-neutralizing antibodies against one serotype, and multitypic indicates DENV-neutralizing antibodies against two or more serotypes. Taken from: Forshey et al. [29].

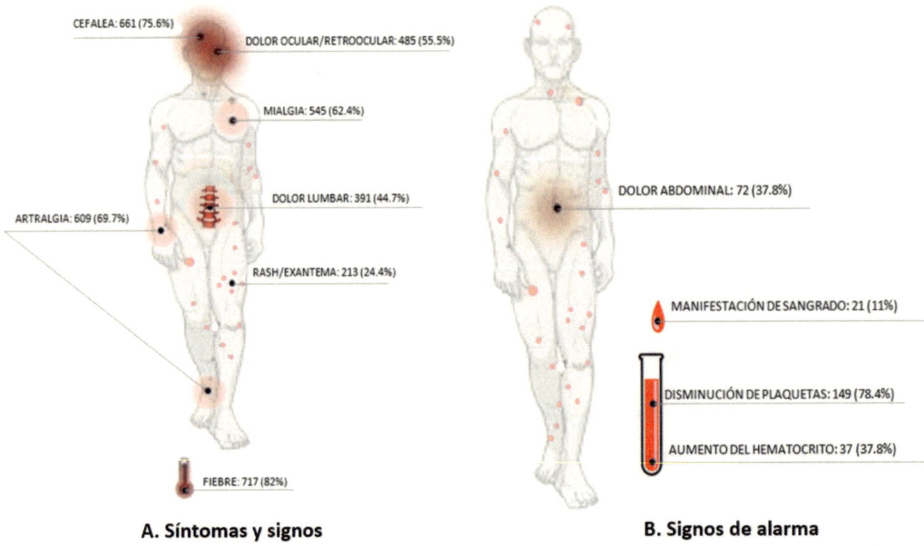

Figure 4.
Symptomatology of patients diagnosed with dengue. (A) Symptoms and signs. (B) Warning signs. Taken from: Perales-Carrasco et al. [28].

2.3 Signs and symptoms in coinfections

In recent years, new viruses such as chikungunya (CHIKV) and Zika (ZIKV) have also been introduced. In recent years after the ZIKV epidemic, cases of ZIKV infection have continued to be observed, and in children, according to Salgado et al. [30], there were found patients with encephalitis with coinfection of DENV and ZIKV.

Another study, also conducted in Peru, showed that the circulating serotypes during the coastal El Niño phenomenon were DENV-2 and DENV-3, as well as confirmed cases of CHIKV and ZIKV, even in high Andean areas; concomitantly, the study revealed that the main symptoms of dengue were headaches, arthralgias, and back pain associated with fever (**Table 1**) [27].

Taken from: Forshey et al. [29].

In Peru, there could be a subdiagnosis or overdiagnosis of dengue and therefore of the clinical variability, on the one hand; the amount of arbovirosis that can give a similar clinical presentation is wide, and within these viruses is oropuche, which can be confused with dengue during the endemic months [31]. The contrary occurs in patients with a second dengue virus infection in which the diagnostic methods have a lower sensitivity of 60%, as is the case of non-structural (NS1), a test widely used in our environment [26].

The Huánuco region, located in the center of Peru, was one of the cities that presented an increase in dengue cases, where about 90% of patients presented with myalgia, headache, and rash; being in these patients a diagnostic confirmation of 92% by PCR. This being an area with low endemicity, but as a result of coastal El Niño, it could mean a majority of primary infection, and therefore this high rate of clinical diagnostic correlation [26]. In addition, it is important to know the behavior in children under 5 years of age, in which many of them have antigens from mothers in endemic areas, which leads to more severe manifestations being possible in this particular age group [32].

Finally, it can be observed that, in the years before the dengue virus infection, the agent (DENV-2) and the clinical manifestations were similar, with the difference in the number of cases and the increase in coinfections of the new circulating

Clinical symptoms	Total n = 496 (%)	PCR real-time confirmed cases		
		DENV (n = 170)	ZIKV (n = 39)	CHIKV (n = 23)
		n (%)	n (%)	n (%)
Chills	3 (0.6)	1 (0.6)	0 (0.0)	0 (0.0)
Headache	444 (89.5)	152 (89.4)	34 (87.2)	20 (87.0)
Dizziness	1 (0.2)	0 (0.0)	1 (2.6)	0 (0.0)
Cough	1 (0.2)	1 (0.6)	0 (0.0)	0 (0.0)
Sore throat	184 (37.1)	50 (29.4)	11 (28.2)	11 (47.8)
Nausea and/or vomits	251 (50.6)	86 (50.6)	20 (51.3)	13 (56.5)
Loss of appetite	312 (62.9)	104 (61.2)	23 (59.0)	18 (78.3)
Back pain	270 (54.4)	105 (61.8)	23 (59.0)	17 (73.9)
Dysuria	1 (0.2)	0 (0.0)	0 (0.0)	0 (0.0)
Myalgia	419 (84.5)	147 (86.5)	35 (89.7)	17 (73.9)
Arthralgia	396 (79.8)	143 (84.1)	32 (82.1)	19 (82.6)
Retro-ocular pain	337 (67.9)	118 (69.4)	27 (69.2)	17 (73.9)
Rash	89 (17.9)	26 (15.3)	8 (20.5)	6 (26.1)
Melena	2 (0.4)	0 (0.0)	0 (0.0)	0 (0.0)
Nasal bleeding	9 (1.8)	3 (1.8)	1 (2.6)	1 (4.3)
Gums bleeding	3 (0.6)	2 (1.2)	1 (2.6)	0 (0.0)
Petechiae	11 (2.2)	3 (1.8)	0 (0.0)	1 (4.3)
Ecchymosis	2 (0.4)	1 (0.6)	1 (2.6)	0 (0.0)
Blood-tinged sputum	1 (0.2)	0 (0.0)	0 (0.0)	0 (0.0)
Abdominal pain	22 (4.4)	7 (4.1)	1 (2.6)	1 (4.3)
Thoracic pain	5 (1.0)	2 (1.2)	0 (0.0)	0 (0.0)
Fatigue	3 (0.6)	0 (0.0)	1 (2.6)	0 (0.0)
Altered mental status	1 (0.2)	1 (0.6)	0 (0.0)	1 (4.3)

Table 1.
Clinical symptoms in patients with positive samples for DENV, ZIKV, and CHIKV.

viruses; this should make the health staff reflect on making proper use of diagnostic tests to provide better care and avoid fatal outcomes, as it was in some cases discussed above in the last phenomenon of the coastal El Niño (**Table 2**).

3. Laboratory in the diagnosis of dengue

Today, there are guidelines established by international organizations for the rational use of dengue diagnostic tests. The World Health Organization (WHO) recommends the use of polymerase chain reaction (PCR) for the early detection of dengue and its complementation with other tests such as immunoglobulin M (IgM), immunoglobulin G (IgG), and NS1 [33]; however, the use according to the clinical picture and the time of the disease will favor the optimal use of the different tests.

The sensitivity and specificity of the NS1 antigen test can range from 49 to 59% and from 93 to 99%, respectively, while that of the IgM antibody test is from 71 to

Characteristics	**Crude analysis**			**Risks for dengue**
	Chikungunya	**Dengue**	**p-value**	**Adjusted odds ratio (95% CI)***
Clinical				
Diarrhea, n (%)	3/37 (8)	13/57 (23)	0.064	2.13 (0.29–15.66)
Ascites, n (%)	0/37 (0)	1/57 (2)	1.000**	N.E.
Pleural effusion, n (%)	0/37 (0)	2/56 (4)	0.516	N.E.
Laboratory				
Hemoglobin (mg/dl) median (interquartile range (IQR)) [n]	10.5 (10–12) [35]	10.5 (10–12) [36]	0.910	
Decrease for age, n (%)	26/36 (72)	25/53 (47)	0.019	1.33 (0.26–6.87)
Increase for age, n (%)	0/36 (0)	1/53 (2)	1.000**	N.E.
Hematocrit (%) median (IQR) [n]	30.9 (29–34) [33]	31.5 (30–35) [37]	a. 0.510	
Decrease for age, n (%)	24/33 (73)	30/52 (58)	0.160	1.04 (0.26–4.19)
Increase for age, n (%)	0/33 (0)	1/52 (2)	1.000**	N.E.
White blood cells (1000 cells/ml) Median (IQR) [n]	6.4 (5–10) [33]	7.4 (5–12) [36]	0.220	
Decrease for age, n (%)	17/33 (52)	16/53 (30)	0.048	0.28 (0.07–1.08)
Increase for age, n (%)	4/33 (12)	5/53 (9)	0.728	1.97 (0.27–14.17)

Note: N.E.: Not estimable. Taken from: Paternina-Caicedo et al. [32].
**Adjusted by age, days with symptoms, and sex.*
***Fisher's exact test.*
****Best fit was the natural logarithm of the exposure variable.*

Table 2.
Clinical and laboratory characteristics of chikungunya and dengue and their relative adjusted risks among children <24 months of age in Colombia.

80% and 46 to 90%, respectively, considering a median of 5 days of fever before the collection of the samples (interquartile range of 3–7 days) for the two tests mentioned. The diagnostic accuracy for the detection of IgM increases for late acute infection (5 days after the onset of symptoms) compared to the early one. The NS1 antigen is an early marker of acute infection, and its combined use with IgM detection can provide a definitive diagnosis of 96.9–100% for samples obtained after 3 days of illness [33]. The reported sensitivity and specificity of IgG for dengue are 92.0 and 100%, respectively [34].

The patient usually has an incubation period of 4–5 days after the bite by mosquitoes of the *Aedes* genus, then presents a clinical picture with variable signs and symptoms for a period of 4–5 days, a period in which he presents the virus of the dengue circulating in the bloodstream and can transmit the disease to other patients through new bites by the aforementioned vector, so techniques based on virus isolation, through cultures, or the detection of genomic material, such as PCR, require samples taken during this time. The end of the patient's clinical picture is usually manifested by a generalized maculopapular rash, which indicates recovery and can guide the use of serological tests, such as the detection of IgM and IgM antibodies, since the viral load values in the patient have disappeared or significantly reduced, which would make the use of molecular tests or culture inefficient. Leukopenia can be found at this stage with normal platelet and transaminase counts [3].

We can summarize the diagnostic tests used for dengue in four groups: (i) virus isolation and characterization, (ii) detection of the genomic sequence through a nucleic acid amplification test, (iii) detection of specific antibodies against the virus, and (iv) identification of dengue virus (glycoprotein) antigens. Isolation of the virus is achieved by cell culture that gives the most specific result, and the sera are usually collected in the first 3–5 days after the fever starts. Virus isolation is highly dependent on viral load, which limits the period during which the virus can be successfully isolated in the patient's serum. In addition, its high cost makes this test little accessible to most laboratories [3]. Viral identification can also be done using dengue-specific monoclonal antibodies by immunofluorescence and reverse transcription-PCR (RT-PCR) [3].

On the other hand, serological tests are relatively inexpensive and easy to perform. These characteristics make them the most used tests for dengue infection. IgM levels begin to rise on the third day of a primary infection and peak at 2 weeks after the onset of fever (**Figure 5**). IgG is detectable at the end of the first week of illness and may persist for life. Enzyme-linked immunosorbent assay (ELISA) tests can analyze the levels of IgM and IgG, and the IgM/IgG ratio is useful to distinguish primary from secondary infections. The IgM/IgG ratio greater than 1.4 is indicative of primary dengue infection, while the IgM/IgG ratio lesser than 1.2 is indicative of secondary dengue infection. The potential cross-reactivity of dengue virus with other flaviviridae when using serological assays remains a significant limitation for its use. Prior vaccination against yellow fever can also lead to a false positive serological test for dengue virus. The prolonged period of seroconversion also results in false negatives [3]. All flaviviruses produce a glycoprotein called NS1 and tests such as antigen capture ELISA and quick tests based on immunochromatography can be used to identify it in the bloodstream; it is detectable from days 0 to 9 after the onset of symptoms, although detection appears to be higher in the samples collected up to 3 days after the onset of symptoms. Quick tests are now available and provide results in 15 min. Rapid tests for NS1 have been estimated to have a significantly higher sensitivity for primary infections (94.7%) than for secondary infections (67.1%; $p < 0.001$) and now appear to be a potential alternative to culture, PCR, and serology [38].

The Brazilian Ministry of Health recommends that samples of patients with suspected dengue fever taken up to 8 days (preferably 5) after the onset of symptoms should be processed using ELISA for the detection of NS1 and qRT PCR for the detection of the DENV genome and the serotype. At 8–15 days after the onset of symptoms, the samples are analyzed for IgM detection using ELISA. After 15 days,

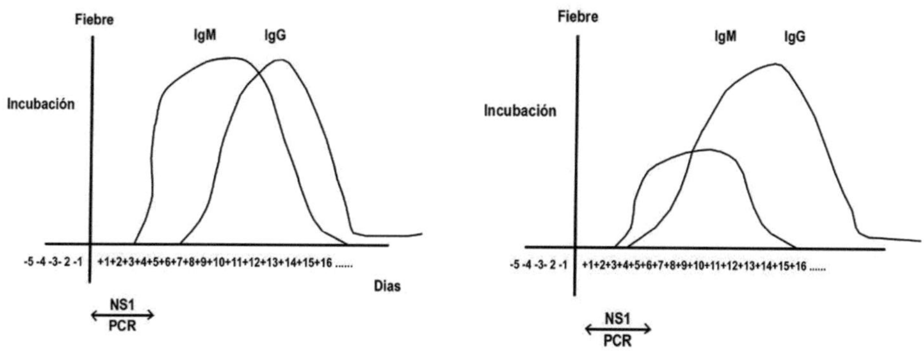

Figure 5.
(A) Primary infection by dengue. (B) Secondary infection by dengue. Source: Clinical Pathology Department, Almanzor Aguinaga Asenjo, Hospital, Essalud.

the sera are selected for IgG using ELISA. Dengue infection cannot be excluded in samples that are negative for the NS1 antigen and must be confirmed by IgM/IgG detection [35].

Cases of DENV-2 had a higher proportion of severe dengue than among those of DENV-1 and DENV-4 [39]. Nevertheless, the secondary infection was not a predictor of severe clinical manifestation in adults, who were primarily infected with serotype DENV-3 [40]; on the other hand, the dengue in children have suggested that infection with secondary DENV-2 is more likely to result in severe disease compared with other serotypes [41].

The fifth variant DENV-5 has been isolated in October 2013. This serotype follows the sylvatic cycle unlike the other four serotypes which follow the human cycle. The likely cause of emergence of the new serotype could be genetic recombination, natural selection, and genetic bottlenecks [42].

4. Diagnosis of dengue and other arbovirosis in the context of the Guillain Barre syndrome epidemic

During the months of June–July of 2019, 35 cases were registered and diagnosed as the Guillain-Barre Syndrome, at the Almanzor Aguinaga Asenjo National Hospital of Chiclayo in Peru, of which 22 had electrophysiology results compatible with the said syndrome, two had a normal result, and 11 were not evaluated with the mentioned diagnostic test. Three cases had IgG for flavivirus, three cases had IgG for flavivirus and IgG for chikungunya concomitantly, four cases had IgG for chikungunya, and one case had IgM for chikungunya. In other words, there were 11 cases of patients with a history of flavivirus or chikungunya infections in the context of the presentation of Guillain-Barre syndrome [43]. These patients were evaluated with the recomLine Tropical Fever IgG and IgM tests, immunoblot of German origin that has a sensitivity for IgG of 100% for primary infection by Zika, 100% for secondary infection for dengue or Zika, and 98.6% for primary infection by dengue; also the IgM has a sensitivity of 72.7% for dengue or Zika, and both tests have a specificity of 96–100%. On the other hand, the mentioned test describes a sensitivity and specificity of 100% for both IgM and IgG for chikungunya's diagnosis [44].

In the literature, there is the case of a dengue patient who developed Guillain-Barre syndrome, who presented the NS1 antigen on the second day of symptoms with subsequent IgM and IgG positive on the sixth day of evolution [45]. There is also another case described with similar laboratory findings, but that developed the syndrome approximately 2 weeks after the onset of dengue symptoms [46]. Therefore, this syndrome could develop early or late in relation to the onset of symptoms due to infection. In our cases, we did not have positive IgM and we did not have the opportunity to evaluate the NS1 antigen, but it is noteworthy that all cases detected with flavivirus antibodies only had positive IgG in their results. The previous cases described in the existing literature may represent primary cases of dengue since they raised IgM values early.

In our cases, the majority of patients did not show joint pain during the diagnosis of Guillain-Barre syndrome, which could suggest that these are non-acute cases, but as described in the case cited, this syndrome may occur during convalescence of the dengue; on the other hand, in an endemic area such as Lambayeque-Peru, the presence of cases with secondary infection that usually have low IgM values and not even increase it (**Figure 5**) should not attract attention [47]. In addition, Ramabhatta et al. [48] conducted a study on a sample of 568 cases diagnosed of dengue and showed that IgG-positive patients were more prone to complications than IgM-positive patients, therefore, the etiological association between dengue and Guillain-Barre syndrome in the Lambayeque region could not be ruled out.

5. Dengue lethality

5.1 Lethality in the context of Peru and Latin America

In 2014, according to WHO and Pan American Health Organization (PAHO), the average fatality rate for the Americas is 0.04%, being among the countries with the highest rate, followed by Dominican Republic with 1.54%, Peru with 0.12%, compared to Guatemala and Colombia that have 0.07% [49]. In Colombia and Peru, the most frequent serotype 2 prevailed, and in the Dominican Republic serotype 4 prevailed [50].

Nationally, the Center for Epidemiology, Prevention and Control of Diseases of the Ministry of Health, reported in 2017, 76,093 cases of dengue in the country (3.03 times more cases in relation to 2016, and the largest number of cases reported in the last 5 years [9, 51] and 92 reports of deaths by dengue, the highest number reported in the last 10 years) (**Figure 6**).

About 43.6% came from Piura, 17.1% from Loreto, 9.9% from Madre de Dios, 8.8% from Ucayali, 4.2% from San Martín, and the remaining 16.4% from other regions; all the age groups were affected, but with a greater proportion in people over 65 (37%) and young adults (21.7%) [9].

In the Piura Healthcare Network, 30 deaths associated with dengue virus were confirmed by laboratory, and occurred between epidemiological weeks Nos. 08 and 35, over 8 months; a similar panorama reported by the Lambayeque Healthcare Network, which reported the death of six dengue-associated patients, until epidemiological week No. 20 [13, 52]; although this information could be underestimated, because in many cases it is attributed to pneumonia, and actually the cases of dengue are not properly diagnosed, causing figures not approximate to reality [53].

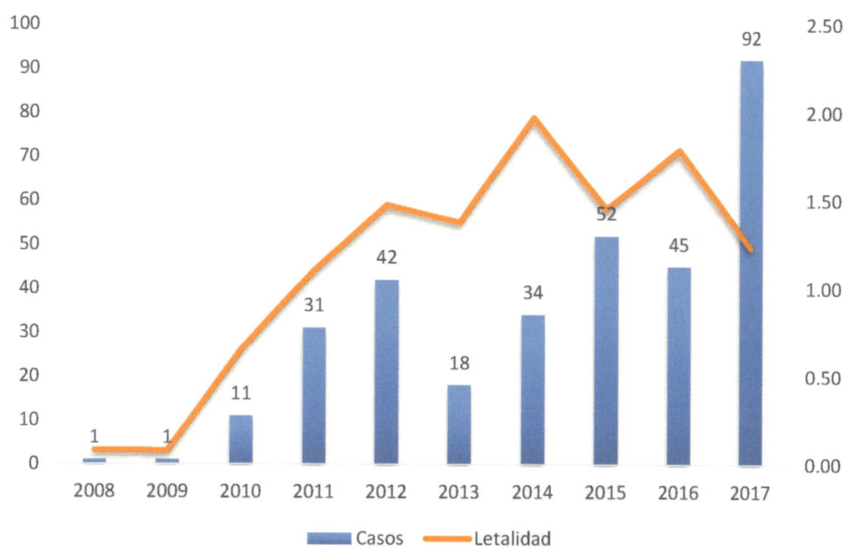

Figure 6.
Death toll and dengue lethality in Peru, 2008–2017. Source: Metaxenic disease surveillance system of the Center for Epidemiology, Disease Prevention and Control of the Ministry of Health (CDC-Perú).

In the departments of the north coast of Peru, such as Piura and Lambayeque, there are several conditions that favor the presence of epidemics, rainfall, and flooding due to the occurrence of the Coastal El Niño phenomenon, population growth at risk (young People, Urban Marginal Neighborhoods, etc) that is associated with the non-existence of basic infrastructure, insufficient water supply that leads to temporary water storage, constant circulation of *Aedes aegypti*, high temperatures and humidity, and poor community empowerment in the integrated control of vector control. Also in the Peruvian jungle, such as Loreto, Madre de Dios, Ucayali, and San Martin, they have a high incidence of death and lethality due to their diverse climatic and sanitary conditions, in addition to their population growth [13].

In the Healthcare Network of Piura, 22,562 cases of dengue were notified, 88 of which were severe dengue and 30 died, with 1.3% of lethality in general and 34.1% of lethality of severe cases; in Lambayeque there were 1384 cases; 13 being cases of severe dengue and nine deaths due to dengue, which makes 9.4% lethality in general and 43.3% lethality of severe cases, showing differences with national figures [37] (**Table 3**).

Although serotypes 2 and 3 were isolated in 94% of the positive cases; in Piura and Lambayeque, it was serotype 3 that was isolated in 90% of the cases and in almost all the deceased cases.

5.2 Delays in the process of health care as a method to identify the causes of mortality

The "delays" proposed by Thaddeus et al. in 1993, considered as the time between the appearance of a complication and its appropriate treatment and

Country	Serotype	N° dengue cases	N° severe cases	Deceased	General lethality (×1000)	Severe cases lethality (×100)
South America		387,669	1476	318	0.8	21.5%
Argentina	DEN 1,3	557	0	0	0.0	0.0%
Bolivia	DEN 1,4	10,842	66	15	1.4	22.7%
Colombia	DEN 1,2,3	26,279	286	15	0.6	5.2%
Chile	DEN 1,3	10	0	0	0.0	0.0%
Ecuador	—	11,387	18	4	0.4	22.2%
Brazil	DEN 1,2,3,4	252,054	378	133	0.5	35.2%
Venezuela	DEN 1	8615	359	16	1.9	4.5%
Paraguay	DEN 1,2	1832	0	0	0.0	0.0%
Uruguay	—	0	0	0	0.0	0.0%
Peru	DEN 2,3	74,648	251	92	1.2	36.7%
Essalud Piura*	DEN 2,3	22,562	88	30	1.3	34.1%
Essalud Lambayeque*	DEN 2,3	1384	30	13	9.4	43.3%

Taken and adapted: Díaz-Vélez et al. [37, 50].

Table 3.
General lethality and severe cases lethality of dengue reported by Social Security of Piura and Lambayeque compared to countries of South America, 2017.

resolution, initiating these concepts in the framework of care for severe maternal mortality and morbidity evaluating them as autonomy factors for the search for medical care, distance, and health services [36]. The use of this approach is considered, since it would allow to identify and classify the barriers and situations related to the search for medical care in patients affected by dengue, which are part of a chain of delays or delays that would hinder risk prevention, limit the access to quality health services, and would result in the lack of timely attention to the complication and, consequently, in death [54].

5.2.1 Delay in the recognition of the health problem

Poor recognition of a clinical disorder is one of the factors that cause the delay in seeking attention. It includes deficiencies in health education for communities and families, which makes it difficult to recognize warning signs (signs and symptoms) in conditions that can be life-threatening [36].

5.2.2 Delay in deciding to get attention

This delay is usually caused by limitations in the understanding of what medical care implies and could lead to a large number of patients arriving at health facilities in poor conditions, including factors such as information on dengue and institutional recognition, social and environmental situation, onset of symptoms, self-medication, gender and initial care, and motivations to make decisions [36, 55].

5.2.3 Delay in arriving at health services

It involves the difficulty of arriving at a health facility, either because of the difficult access to services or because it takes too long to reach the place of care, which can discourage the patient from seeking care, even when he has decided to seek care opportunely. It is generally the result of the lack of access to health services and economic, organizational, and sociocultural barriers which control the use of services. It is also possible to mention travel time, transport system used, and the socioeconomic impact of the delay [36, 55].

5.2.4 Delay in receiving the appropriate treatment

The cumulative effect of the first and second delays helps increase the risk of arrival at the health facility in serious conditions. Some never arrive at the hospital, and even if they do, it is possible that the treatment given to them is not adequate and poor surveillance or administrative procedures hinder the care. Other studies have shown more causes for inadequate treatment: chronic lack of trained personnel and essential supplies. Other factors mentioned are: failures in the operation of the public network, which determines waiting, reconsultation, and family movements between institutions; poor staff training and high emergency saturation [36, 55].

In relation to the first delay, aspects such as the delay in recognizing the health problem, absence of preventive-promotional talks, and lack of recognition of risk situations are described as the main ones, similar to studies that describe the population ignorance about the possibility of disease severity [56]. This last point reflects the poor knowledge by the population of less frequent dengue symptoms that in turn are associated with severity [57]. In the second delay, there are cases that went to non-health personnel and even self-medicating that are associated with delay as an explanation of serious or fatal cases [55, 58, 59] (**Figure 7**).

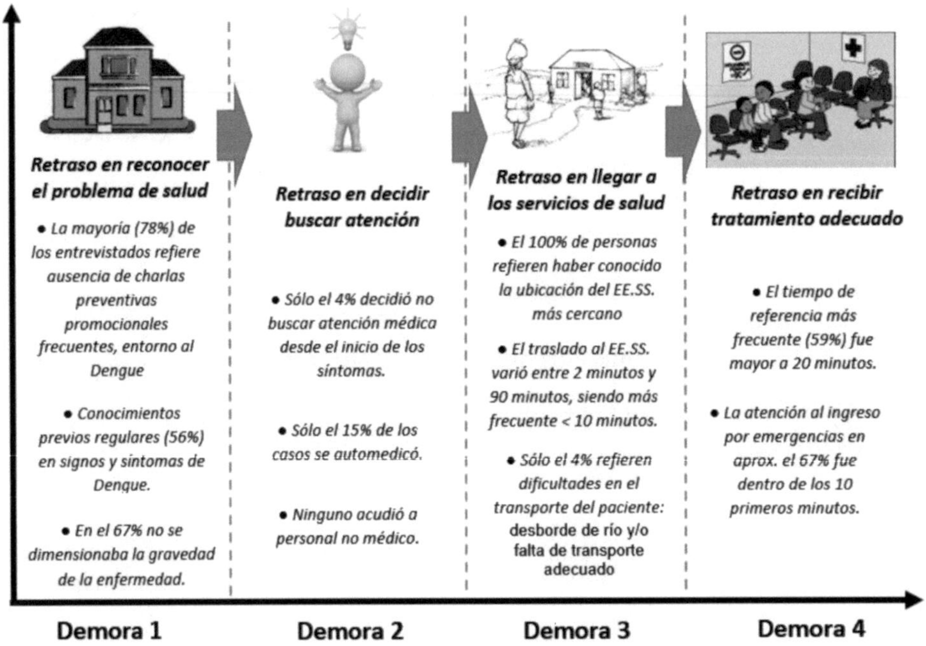

Figure 7.
Timeline of delays in the process of care of lethal cases care of dengue in two hospitals of EsSalud, in the Departments of Piura and Lambayeque, during 2017. Taken from: Burga-Cueva et al. Analysis of Lethality by Dengue in two Essalud Hospitals, in the Departments of Piura and Lambayeque. 2017. [64].

In the third delay, limitations for access to health services are evidenced, and some are given references, but lack of economic resources or available transportation is evidenced, thus also describing the distance of health facilities (to go to the nearest one) [60]. Finally, the fourth delay involves aspects such as the time of transfer to establishments of greater resolving capacity and the waiting time of cases upon arrival in emergencies, as mentioned by Ardila et al. [55], who describe the feeling of discomfort generated by a new interrogation and the waiting time that involves admission to a health facility of greater complexity (**Figure** 7).

6. Preventive measures against dengue

A study conducted in a population with a recent dengue outbreak showed that the level of knowledge was low in 76.2% of the population, 45% did not recognize the bite of the vector as the form of disease transmission, and 34% did not recognize the etiologic agent; of the most recognized clinical manifestations were fever, followed by headache, and musculoskeletal pain. Overall, 74.9% have a low level of knowledge about warning signs and about 93% were intermediate/low in prevention, and 43% of them are unaware of the reproduction of the vector, and 71% are unaware of the role of abate; results that show that the population despite having been exposed still does not know the prevention measures [61].

PAHO has planned to cooperate with member countries to stimulate the search for concrete solutions through a communication methodology to impact behavior (COMBI) [62, 63]. It should be noted that, since the introduction of dengue in America, attempts have been made to propose some integrated programs, with a community approach to the control of *Aedes aegypti*. This approach has been to educate the community about dengue disease and how to prevent transmission by controlling the *Aedes aegypti* vector in the domestic and community environments; in this context, it has been documented that many of these programs were successful in educating the community about dengue and its prevention [65].

Nevertheless, this improvement of the cognitive level related to the disease has not resulted in the action of preventing the disease. In this sense, even though people in a region with dengue endemicity are very well versed in the disease, they do not implement these measures that they know control vector proliferation and therefore the transmission of dengue; therefore, it is essential to reorient educational programs focused on the behavioral change of the population [66].

Likewise, historically in the region, efforts to control dengue vectors resulted in the elimination of populations of *Aedes aegypti* in many of the tropical and subtropical countries by the 1970s. However, vector populations were reintroduced through the emergence of new serotypes [67]. Therefore, currently, the main purpose of most programs is to reduce the densities of vector populations as much as possible and keep them at low levels. When feasible, efforts should also be made to reduce the longevity of adult female mosquitoes through the use of insecticidal methods in order to reduce the risk of virus transmission [65].

It should be noted that keeping infestation with *A. aegypti* low carries significant economic costs to society; however, when an outbreak of dengue occurs, the cost increases considerably in vector control and patient care; so, from this perspective, effectiveness and profitability could be maximized by intervening in the vector habitat (potential hatcheries) through promotion and prevention actions [68–70]. Although the concept of vector control is reasonable, control should be early in an outbreak or applied strategically during periods between epidemics to avoid escalation in transmission [71].

Another preventive measure to control the rapid spread of an outbreak is to manage the infected human host and prevent it from infecting *Aedes* mosquitoes, this in turn would reduce the amount of new infections to humans, breaking the epidemiological chain of dengue transmission [72]. So, meanwhile, there is no vaccine with proven efficacy for dengue prevention in all population groups, and the main strategy to prevent transmission and disease is vector control through the elimination of larval habitats (elimination of potential hatcheries) and prevention of mosquito-human contact [73]. Some well-documented successes indicate that rigorously applied vector control can reduce the transmission of DENV and the disease [74].

In that sense, success in reducing the burden of dengue on public health will require an integrated multiple approach; although the concept of integrated intervention for dengue prevention is gaining increasing acceptance, to date, no consensus has been reached regarding the details of how and what combination of approaches can be implemented most effectively to control the disease [75].

Integrated vector management, the strategic method promoted by WHO, is defined as, "a rational decision-making process for the optimal use of resources for vector control," which includes lobbying, social mobilization, and legislation; planning and delegated decision-making at the lowest possible administrative level; guaranteeing the rational use of available resources; adaptation of strategies and interventions based on vector habitat, epidemiology, and local resources; and development of an essential infrastructure for integrated vector management based on the situation analysis [67].

However, the discipline of vector control has been strongly influenced by the theory developed by Ronald Ross and George Macdonald (i.e., the Ross-Macdonald model), which states that the potential for transmission of mosquito-borne pathogens depends largely on the abundance of adult vector mosquitoes, survival through the incubation period of the pathogen, and the rate of human infection [76].

Therefore, with this approach, interventions that reduce the population density of adult mosquitoes, the daily probability of survival, and the contact of the mosquito with humans are expected to have the greatest impact on decreasing virus transmission. It should be noted, however, that the Ross-Macdonald model was not formulated to specifically explore larval mosquito control. Recent quantitative assessments indicate that, under certain circumstances, control of the larvae may lead to greater than expected reductions in the transmission of pathogens [77]. In the context of larval control of *Aedes aegypti*, there should be the large-scale elimination of potential hatcheries.

In this context, taking into account that there is limited efficacy and intensity of the interventions used for dengue vector control, other alternatives to combat dengue endemic persistence are explored. Sustainable community participation and school-based health education interventions have finally evolved as an effective tool in reducing the larval source over other interventions [78], since children have inherent curiosity and enthusiasm to learn new things. Therefore, they can serve as an effective change agent to achieve a change in behavior in the family and community.

Methods for vector control include elimination or management of larval habitats, eliminating larvae with insecticides, the use of biological agents, and the application of adulticides; being for our conviction the elimination and management of larval habitats. Habitats are eliminated by preventing the access of mosquitoes to these containers or by emptying and cleaning them frequently, eliminating the evolutionary stages with the use of insecticides or biological control agents, eliminating adult mosquitoes with insecticides, or by combining these methods [79].

Habitat management seeks to change the environment in order to prevent or minimize the propagation of vectors and human contact with the vector pathogen, destroying, altering (proper conservation of disused material), and eliminating or recycling nonessential containers that serve as larval habitats. Efforts to reduce solid waste should be directed against disposable or nonessential containers [78].

However, the main method of *Aedes* control (and, generally, the only one) used in many countries, remains the spatial application of ultralow volume insecticides (ULVs) for the control of adult mosquitoes [63]. This strategy has to be repeated constantly, its cost is high, and its effectiveness is limited. *Aedes aegypti* prefers to stay inside the houses, therefore, the insecticide aerial application or from trucks simply does not reach the mosquitoes that stay in hidden places, such as wardrobes. There have been several cases of homeowners in various countries who have not allowed the entry of home spraying equipment or have closed windows and doors well to prevent outside fog produced by the insecticide from entering their homes, reducing in this way the effectiveness of the intervention [65] (**Table 4**).

Due to inadequate dengue surveillance systems, spraying does not arrive in time to prevent epidemic transmission, and adult mosquito populations return quickly after spraying. Public confidence and complacency regarding such an ineffective approach have only made the challenge of explaining the need for community participation in hatchery control greater [79].

Therefore, our approach, which is the most cost-effective measure to control the transmission of dengue, would be based on the design and execution of activities aimed at eradicating vector proliferation through the elimination of favorable habitats (potential hatcheries: tires, bottles, and buckets) for oviposition and allowing the development of the aquatic stages of the vector; with a participatory methodology based on the sociocultural characteristics of the population under study, with the local schools as main actors; for which, at first, the level of knowledge, attitude, and practice of dengue prevention measures of the population must be determined and from which it will design and carry out promotional, prevention interventions, with emphasis on behavioral changes.

	***Aedes* mosquito breeding prevention**	**Prevention of exposure to *Aedes* mosquito bites**	**Search for medical attention**
Individuals and households	• Water storage practices • Home plant care • Animal care • Garbage disposal • Storage of daytime materials in the yard	• Use of insecticides and spray repellents • Placing wire mesh on windows and doors • Sleep protected by a mosquito net during naps	• Disease recognition • Home treatment • Search for medical attention
Communities, community groups, schools, NGOs	• Communication with behavioral impact • Community cleaning • Promotion or organization of essential services: water, garbage collection • Promotion of the recycling of tires, cans, bottles, etc.	• Housing improvement	• Facilitation of patient transport to health facilities

Table 4.
Comprehensive behavioral monitoring of mobilization and social communication for dengue prevention and control.

Finally, the need for a good understanding and emphasis on behaviors related to the management of *Aedes aegypti* hatcheries, the main dengue vector; it should be the promotion and prevention approach at the community level, divided into individual and collective activities for the prevention of *Aedes aegypti* reproduction, prevention of exposure to *Aedes* mosquitoes, and seeking medical attention.

Taken from: Parks W, Lloyd L. COMBI. Planning social mobilization and communication for the prevention and control of dengue. Ginebra; 2004 [65].

Author details

Cristian Díaz-Vélez[1,2,3]*, Jorge Luis Fernández-Mogollón[1,3], John Alexis Cabrera-Enríquez[4], Stalin Tello-Vera[5], Oscar Medrano-Velásquez[6,7] and Elmer Córdova-Calle[8]

1 Médico Epidemiólogo, Oficina de Inteligencia Sanitaria, Hospital Nacional Almanzor Aguinaga Asenjo, EsSalud, Chiclayo, Peru

2 Facultad de Medicina, Universidad Nacional Pedro Ruiz Gallo, Chiclayo, Peru

3 Facultad de Medicina, Universidad de San Martín de Porres, Chiclayo, Peru

4 Médico Infectólogo, Unidad de Infectología Pediátrica, Hospital Nacional Almenara Irigoyen, EsSalud, Lima, Peru

5 Médico Patólogo Clínico, Laboratorio de Biología Molecular y Citometría de Flujo, Hospital Nacional Almanzor Aguinaga Asenjo, EsSalud, Chiclayo, Peru

6 Licenciado en Enfermería, Servicio de Enfermería, Hospital III José Cayetano Heredia, EsSalud, Piura, Peru

7 Auxiliar, Facultad de Enfermería, Universidad Nacional de Piura, Piura, Peru

8 Licenciado en Enfermería, División de Inteligencia Sanitaria, Hospital III José Cayetano Heredia, EsSalud, Piura, Peru

*Address all correspondence to: cristiandiazv@hotmail.com

References

[1] IMARPE. Definición de "El Niño Costero" [Internet]. Available from: http://www.imarpe.pe/imarpe/index.php?id_seccion=I0175040200000000000000

[2] IMARPE. Informe Técnico Extraordinario N°001-2017/ENFEN EL NIÑO COSTERO 2017 [Internet]. Lima, Perú: Comisión Multisectorial encargadada del estudio Nacional Fenómeno "El Niño Costero 2017"; 2017. Available from: http://www.imarpe.pe/imarpe/archivos/informes/imarpe_inftco_informe__tecnico_extraordinario_001_2017.pdf

[3] Maguiña-Vargas C, Gastelo-Acosta R. Leptospirosis a silent disease in the El Niño phenomenon. Rev Cuerpo Méd HNAAA. 2017;**10**(1):4-6

[4] Espinoza-Neyra C, Jara-Pereda M, Díaz-Vélez C. Post-traumatic stress disorder in a population affected by floods caused by El niño in Peru. 2017;**34**:751-752

[5] Mitchell C. OPS/OMS Perú-El Niño Costero–2017 Perú | OPS/OMS [Internet]. Pan American Health Organization/World Health Organization. 2017. Available from: https://www.facebook.com/pahowho. https://www.paho.org/per/index.php?option=com_content&view=article&id=3710:emergencia-por-impacto-del-fenomeno-el-nino-costero-2017-peru&Itemid=1060

[6] Peruvian Ministry of Health. Boletín Epidemiológico del Perú 2017 SE 29 [Internet]. Lima, Perú: Ministerio de Salud del Perú; 2017. Available from: https://www.dge.gob.pe/portal/docs/vigilancia/boletines/2017/29.pdf

[7] Peruvian Ministry of Health. Boletín Epidemiológico del Perú 2017 SE 52 [Internet]. Lima, Perú: Ministerio de Salud del Perú.; 2017. (https://www.dge.gob.pe/portal/docs/vigilancia/boletines/2017/52.pdf)

[8] Peruvian Ministry of Health. Sala situacional del dengue, Perú SE 1 2018 [Internet]. Lima, Perú: Ministerio de Salud del Perú; 2018. Available from: http://www.dge.gob.pe/portal/docs/vigilancia/sala/2018/SE01/dengue.pdf

[9] Peruvian Ministry of Health. Análisis de la Situación de Salud: Dengue 2017 [Internet]. 2018. Available from: http://www.dge.gob.pe/portal/docs/vigilancia/sala/2017/SE51/dengue.pdf

[10] Ruiz EF, Vasquez-Galindo CM, Aquije-Pariona XM, Torres-Roman JS. Outbreaks caused by *Aedes aegyptis* due to El Niño in a coastal area of Peru. Travel Medicine and Infectious Disease. 2018;**21**:78-79

[11] Rohani P. The link between dengue incidence and El Niño Southern Oscillation. PLoS Medicine. 2009;**6**(11). Available from: https://www.ncbi.nlm.nih.gov/pmc/articles/PMC2770118/

[12] Ministry of Health of Peru MINSA. Dengue Situation Room in Peru. DGE SE 1; 2018

[13] Medrano-Velásquez O, Córdova-Calle E, Ojeda-Gallo PM, Díaz-Vélez C. Clinical, epidemiological of the epidemic outbreak of dengue during the Phenomenon Niño Costero 2017, Red Asistencial de Piura, Peru. Rev Cuerpo Méd HNAAA. 2018;**11**(1):52-60. Available from: http://cmhnaaa.org.pe/ojs/index.php/rcmhnaaa/article/view/60

[14] Chretien J-P, Anyamba A, Bedno SA, Breiman RF, Sang R, Sergon K, et al. Drought-associated chikungunya emergence along coastal East Africa. American Journal of Tropical Medicine and Hygiene. 2007;**76**(3):405-407.

Available from: https://pubag.nal.usda.gov/download/55909/PDF

[15] Flahault A, Aumont G, Boisson V, de Lamballerie X, Favier F, Fontenille D, et al. An interdisciplinary approach to controlling chikungunya outbreaks on French islands in the south-west Indian ocean. Med Trop Rev Corps Sante Colon. 2012;**72**:66-71

[16] Flahault A, de Castaneda RR, Bolon I. Climate change and infectious diseases. Public Health Review. 2016;**37**. Available from: https://www.ncbi.nlm.nih.gov/pmc/articles/PMC5810060/

[17] Ministry of Health of Peru MINSA. Dengue situation room in Peru. DGE SE 29; 2017

[18] Herrera-Pérez D, Saavedra-Barón A, Fernández-Mogollón J. Leptospirosis and co-infections during the coastal "el niño" in a hospital in northern peru. Rev Peru Med Exp Salud Pública. 2019;**36**(1):148. Available from: https://rpmesp.ins.gob.pe/index.php/rpmesp/article/view/4068

[19] Sippy R, Herrera D, Gaus D, Gangnon RE, Patz JA, Osorio JE. Seasonal patterns of dengue fever in rural Ecuador: 2009-2016. PLoS Neglected Tropical Diseases. 2019;**13**(5):e0007360

[20] Ecuadorian Ministry of Health. Ministerios de salud y defensa articulan acciones frente alerta de dengue emitida por autoridades sanitarias del Perú [Internet]. Ecuador; 2018 feb. Available from: https://www.salud.gob.ec/ministerios-de-salud-y-defensa-articulan-acciones-frente-alerta-de-dengue-emitida-por-autoridades-sanitarias-del-peru/

[21] Valdés Miró V, Díaz Castillo AO, Borrell Ferrer MC, Cabreras Cabreras AV. Estratificación para la vigilancia entomológica del dengue. Rev Cubana Med Trop. 2009;**61**(2) 0-0. Available from: http://scielo.sld.cu/scielo.php?script=sci_abstract&pid=S0375-07602009000200009&lng=es&nrm=iso&tlng=es

[22] Schaber KL, Paz-Soldan VA, Morrison AC, Elson WHD, Rothman AL, Mores CN, et al. Dengue illness impacts daily human mobility patterns in Iquitos, Peru. Barrera R, editor. PLoS Neglected Tropical Diseases. 2019;13(9):e0007756. DOI: 10.1371/journal.pntd.0007756

[23] Paico-Romero C, Polo-Capuñay A, Díaz-Exebio G, Díaz-Vélez C. Validation and development of an instrument: Level of knowledge for the diagnosis and treatment of dengue fever in Lambayeque region. Acta Médica Peru. 2012;**29**(3):143-147. Available from: http://www.scielo.org.pe/scielo.php?script=sci_abstract&pid=S1728-59172012000300003&lng=es&nrm=iso&tlng=es

[24] Paico-Romero CN, Paico-García JA, Díaz-Vélez C. Associated factors with the level of knowledge in diagnosis and treatment of dengue in physicians of the First Attention level of the Lambayeque Region. Rev Cuerpo Méd HNAAA. 2016;**9**(4):214-218

[25] Mandell GL, Bennett JE, Douglas RG. Enfermedades infecciosas: principios y prácticas. Médica Panamericana. 1991

[26] Palomares-Reyes C, Silva-Caso W, Del Valle LJ, Aguilar-Luis MA, Weilg C, Martins-Luna J, et al. Dengue diagnosis in an endemic area of Peru: Clinical characteristics and positive frequencies by RT-PCR and serology for NS1, IgM, and IgG. International Journal of Infectious Diseases. 2019;**81**:31-37

[27] Sánchez-Carbonel J, Tantaléan-Yépez D, Aguilar-Luis MA, Silva-Caso W, Weilg P, Vásquez-Achaya F, et al. Identification of infection by

Chikungunya, Zika, and Dengue in an area of the Peruvian coast. Molecular diagnosis and clinical characteristics. BMC Research Notes. 2018;**11**(1):175

[28] Carrasco TP, Carlos J, Cabrera P, Luis P, Cabrejos Sampen G, Díaz-Vélez C. Clinical, epidemiological and geographic profile of dengue cases during El Niño Costero Phenomenon 2017, Lambayeque-Perú. Rev Habanera Cienc Médicas. 2019;**18**(1):97-113

[29] Forshey BM, Reiner RC, Olkowski S, Morrison AC, Espinoza A, Long KC, et al. Incomplete protection against dengue virus type 2 re-infection in Peru. PLoS Neglected Tropical Diseases. 2016;**10**(2)

[30] Salgado DM, Vega R, Rodríguez JA, Niño Á, Rodríguez R, Ortiz Á, et al. Clinical, laboratory and immune aspects of Zika virus-associated encephalitis in children. International Journal of Infectious Diseases. 2020;**90**:104-110

[31] Atamari-Anahui N, Ccorahua-Ríos MS, Cabrera-Enríquez JA, Vilcarromero S. La implicancia del reordenamiento genético en el diagnóstico y la epidemiología del virus Oropuche en el Perú. Salud Pública México. 2018;**60**(5, sep-oct):487. Available from: http://www.saludpublica.mx/index.php/spm/article/view/9215

[32] Paternina-Caicedo A, De la Hoz-Restrepo F, Díaz-Quijano F, Caicedo-Torres W, Auxiliadora Badillo-Viloria M, Bula-Anichiarico D, et al. Features of dengue and chikungunya infections of Colombian children under 24 months of age admitted to the emergency department. Journal of Tropical Pediatrics. 2018;**64**(1):31-37. Available from: https://academic.oup.com/tropej/article/64/1/31/3748255

[33] Bhaskaran D, Chadha SS, Sarin S, Sen R, Arafah S, Dittrich S. Diagnostic tools used in the evaluation of acute febrile illness in South India: A scoping review. BMC Infectious Diseases. 2019;**19**(1). Available from: https://bmcinfectdis.biomedcentral.com/articles/10.1186/s12879-019-4589-8

[34] Valero N, Montiel M, Arias J, Fuentes B, Mavarez A, Nava L, et al. Comparison between inmunochromatographic and enzyme linked immunosorbent assay (ELISA) in the dengue diagnosis. Kasmera. 2006;**34**(1):53-60. Available from: http://ve.scielo.org/scielo.php?script=sci_abstract&pid=S0075-52222006000100007&lng=es&nrm=iso&tlng=es

[35] Salles TS, Da Encarnação Sá-Guimarães T, De Alvarenga ESL, Guimarães-Ribeiro V, De Meneses MDF, De Castro-Salles PF, et al. History, epidemiology and diagnostics of dengue in the American and Brazilian contexts: A review. Parasite Vectors. 2018;**11**(1):264

[36] Dávila-Gonzales JA, Guevara-Cruz LA, Díaz-Vélez C. Nivel de conocimientos de dengue, signos de alarma y prevención en distrito de reciente brote. Rev Biomedica. 2020

[37] Gutiérrez C, Montenegro-Idrogo JJ. Knowledge about dengue in an endemic Peruvian region. A population-based study. Acta Médica Peru. 2017;**34**(4):283-288

[38] Otu A, Ebenso B, Etokidem A, Chukwuekezie O. Dengue fever—An update review and implications for Nigeria, and similar countries. African Health Sciences. 2019;**19**(2):2000-2007. Available from: https://www.ncbi.nlm.nih.gov/pmc/articles/PMC6794512/

[39] Rodríguez-Morales AJ, Failoc-Rojas VE, Díaz-Vélez C. Gastrointestinal, respiratory and/or arboviral infections? What is the cause of the Guillain-Barré syndrome epidemics in Perú? Current status–2019. Travel Medicine

and Infectious Diseases. 2019;**30**:114-116. Available from: https://linkinghub.elsevier.com/retrieve/pii/S1477893919301127

[40] Mikrogen-recomLine Tropical Fever IgG/IgM [Internet]. [citado 17 de febrero de 2020]. Available from: https://www.mikrogen.de/english/deutschland/products/product-overview/testsystem/tropical-fever-igg.html

[41] Dalugama C, Shelton J, Ekanayake M, Gawarammana IB. Dengue fever complicated with Guillain-Barré syndrome: A case report and review of the literature. Journal of Medical Case Reports. 2018;**12**. Available from: https://www.ncbi.nlm.nih.gov/pmc/articles/PMC5952700/

[42] Ralapanawa DMPUK, Kularatne SAM, Jayalath WATA. Guillain-Barre syndrome following dengue fever and literature review. BMC Research Notes. 2015;**8**:729

[43] De Paula SO, Fonseca BAL. Dengue: A review of the laboratory tests a clinician must know to achieve a correct diagnosis. Brazilian Journal of Infectious Diseases. 2004;**8**(6):390-398

[44] Ramabhatta S, Palaniappan S, Hanumantharayappa N, Begum SV. The clinical and serological profile of pediatric dengue. Indian Journal of Pediatrics. 2017;**84**(12):897-901

[45] Sanchez JD. OPS/OMS|Descripción de la situación epidemiologica actual del dengue en las Américas [Internet]. Pan American Health Organization/World Health Organization; 2020. Available from: https://www.paho.org/hq/index.php?option=com_content&view=article&id=4494:2010-descripcion-situacion-epidemiologica-actual-dengue-americas&Itemid=40370&lang=es

[46] Dengue y dengue grave [Internet]. [citado 16 de febrero de 2020]. Available from: https://www.who.int/es/news-room/fact-sheets/detail/dengue-and-severe-dengue

[47] Guzmán J. Situación Epidemiológica de dengue en el Perú. Bol Epidemiológico Perú Lima Minist Salud. 2017;**26**(14):429-432

[48] Perales Carrasco JCT, Cabrera P, Luis P. Perfil Clínico, Epidemiológico y Geográfico de Casos de Dengue durante el Fenómeno El Niño Costero en La Red Asistencial Essalud, Lambayeque 2017 [Clinical, epidemiological and geographic profile of dengue cases during the coastal El Niño phenomenon in the Essalud Healthcare Network]; 2018

[49] Huamanchumo Effio ED. Análisis de la Mortalidad en el Hospital Nacional Almanzor Aguinaga Asenjo Chiclayo 2009-2017 [Internet]. Lambayeque-Perú: Universidad Nacional Pedro Ruiz Gallo; 2018. Available from: http://190.108.84.117/handle/UNPRG/1913

[50] Díaz-Vélez C, Leguía-Cerna JA, Puescas-Sánchez PR, Medrano-Velásquez O. Dengue lethality in social security assistance centers in Peru during Coastal El Niño, Northern Peru, 2017. Rev Cubana Med Trop. 2019;**71**(2)

[51] Pacagnella RC, Cecatti JG, Osis MJ, Souza JP. The role of delays in severe maternal morbidity and mortality: expanding the conceptual framework. Reprod Health Matters. 2012;**20**(39):155-163

[52] Rodríguez-Angulo E, Aguilar-Pech P, Montero-Cervantes L, Hoil-Santos J, Andueza-Pech G. Demoras en la atención de complicaciones maternas asociadas a fallecimientos en municipios del sur de Yucatán, México. Rev Bioméd. 2012;**23**(1):23-32

[53] Ardila Pinto F, Martínez S, Fuentes M, Borrero E. Análisis de las demoras en salud en personas que

enfermaron de gravedad o fallecieron por dengue en cinco ciudades de Colombia. Physis Rev Saúde Coletiva. 2015;**25**:571-592

[54] Carabali M, Hernandez LM, Arauz MJ, Villar LA, Ridde V. Why are people with dengue dying? A scoping review of determinants for dengue mortality. BMC Infectious Diseases. 2015;**15**(1):301

[55] Arauz MJ, Ridde V, Hernández LM, Charris Y, Carabali M, Villar LÁ. Developing a social autopsy tool for dengue mortality: A pilot study. PLoS One. 2015;**10**(2):e0117455

[56] Charette M, Berrang-Ford L, Coomes O, Llanos-Cuentas EA, Cárcamo C, Kulkarni M, et al. Dengue incidence and sociodemographic conditions in Pucallpa, Peruvian Amazon: What role for modification of the dengue-temperature relationship? American Journal of Tropical Medicine and Hygiene. 2020;**102**(1):180-190

[57] Burga Cueva JJ, Campos Milián LJ, et al. Análisis de la Letalidad por Dengue en dos Hospitales de Essalud, de los Departamentos de Piura y Lambayeque [Analysis of lethality by Dengue in two Essalud Hospitals, in the Departments of Piura and Lambayeque. 2017]. 2018

[58] Dávila-Gonzales JA, Guevara-Cruz LA, Peña-Sánchez ER, Díaz-Vélez C. Validation of an instrument to measure the level of knowledge in people about dengue, alarm signs and prevention in a district with a recent outbreak of dengue. La Revista Hispanoamericana de Ciencias de la Salud. 2018;**4**(3):119-128

[59] Mosquera M, Obregón R, Lloyd LS, Orozco M, Peña A. Comunicación, movilización y participación: lecciones aprendidas en la prevención y control de la fiebre dengue (FD). Revista de Investigación Desarrollo e Innovación. 2010;**14**(1)

[60] Orozco M, Peña A, Arroyave J. Sistematización de lecciones aprendidas en proyectos COMBI en dengue en la región de las Américas. Organ Panam Salud Costa Rica

[61] Stefany Niño-Effio B, Yong-Cadena HA, Díaz-Vélez C. Knowledge and practices regarding dengue prevention in a Peruvian city affected by a dengue epidemic following the 2018 Coastal Child 2018. Revista Cubana de Medicina Tropical. 2019;**71**(2)

[62] WHO. Dengue Guidelines for Diagnosis, Treatment, Prevention and Control: New Edition [Internet]. World Health Organization; 2009 [citado 16 de febrero de 2020]. Available from: https://apps.who.int/iris/handle/10665/44188

[63] Bisso-Andrade A. The Niño Costero and the high cost of lack of prevention Aland Bisso-Andrade. Revista de la Sociedad Peruana de Medicina Interna. 2017;**30**(2):70-70

[64] Parks W, Lloyd L. Planificación de la movilización y comunicación social para la prevención y el control del dengue: guía paso a paso. Ginebra: Organización Mundial de la Salud; 2004

[65] Torres JR, Castro J. The health and economic impact of dengue in Latin America. Cad Saude Publica. 2007;**23**(Suppl 1):S23-S31

[66] Shepard DS, Coudeville L, Halasa YA, Zambrano B, Dayan GH. Economic impact of dengue illness in the Americas. American Journal of Tropical Medicine and Hygiene. 2011;**84**(2):200-207

[67] Palma-Pinedo H, Cabrera R, Yagui-Moscoso M. Factors behind people's reluctance towards dengue vector control actions in three districts in northern Peru. Revista Peruana de Medicina Experimental y Salud Pública. 2016;**33**:13-20

[68] Dengue Control in North Queensland, Australia: Case Recognition and Selective Indoor Residual Spraying [Internet]. [citado 16 de febrero de 2020]. Available from: https://apps.who.int/iris/handle/10665/163762

[69] Eisen L, Beaty BJ, Morrison AC, Scott TW. Proactive vector control strategies and improved monitoring and evaluation practices for dengue prevention. Journal of Medical Entomology. 2009;**46**(6):1245-1255 Available from: https://academic.oup.com/jme/article-lookup/doi/10.1603/033.046.0601

[70] Gunther VJ, Putnak R, Eckels KH, Mammen MP, Scherer JM, Lyons A, et al. A human challenge model for dengue infection reveals a possible protective role for sustained interferon gamma levels during the acute phase of illness. Vaccine. 2011;**29**(22):3895-3904

[71] Baly Gil A, Abadi González A, Cabrera Junco P, Martínez Rodríguez A, Van der Stuyft P. Loss of quality of life and economic burden caused by dengue fever from the perspective of patients and their families. Revista Cubana de Medicina Tropical. 2019;**71**(1)

[72] Smith DL, Battle KE, Hay SI, Barker CM, Scott TW, McKenzie FE. Ross, Macdonald, and a theory for the dynamics and control of mosquito-transmitted pathogens. Chitnis CE, editor. PLoS Pathogens. 2012;**8**(4):e1002588. DOI: 10.1371/journal.ppat.1002588

[73] Smith DL, Perkins TA, Tusting LS, Scott TW, Lindsay SW. Mosquito population regulation and larval source management in heterogeneous environments. Vasilakis N, editor. PLoS One. 2013;8(8):e71247. DOI: 10.1371/journal.pone.0071247

[74] Alok S, Nessa S, Ahil SB. School training strategies for prevention and control of dengue. Indian Journal of Community Medicine. 2020;**45**(1):106-107

[75] PAHO. Dengue: guías para la atención de enfermos en la Región de las Américas. 2. ed. [Internet]. OPS; 2016. Available from: http://iris.paho.org/xmlui/handle/123456789/28232

[76] WHO. Manejo ambiental para el control de vectores [Internet]. WHO [citado 16 de febrero de 2020]. Available from: https://www.who.int/water_sanitation_health/resources/envmanagement/es/

[77] Weeratunga P, Rodrigo C, Fernando SD, Rajapakse S. Control methods for «*Aedes albopictus*» and «*Aedes aegypti*». Cochrane Infectious Diseases Group, editor. Cochrane Database Systemic Review. 2017. DOI: 10.1002/14651858.CD012759

[78] Bowman LR, Donegan S, McCall PJ. Is dengue vector control deficient in effectiveness or evidence?: Systematic review and meta-analysis. PLoS Neglected Tropical Diseases. 2016;**10**(3):e0004551

[79] Díaz-Vélez C. Prevention of metaxenicas diseases: Repellents, important but little used weapon. La Revista del Cuerpo Médico del Hospital Nacional Almanzor Aguinaga Asenjo. 2018;**11**(2):67-68

Section 2

Immunopathogenesis

Chapter 4

Dengue Immunopathogenesis: A Crosstalk between Host and Viral Factors Leading to Disease: Part I - Dengue Virus Tropism, Host Innate Immune Responses, and Subversion of Antiviral Responses

Henry Puerta-Guardo, Scott B. Biering, Eva Harris, Norma Pavia-Ruz, Gonzalo Vázquez-Prokopec, Guadalupe Ayora-Talavera and Pablo Manrique-Saide

Abstract

Dengue is the most prevalent emerging mosquito-borne viral disease, affecting more than 40% of the human population worldwide. Many symptomatic dengue virus (DENV) infections result in a relatively benign disease course known as dengue fever (DF). However, a small proportion of patients develop severe clinical manifestations, englobed in two main categories known as dengue hemorrhagic fever (DHF) and dengue shock syndrome (DSS). Secondary infection with any of the four dengue virus serotypes (DENV1, -2, -3, and -4) is a risk factor to develop severe forms of dengue disease. DSS is primarily characterized by sudden and abrupt endothelial dysfunction, resulting in vascular leak and organ impairment, which may progress to hypovolemic shock and death. Severe DENV disease (DHF/DSS) is thought to follow a complex relationship between distinct immunopathogenic processes involving host and viral factors, such as the serotype cross-reactive antibody-dependent enhancement (ADE), the activation of T cells and complement pathways, the phenomenon of the *cytokine storm*, and the newly described viral toxin activity of the nonstructural protein 1 (NS1), which together play critical roles in inducing vascular leak and virus pathogenesis. In this chapter that is divided in two parts, we will outline the recent advances in our understanding of DENV pathogenesis, highlighting key viral-host interactions and discussing how these interactions may contribute to DENV immunopathology and the development of vascular leak, a hallmark of severe dengue. *Part I* will address the general features of the DENV complex, including the virus structure and genome, epidemiology, and clinical outcomes, followed by an updated review of the literature describing the host innate immune strategies as well as the viral mechanisms acting against and in favor of the DENV replication cycle and infection.

Keywords: dengue, immunopathogenesis, dengue shock syndrome, severe dengue, virus replication, cell tropism, innate immune response, antiviral response, immune evasion, complement, endothelial dysfunction, vascular leak

1. Introduction

Dengue is still considered the most prevalent viral disease transmitted by arthropod mosquitoes (e.g., *Aedes* mosquitoes), with 50–100 million dengue infections occurring annually, and a global incidence of 30-fold increase observed over the past 50 years [1–3]. Most of the dengue infections with any of the four dengue virus (DENV) serotypes [1–4] result in inapparent, subclinical illness, or mild disease symptoms known as dengue fever (DF). However, some DENV infections can potentially evolve into more severe and fatal disease outcomes known as dengue hemorrhagic fever (DHF) and dengue shock syndrome (DSS) [2]. DHF and DSS are mainly characterized by low numbers of circulating platelets (thrombocytopenia) associated with hemorrhagic manifestations and increased vascular permeability associated with endothelium hyperpermeability, resulting in plasma leakage, low blood pressure, and shock that can lead to death [2]. DENV infections frequently occur in the context of preexisting immunity, where the immune responses to prior DENV infection play an important role in determining the outcome of dengue epidemics and disease severity via antibody-dependent enhancement (ADE) and potentially harmful T cell responses in an *original antigenic sin*-dependent manner [4–8]. Both mechanisms lead to increased activation of immune cells, resulting in exacerbated immune responses or *cytokine storms* that cause endothelium dysfunction and vascular leak [9, 10]. Collectively, these host immunological responses are thought to create a physiological environment that promotes vascular permeability. However, the exact mechanisms underlying the capillary leak are probably more complex than a *cytokine storm*, and the risk of severe disease upon DENV infection cannot be explained completely by a misdirected host immune response to a prior infecting serotype; rather, disease severity appears to be determined by a combination of multiple host and viral factors leading to favorable and unfavorable interactions that regulate viral pathogenesis.

Despite considerable advances in understanding the immunological mechanisms activated during DENV infection, the pathogenic mechanisms underlying the alterations in permeability of the microvasculature remain unclear. The absence of a good animal model faithful to human disease and the limited knowledge of the factors regulating the intrinsic microvascular permeability in health have seriously hampered the research progress in this area. However, in the last decades, significant progress has been made regarding viral and host cellular components involved in DENV infection and disease [8]. The nonstructural protein 1 (NS1) protein of DENV and other related flaviviruses has been described as an essential cofactor in virus replication and assembly [11, 12]. Interestingly, the secreted form of NS1 is also implicated in immune evasion strategies via interaction with several proteins of the complement pathways that protect the virus-infected cells from the immune system processing [12–14]. Contrary, NS1 and anti-NS1 antibodies can also mediate complement activation that may alter capillary permeability [15]. Additionally, the soluble NS1 from DENV can interact with the surface of endothelial cells, immune cells, and platelets to cause endothelial barrier dysfunction and vascular leakage, and potentially hampers the coagulation cascades leading to hemorrhagic manifestations during DENV infection. These phenomena occur via activation of endothelial-intrinsic mechanisms leading to the disruption of the EGL and the integrity of the cell-to-cell contacts and/or induction of pro-inflammatory cytokines, chemokines, and proteases via the TLR4 activation of monocytes/macrophages that may act also on endothelial cells leading to endothelial hyperpermeability and vascular leak [16–22]. Furthermore, NS1 is highly immunogenic and conserved between the *Flavivirus* genus; thus, NS1 from other flaviviruses have been also reported to activate endothelial-intrinsic mechanisms causing vascular leakage in a tissue-dependent manner that mimics each flavivirus disease pathophysiology [17, 23–25]. Additionally, NS1 immunization using mouse models and DENV vaccination or natural DENV infection in humans can elicit antibodies' responses that have been implicated in the contradictory roles of protection and pathogenesis in the infected host [25–42]. Today, no specific and effective vaccine candidate, antiviral therapy, or anti-inflammatory therapeutics have been licensed to combat dengue disease. An effective dengue vaccine is surely needed to avert the millions of dengue cases that occur around the world, continuously threatening with fatal outcomes. For decades, numerous experts in infectious diseases including clinicians, epidemiologists, basic scientists, and vaccine and drug developers have been trying to elucidate the ultimate mechanism of DENV pathogenesis leading to severe dengue disease. The NS1 protein of flaviviruses constitutes a unique "viral toxin" that seems to connect many of the already described DENV immunopathogenic mechanisms leading to severe dengue disease; thus, NS1 might represent the corner piece that completes the elusive dengue pathogenesis puzzle. Therapeutic approaches and vaccine development targeting NS1 may provide different opportunities for the future defeating of the global dengue disease. A better understanding of DENV immunopathogenesis will assist not only in the development of therapeutic interventions but also in the understanding of dengue vaccine efficacy or vaccine adverse events. This chapter briefly summaries the key clinical, virological, and epidemiological facts about DENV innate and humoral responses and gives an extensive update of insights about the viral and host factors that contribute to DENV pathogenesis leading to the development of severe dengue manifestations during DENV infection.

2. Dengue virus features: genomic organization, structure, and life cycle

Dengue virus (DENV) belongs to the genus *Flavivirus* (family *Flaviviridae*), a group of small (50-nm virion diameter) viruses containing a single-positive-stranded RNA genome [5′ capped, not 3′ poly(A) tail] which encodes for three structural proteins: capsid (C), membrane (M), and envelope (E) and seven nonstructural (NS) proteins named NS1, NS2A, NS2B, NS3, NS4A, NS4B, and NS5 (**Figure 1A**, **B**) [43]. The DENV group is comprised of four evolutionary distinct but antigenically and genetically related viruses better known as DENV serotypes -1, -2, -3, and -4 (DENV-1-4), [44, 45]. These four established serotypes (DENV 1–4) share a high degree of sequence similarity between the genomes (~65–70%) [46], with average sequence identity between proteomes of 39–79% [47]. DENV is transmitted to humans by *Aedes* mosquitoes, mainly *Aedes aegypti*. However, the global distribution of *Aedes albopictus* (the Asian tiger mosquito), considered a secondary vector for DENV transmission, is changing rapidly and it is now becoming an increasingly important vector and a common cause of epidemics in *Aedes aegypti*-free countries [48–50]. Human-to-mosquito transmission occurs once the mosquito takes a blood meal from DENV-infected people who are viremic, which is normally up to 2 days before someone shows symptoms of the illness or up to 2 days after the fever has resolved. High viremia and high fever in patients are positively associated with a high rate of DENV transmission from humans to mosquitoes [51]. After feeding on a DENV-infected person, depending mainly on temperature, the virus rapidly replicates in the mosquito's midgut, and within an average of 5.9 days, it disseminates to secondary tissues, including the salivary glands where the virus can be transmitted to the new host (extrinsic incubation period) [52]. Once infectious, the mosquito is capable of transmitting the virus for the rest of its life [53].

After a mosquito bites a human, DENV is delivered into the dermis where it can infect/replicate in dendritic cells (DCs) (Langerhans cells) and keratinocytes residing in the basal and suprabasal layers of the epidermis [54–56] (**Figure 2**). Virus dissemination to the local lymph nodes occurs in association with infected migratory dendritic cells or as free viruses of the lymphatic fluid leading to viremia [57]. At this stage, mosquito saliva has shown to enhance the replication and

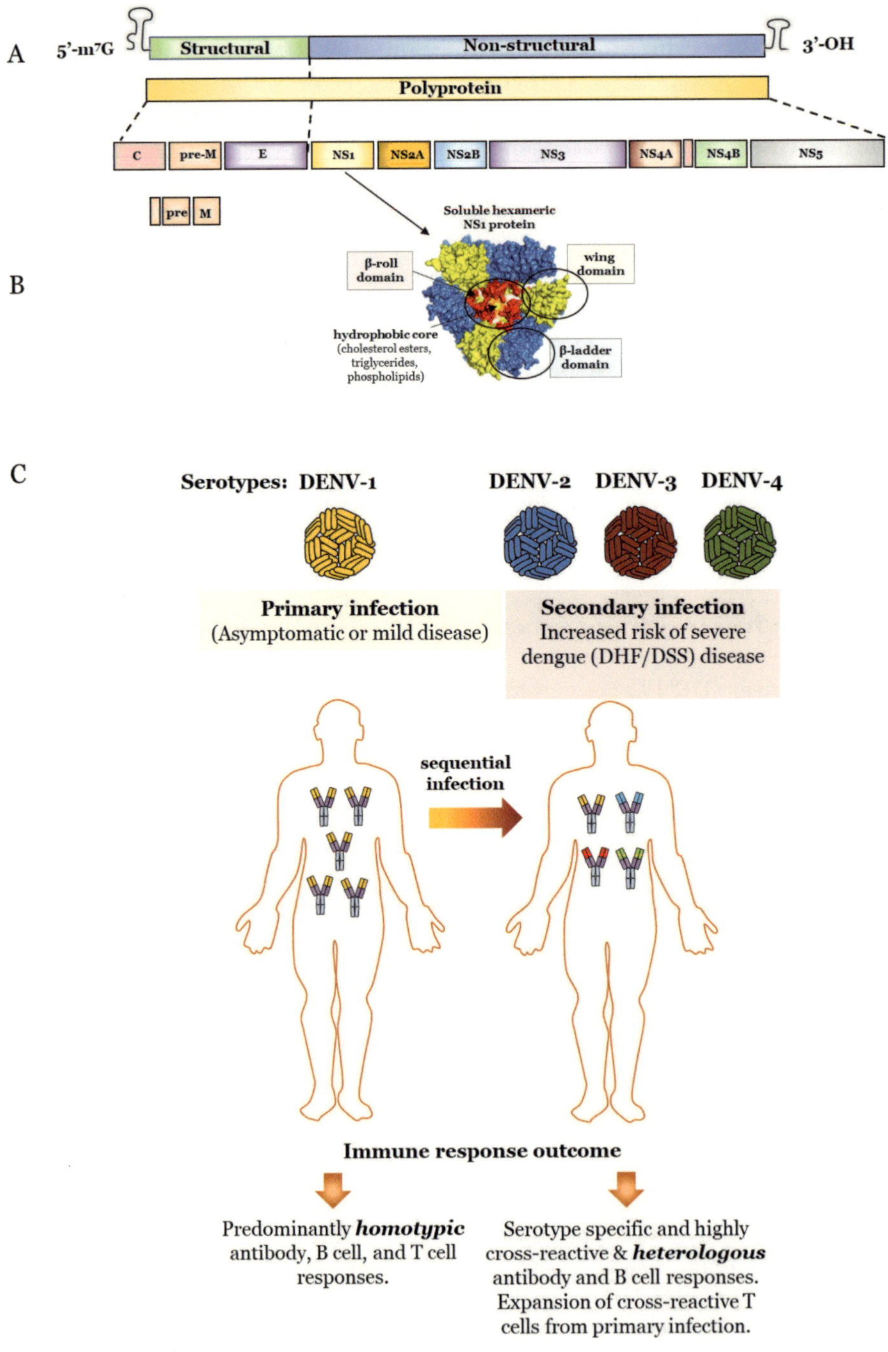

Figure 1.
Dengue virus genome organization, NS1 structure, and dengue epidemiology and disease outcome. (A) Schematic representation of the DENV genome and polyprotein. Dengue virus (DENV; genus Flavivirus, family Flaviviridae) is a positive-sense, single-stranded (~11-kb length), and RNA-enveloped virus with an icosahedral capsid protecting the virus genome, which is transmitted by mosquitoes of the Aedes genus (Aedes aegypti, Ae. albopictus) and affects more than 40% of the human population worldwide living in tropical and subtropical areas. The viral RNA genome poses one single open reading frame encoding for one single polyprotein, which after being processed by cellular and viral proteases generates three structural proteins known as the capsid (C), the membrane (M), and the envelope (E) and seven nonstructural (NS) proteins known as NS1, NS2A, NS2B, NS3, NS4A, NS4B, and N5. The viral RNA contains a cap in the 5′-end, and it has no poly-a tail in the 3′-end. Several secondary structures or UTRs (untranslated regions) are found in both ends which have been shown to participate in viral replication as well as host adaptation. Of the structural proteins, the envelope (E) is the major protein on the virion, which participates in cellular receptor recognition to infect the host cells and the main target for adaptive immune responses in humans. On the other hand, the NS proteins play critical roles in the virus replication cycle and the subversion of the host antiviral responses, particularly those triggered by the innate immune response against DENV infection. (B) Of these NS proteins, NS1 is the only viral protein secreted by DENV-infected cells in which the plasma circulating levels are increased during the acute phase of DENV-infected patients undergoing severe disease. The NS1 protein circulates as a lipoprotein-like particle with a hexameric conformational structure containing three domains termed as the wing domain (here in yellow), the β-ladder domain (in blue), and the β-roll domain (in red) (NS1 hexamer is depicted in this figure). NS1 has been demonstrated to play critical roles in the formation of new viral particles, the evasion of the immune system, and very recently, it was implicated in modulating the virus pathogenesis of DENV that is mainly associated to its potential role in acting as a pathogen-associated pattern molecule (PAMP) which activates the production of pro-inflammatory host soluble factors such as cytokines, chemokines, proteases, etc. from the immune cells and directly triggers the barrier dysfunction of endothelial cell cultures in vitro and vascular leak in the mouse models in vivo. Taking these together, NS1 is now considered as a viral toxin not only of the DENV complex but of many of the closely related flaviviruses, including ZIKV, WNV, and YFV among others. (C) The DENV complex is composed of four serologically but antigenically related types of viruses, known as DENV serotypes (1, 2, 3, and 4). The primary infection with any of the four serotypes often cause inapparent, asymptomatic, or mild diseases that prime the immune system for a long-life immunity against the infecting DENV serotype (here DENV-1, in yellow) which is dominated by homotypic immune responses at mostly all levels, including antibody-B cells' and T cells' responses. During secondary infections, things get more complicated as infection with a different DENV serotype as the one from the primary infection; here DENV-2 (blue), DENV-3 (red), and DENV-4 (green) results in cross-reactive and heterologous immune responses that are considered the main risk factor to develop severe manifestations of DENV infections, including dengue hemorrhagic fever and dengue shock syndrome (DHF/DSS), which may lead to life-threatening health complications and sometimes, death. In the course of this chapter, we will explain how these epidemiological factors may be associated with the development of severe dengue disease that may be a consequence of a combined interplay set of immunopathogenic mechanisms triggered by the host immune response having DENV infection as the main trigger. The model of NS1 hexamer was built based on the crystal structure deposited in the Protein Data Bank (PDB4O6B). Molecular graphics were performed using the PyMOL molecular graphics.

pathogenesis of numerous arthropod-borne viruses, including DENV [58–62]. DENV infection cycle initiates with the virus attachment to the target cells [63]. The current model suggests that DENV uses both attachment factors and primary receptor(s) that facilitate virus recruitment on the cell surface, and later, internalization inside host cells via receptor-mediated endocytosis including clathrin-mediated and nonclassical clathrin-independent endocytosis [64, 65]. Despite this, the single definitive receptor mediating this critical step in the DENV replication cycle continues to be elusive. So far, numerous candidates have been described in the mammalian and mosquito cells, including glycosaminoglycans such as heparan sulfate and lectins, the adhesion molecule of dendritic cells (DC-SIGN), the mannose receptor (MR) of macrophages, the lipopolysaccharide (LPS) receptor CD14, and stress-induced proteins such as the heat-shock proteins 70 and 90 and the endoplasmic reticulum (ER) chaperonin GRP78 [64–68]. This suggests that DENV may not use a unique, specific receptor to enter cells, but recognizes diverse molecules, both in the vertebrate and mosquito hosts, which can potentially explain the broad tissue range that defines DENV tropism and infection.

After the internalization of the virion, a fusion between the viral E protein and the endosomal membrane mediates the access of the viral genome into the cytoplasm [43, 65]. The E protein is a glycosylated viral protein and a member of class II viral membrane fusion protein family [43, 69]. The crystal structure of

E glycoprotein ectodomain revealed three domains contributing to the β-barrel central structure of the protein (domain I, DI), permitting the fusion of viral and cellular membranes during virus entry (domain II, DII, and *fusion loop*), and a structural basis for immune recognition and cellular receptor binding (domain III, DIII) [43, 70]. The low pH of the endosomal compartment induces conformational changes in the E glycoprotein, which allows the fusion of the viral and host membranes [43, 69]. This results in the release of the viral RNA genome into the cytoplasm. The single-stranded positive-sense RNA immediately acts as a messenger RNA, which can be subsequently translated by cellular machinery to generate viral polyproteins, subsequently processed by both cellular and viral proteases to generate mature viral proteins [69, 70]. In this stage, the nonstructural proteins have been shown to induce massive remodeling of ER membranes, manifesting as convoluted membranes and vesicle packets (VPs) to form a dynamic and membrane-bound multi-protein assembly, named the replication complex (RC) where the genome is replicated, and new viral RNA copies are incorporated into nascent particles [71, 72]. Viral RNA synthesis relies on NS5, the RNA-dependent RNA polymerase as well as on critical RNA secondary and tertiary structures [73–75]. NS3 is a

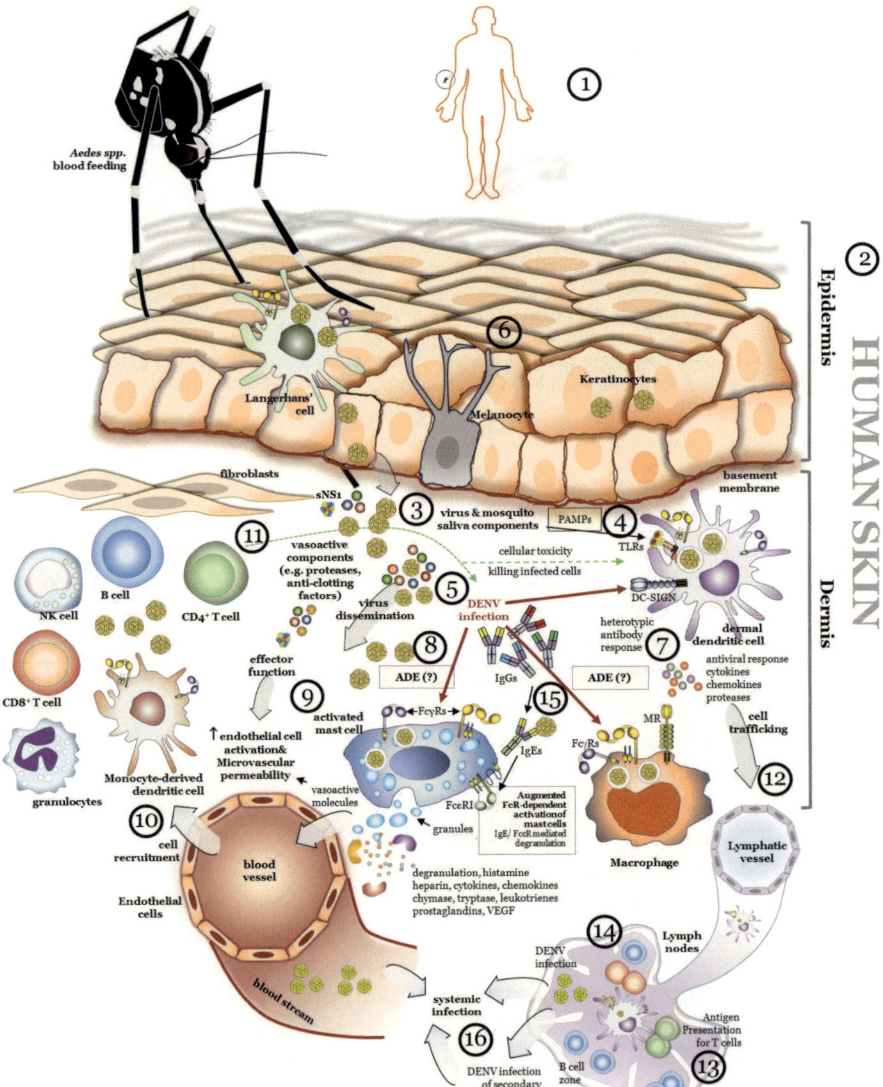

Figure 2.
Dengue virus infection, pathogenesis, and immune responses in the skin. The skin represents the first line of defense of the human body against pathogens such as viruses, as it generates early immune responses, aiming to protect humans against cutaneous and systemic infection (1). The human skin constitutes a complex organ nicely structured in three escalated layers known as the epidermis, which is composed of closely packed epithelial cells including keratinocytes, melanocytes, and Langerhans cells (LCs), a specialized type of dendritic cell (DC) that constantly probes for antigen in the most exposed, superficial layer of the skin; the dermis, which is made of dense, irregular connective tissue, blood vessels, and other structures; and the inner hypodermis, which is composed mainly of loose connective and fatty tissues (2). Upon disturbance of the epidermal barrier by mosquito blood-feeding, DENV-infected mosquitoes inoculate newly generated infectious virus particles along with mosquito saliva in which a complex mixture of proteins that exerts profound effects in the human immune system allows the acquisition of the mosquito blood meal from its host by circumventing vasoconstriction, platelet aggregation, coagulation, and inflammation or hemostasis (3). In the skin, major constituents of the innate immune system include phagocytic cells such as macrophages, neutrophils, and DCs as well as innate leukocytes such as natural killer (NK) cells, mast cells (MCs), basophils, and eosinophils. Also, epidermal keratinocytes act as active innate immune cells. In response to sensing pathogen-associated molecular patterns (PAMPs) expressed by microbes and host danger molecules, innate immune receptors present on keratinocytes and APCs become activated, causing the release of inflammatory cytokines and antimicrobial peptides (4). At the site of inoculation in the skin, the key targets of DENV infection are immune cells of the myeloid lineage, including various subsets of DCs, monocytes/macrophages, and MCs (5). Despite this, limited virus particles are thought to be deposited in the epidermis during mosquito blood-feeding (3), and in that location, Langerhans cells as well as keratinocytes are considered target cells (6). In the dermis, DCs and monocytes/macrophages are also prime infection targets (7). MCs are not substantially infected in the skin (8). However, exposure to DENV triggers an augmented activation of MCs leading to degranulation and release of de novo-synthesized inflammatory and vasoactive mediators, including proteases, leukotrienes, and histamine that, along with some vasoactive molecules and maybe the secreted NS1 originated from infected mosquito cells in the salivary glands, promote edema within the site of infection as a consequence of the increased microvascular permeability (9). Activation of MCs also induces the secretion of cytokines and chemokines that leads to the recruitment of NK cells, neutrophils, and monocyte-derived dendritic cells (mDCs) to the site of infection (10). Already in the skin, mDCs can serve as targets of infection, allowing the amplification of the virus in the skin, while natural killer (NK) cells, natural killer T (NKT) cells, and CD8+ T cells can kill DENV-infected cells and promote virus clearance in a cellular cytotoxic-dependent manner (11). Once human skin is infected, DENV-infected DCs take virus into the draining lymph nodes using afferent lymphatic vessels where they spread DENV infection and most importantly activate antigen-specific $CD4^+$ and $CD8^+$ T cells which initiates the adaptive immune response (12, 13). In the T cell zones, activated T cells become effectors cells to promote the development of DENV-specific memory B cells and plasma cells in the germinal center of LN. Activated T cells can reenter circulation and potentially return to the skin for virus clearance during subsequent DENV infections, playing an important role in protecting against DENV (14). In the skin, in addition to the mosquito saliva, DENV infection of target cells such as DCs, monocytes/macrophages, and MCs can be also modulated by the presence of preexisting antibody responses against previous infections with distinct DENV serotypes or other closely related flaviviruses, in an antibody-dependent enhancement (ADE) manner (See DENV-ADE in Part II for more details). For MCs and DCs, DENV-ADE is possible through Fc-γ-receptors (FcγRs). Besides, MCs degranulation can be enhanced through cross-linking of FcεRs when bound to DENV-specific IgE, leading to augmented MC activation and presumably immune-mediated vascular injury (15). After skin infection, DENV must achieve systemic infection to complete its transmission cycle by infecting new mosquito hosts. Infection of secondary LNs following infection of the draining LN are considered the amplification centers for DENV that contributes to the systemic infection and virus transmission (16).

protease-helicase which together with its cofactor NS2B, participates in the processing, efficient RNA synthesis, and capping of the viral polyprotein [72, 76, 77]. NS2A recruits nascent RNA as well as C-pre-M-E [78]. NS1 interacts with structural proteins and NS4A-2 K-4B to facilitate the production of infectious virus particles [11, 79]. Because of their critical roles in the DENV replication cycle, NS2B, NS3, and NS5 along with NS4B are the main focus to design new inhibitors for antiviral therapy against DENV and other related flaviviruses [80–83]. Assembled viruses are transported through the trans-Golgi network (TGN) where under acidic conditions, a cellular protease, *furin*, cleaves pre-M, allowing full maturation of infectious virions that will be finally released via exocytosis [84].

3. Dengue virus infection, epidemiology, and clinical features

Dengue is the arboviral infection with the highest disease incidence worldwide, with 2.5 billion people living in dengue-endemic tropical and subtropical regions [1, 85, 86]. In the last four decades, the geographical spread and intensity of dengue have grown dramatically around the world accompanied by the wide distribution of the two main vector mosquitoes, *Aedes aegypti* and *Aedes albopictus*, which today are fully adapted to human dwellings creating new opportunities not only for DENV but also for other arthropod-transmitted viruses (arboviruses) transmission, such as Zika virus (ZIKV) and chikungunya virus (CHIKV), within human populations. These features along with the continuous growing of urbanization, globalization, and the lack of effective mosquito control represent some of the critical factors that have contributed to the emergence and reemergence of mosquito-transmitted viruses around the world [48, 87, 88].

Infection with any of the four DENV serotypes results in a diverse range of symptoms going from mild undifferentiated fever to life-threatening manifestations, which are characterized by increased vascular permeability, hemorrhage, and shock [89] (**Figure 1C**). In 1997, the World Health Organization (WHO) classified symptomatic DENV infections into three categories and subcategories known as dengue fever (DF), dengue hemorrhagic fever (DHF), and dengue shock syndrome (DSS). After an incubation period of 3–7 days, symptoms start suddenly and follow three phases: an initial febrile phase, a critical phase around the time of defervescence, and a spontaneous recovery phase [89]. Classical DF is an incapacitating disease that affects older children, adolescents, and adults, mainly characterized by the abrupt onset of fever (up to 40°C) and severe headache, accompanied by retro-orbital pain, myalgia, arthralgia, gastrointestinal discomfort, and transient rash [89]. In turn, DHF and DSS can rapidly deteriorate, progressing to hemorrhage with or without vascular leak after an early acute-onset febrile period, particularly during defervescence, where the symptoms are similar to those presented during classical DF. DHF and DSS are classified into four subcategories or grades (I–IV), where grades I and II (DHF) are represented by mild cases presenting some bleeding manifestations without shock (petechiae, purpura, ecchymosis, bruising, epistaxis, etc.), whereas III and IV (DSS) are more severe and accompanied by severe hemorrhagic manifestations and thrombocytopenia (platelets counts: <100,000 platelets/μL) and evidence of increased vascular permeability (ascites, pleural effusion, increased hematocrit concentrations, and severe abdominal pain) during a critical period, sometimes accompanied with a profound and prolonged shock that potentially leads to death [90]. In this critical stage, liver failure, myocarditis, and encephalopathy often occur with minimal associated plasma leakage [89]. In 2009, the WHO revised the classification system for dengue and established new guidelines that replaced the more complicated dengue fever/dengue hemorrhagic fever (DF/DHF) system to separate patients enduring severe disease from those with non-severe manifestations. This new guideline defined two new major entities—dengue and severe dengue—which encompasses a set of "warning signs" intended to help clinicians identify the patients likely to develop complications during the critical phase of the illness [89].

Currently, there is no effective and safe vaccine or FDA-approved specific antiviral drug options to combat dengue disease, with treatment being purely supportive [91]. Prevention or reduction of DENV transmission by implementing combined effective control strategies remains as the primary approach to be used to prevent DENV transmission within human populations [92]. With the majority of DENV infections being asymptomatic (70–80%), and most symptomatic infections not progressing to severe disease [3], the global distribution of dengue remains highly uncertain as the actual numbers of dengue cases are underreported and many cases are misclassified. One recent study estimate indicates that 390 million DENV infections occur annually with more than 500,000 cases of hospitalizations and more than 25,000 deaths (2.5% case fatality, annually) [1]. A different study estimated that 3.9 billion people living in 128 countries are at risk of being infected with dengue viruses [85]. These studies demonstrate the worldwide expansion of the dengue disease and the establishment of an increasingly important infectious disease of global public health significance.

4. Dengue immunopathogenesis and severe disease: host and viral factors

The hallmark of severe dengue is the transient perturbation in the integrity of the endothelium lining the inner side of blood vessels as well as the alteration in the coagulation cascade leading to shock and severe hemorrhage manifestations [9, 89]. Increased vascular permeability in severe dengue results in decreased circulating plasma volume, haemoconcentration, and pleural and peritoneal effusions that result in severe life-threatening shock [93–96]. Numerous epidemiological pieces of evidence indicate that appearance of the life-threatening manifestations during severe dengue occurs shortly after the defervescence stage of dengue disease, when the peak of viremia passed, meaning that host innate and adaptive immune responses have cleared the virus from host tissues [97, 98]. At this time, a transient vascular leakage pathology is observed followed by a rapid recovery in association with the late febrile phase. This association led to the suggestion that the key biological mechanisms such as alterations on the vasculature that leads to the pathogenesis of clinical complications during DENV infection are rather functional than the structural changes in the endothelium and are primarily a consequence of short-lived biological mediators closely linked to the host immune responses [93–96].

Although many severe infections occur upon secondary encounters with heterologous DENV serotypes [9, 99], suggesting an immune-mediated process is involved, the multifactorial immunopathogenic process of DENV infection implies a complex interaction between distinct viral and host processes that sometimes leads to increased virus infection, exacerbated immune responses, and the appearance of life-threatening severe manifestations such as severe plasma leakage, hemorrhage, and organ failure. Higher virus pathogenicity (virulence), preexisting serotype cross-reactive antibodies, activation of DENV-infected immune cells [e.g., monocytes and mast cells (MCs)], T cell responses, activation of complement pathways, the potential infection of endothelial cells, and the new pathogenic roles of the secreted NS1 of DENV may work synergistically to induce the release of vasoactive cytokines which results in increased endothelial permeability causing vascular leakage and pleural effusion, which are still considered pathognomonic features of severe dengue that leads occasionally to shock and death [8, 9, 35, , 96, 99–110]. In this section, we highlight in two parts I and II, the immunological events elicited by DENV infection, which have been suggested to play a key role in the development of severe dengue manifestations.

4.1 Dengue virus tropism and infection of immune cells

Numerous *in vitro* studies have shown that DENV is able to infect a variety of cell types including epithelial cells, endothelial cells, hepatocytes, muscle cells, dendritic cells, monocytes, B cells, and mast cells [65, 66, 111–117]. Several autopsies and *ex vivo* studies have found the presence of DENV antigens (e.g., envelope protein, NS3) in some tissues such as the skin, liver, spleen, lymph node, kidney, bone marrow, lung, thymus, and brain [56, 67, 68, 118–122]. However, infectious virus particles have not always been isolated from all these organs but only from the liver and peripheral blood mononuclear cells (PBMCs), suggesting that: (a) the presence of DENV antigens such as the structural proteins E, pre-M, and C in several organs may not always be associated with the evidence of productive viral infection and severe organ pathology and (b) the immune cells and liver may be the main targets for DENV replication during the dengue disease [67].

In animal models such as the alpha/beta (IFN-α/β)-deficient mice (*Ifnar*$^{-/-}$) and nonhuman primates, DENV has been recovered from the spleen, liver, peripheral lymph nodes, and the central nervous system [123–127]. However, the absence of an appropriate animal disease model has largely hampered with the understanding of the role played by DENV tropism *in vivo*. Sustained viral replication and severe manifestations have been observed in *Ifnar*$^{-/-}$ mice after infection with DENV, which gives a clear advantage to study DENV pathogenesis *in vivo*, but the absence of intact IFN signaling is a limitation that must be considered when interpreting data [128].

The fact that DENV can infect many mammalian and insect cell types *in vitro* and *in vivo* suggest there are different molecules or cellular routes that might be controlling virus attachment and internalization, resulting in productive infection [63]. Numerous studies have shown that C-type lectins including DC-SIGN (CD209) and C-type lectin domain family 5, member A (CLEC5A) expressed on dendritic cells and macrophages act as cellular receptors for DENV [129–131]. Other extensively studied DC receptors are the mannose receptor (MR), Langerins, Fc-receptors, TIM3, TIM4, and AXL [63, 65, 132, 133]. Contrary to the DC-SIGN that may primarily function as a viral attachment factor, DENV binding to CLEC5A (C-type lectin domain family 5, member A), highly expressed by monocytes, macrophages, neutrophils, and dendritic cells, has been shown to induce the production of antiviral and pro-inflammatory cytokines suggesting that this C-type lectin may act as a cognate receptor for dengue virion [131, 134]. These cytokines include type I IFNs and chemotactic factors such as migration inhibition factor (MIF), monocyte chemotactic factor (MCP), and IL-8 [102, 134]. DENV infection of DCs also induces the production of matrix metalloproteinases (MPPs), MMP-2 and MMP-9, which induces migration of DCs to lymph nodes where virus further replicates before it disseminates into the blood circulation [135]. In the skin, DENV also infects mast cells that can be activated leading to degranulation and increased secretion of various inflammatory cytokines (IL-1, IL-6, TNF-α, and IFN-α), chemokines (CCL5, CXCL12, and CX3CL1), and chymase, the latter being a protease found circulating at high levels in the blood of dengue patients, suggesting a potential role in the development of severe dengue that contributes to vascular leakage [115, 136–140]. All these innate immune processes together lead to an antiviral state in nearby cells, generating an inflammatory response and recruitment of natural killer (NK) cells to combat DENV infection [54, 141].

Along with DCs, monocytes and macrophages are also the primary targets of DENV infection [142, 143]. In lymphoid and nonlymphoid tissues, macrophages are considered the primary reservoirs of DENV after its dissemination from the skin [144]. Macrophages susceptible to DENV have been found in different organs in the mouse models or human autopsies, namely, Kupfer cells in the liver, alveolar macrophages in the lungs, dermal macrophages, microglial cells (brain and spinal cord), and monocytes in the peripheral blood [118, 120, 122, 145–147]. Comparable to DENV infection of DCs, DENV can use an array of cell surface receptors to infect monocytes and macrophages, including mannose receptor (CD205), CD14-associated protein, heat shock proteins (HSP70/HSP90), DC-SIGN (CD209), CD300a, AXL, TIM4, PD1, and the Fc receptors, particularly FcγRI (CD64) and FcγRII (CD32, 63). These two Fc-Rs play major roles in enhancing DENV infection of monocytes and macrophages, particularly during secondary infections [148–151].

Other populations of immune cells including NK cells can also be activated during DENV infection, particularly in patients with DHF compared to those with DF [141, 152, 153]. Additionally, B cells and T cells have been studied to test permissiveness to DENV, but these studies have resulted in contradictory results [154–156]. *In vitro* studies using B cell and T cell lines (e.g., *Raji* cells, Daudi, and Jurkat) and primary B cells derived from healthy human peripheral blood mononuclear cells

(PBMCs) have revealed the potential role of these cells in DENV replication, both in presence and absence of heterologous antibodies [67, 155, 157–159]. Additional studies using a humanized mouse model found that DENV infected both B and T cells accompanied by an important production of pro-inflammatory cytokines such as IL-6 and TNF-α, like monocytes and macrophages [160]. Despite this evidence, the role of lymphoid cells such as B and T cells in DENV tropism and replication needs further exploration.

4.2 DENV infection and the host innate immune responses

Although plasma leakage in severe dengue occurs at the end of the acute illness, there is substantial evidence that the pathophysiologic processes start at the earliest stages of DENV infection [95, 96]. Introduction of DENV particles along with mosquito saliva triggers a variety of host innate immune responses leading to the production of antiviral and pro-inflammatory cytokines mostly from the immune cells exposed to DENV [57, 62, 138]. At this stage, innate immune cells are the first to respond to infection through stimulation of patterns recognition receptors (PRRs) recognizing pathogen-associated molecular patterns (PAMPs) as well as endogenous molecules released from damaged cells, termed damage-associated molecular patterns (DAMPs) [161, 162]. PRR recognition triggers the production of cytokines and chemokines, which induces a local antiviral state [54, 55]. This local innate response could potentially play an important role in modulating local viremia and virus dissemination by recruiting susceptible target cells for DENV infection at the inoculation site [57, 62, 144].

PRRs include transmembrane proteins such as the Toll-like receptors (TLRs) and C-type lectin receptors (CLRs) as well as cytoplasmic proteins such as the retinoic acid-inducible gene (RIG)-I-like receptors (RLRs) and NOD-like receptors (NLRs) [161]. These are an essential part of the innate immune response against the virus, sensing viral replication in the cytoplasm [161, 163]. The PRRs that are associated with DENV recognition after infecting target cells are the cytoplasmic retinoic acid-inducible gene I (RIG-I) and the melanoma differentiation-associated protein 5 (MDA5) and the endosomal Toll-like receptor 3 (TLR3) and TLR7 [164–166]. Recognition of DENV RNA by TLR-3 results in the production of type I IFN and chemokines such as IL-8 via sensing of phosphate-containing RNA and long double-stranded RNA (dsRNA) in the cytoplasm or inside endosomal compartments [167, 168]. DENV infection in nonhuman primates demonstrated that the administration of TLR-3 and TLR7 agonists resulted in significantly decreased viral replication and increased production of pro-inflammatory chemokines as well as increased production of antibodies targeting DENV [169], indicating a protective role for TLRs during DENV infection.

Additional pathways such as the cyclic GMP-AM synthase (cGAS), a DNA-sensor pathway which triggers the simulator of IFN genes (STING) pathway are also activated during DENV infection leading to the production of type I IFN and activation of TLRs (TLR9), an endosomal PRR that recognizes cytoplasmic DNA originated from mitochondrial damage [170–172]. In addition to type I IFN production, small RNAs such as micro RNAs (miRNA) and the complement system are important components of the innate immune response against viral infections [173, 174]. miRNAs are processed by and interact with the proteins in the RNA interference (RNAi) pathway, such as Dicer, Drosha, Argo1, and Argo2 [175]. RNA interference (RNAi) is an important antiviral defense response in plants and invertebrates [176]. In DENV infection, knockdown of these components resulted in increased DENV replication in mammalian cells, suggesting that the RNAi pathways may play important roles in the cellular anti-DENV responses [177, 178]. Additional evidence showed that DENV can interfere with RNAi pathways in human hepatocytes cells via NS4B and subgenomic flavivirus RNA (sfRNA) interactions with Dicer's ability to process small

RNA *in vitro* [179]. sfRANs are abundant noncoding RNA sequences derived from the stalling of the host 5′-3′ exoribonuclease XRN1/Pacman in the 3′-untranslated regions (3′UTRs) of the viral genomic RNA [180]. sfRNAs have been shown to block exonuclease XRN1, increasing the overall messenger RNA stability within the host cell which may also benefit the viral RNA [181–183]. However, evidence for RNAi contribution to mammalian antiviral defense are few and still controversial [179]. miRNAs have been shown to regulate TLRs and IL-1 signaling pathways in response to viral infection, which provides control of host innate immune responses [184]. So far, there have been reported several cellular miRNAs (miRNAome) that are modulated during DENV infection of mammalian cells, mainly related to the regulation of IFN-β signaling pathways [185–188]. Some of these miRNAs have been proposed to be used as biomarkers in dengue-infected patients [189, 190]. Interestingly, modulation of microRNA expressions have been also described upon DENV infection of insect cells (e.g., C6/36 cells) as well as adult vector mosquitoes such as *Aedes albopictus* [191–193], suggesting that DENV might also regulate the activation of these antiviral RNAi pathways in vector mosquitoes, potentially avoiding viral clearance that promotes viral replication and transmission [194]. Despite RNAi constituting an evolutionarily conserved phenomenon of the mosquito-innate immune response to virus infections [195], viruses have found ways to subvert the RNAi-mediated antiviral responses in vector mosquitoes to manipulate miRNA profiles to their own benefit [196].

Regarding the complement system, this multifaceted pathway has been shown to limit DENV replication; however, excessively activated complement components have been also associated with disease severity [197]. The complement cascade constitutes an integral component of the immune system, composed of many plasma proteins that once activated can initiate a proteolytic cascade, resulting in the release of chemokines, facilitation of particle phagocytosis via opsonization, and deposition of the cell-killing membrane attack complex (MAC) designed to target and destroy foreign pathogens such as viruses [174]. Activation of the complement system occurs via three convergent pathways: the classical, the lectin, and the alternative pathways [174]. *In vitro* experiments showed that DENV replication enhances complement activation [197–199]. Additionally, clinical and *in vivo* studies have shown that excessive consumption of some complement components (e.g., C3, C4, and factor B) contributed to severe manifestations by increasing the levels of complement-activated products which enhance vascular permeability to cause severe dengue disease [9, 108, 109, 200]. In fact, increased circulation of anaphylatoxins (C3a, C4a, and C5a) in the blood of severe patients correlated with symptoms of vascular leakage [109, 200]. In autopsy studies from children who died of acute severe dengue manifestations (DHF/DSS), augmented deposition of complement components from both classical and alternative pathways were found on hepatocytes which results in severe liver damage and death [120]. Altogether, these data support the hypothesis that exacerbated complement activation influences dengue disease immunopathogenesis leading to disease severity [197].

4.3 DENV subversion of antiviral responses

The first barrier to overcome for successful viral infection is the rapid innate immune responses of the host, including type I IFNs, inflammatory cytokines, complement responses, NK cells, apoptosis, and autophagy [201, 202]. These innate immune responses are meant to defeat viral infections by engaging specific viral components (e.g., RNA and DNA) leading to activation of immediate protective defense mechanisms such as the rapid recognition of PAMP in nonimmune and innate immune cells [161]. IFN production is a key goal of PRR activation for viral pathogens, and DENV is highly susceptible to effective induction of both type

I (IFN α/β) and type II (IFN γ) interferons [124, 203, 204]. Accordingly, *in vivo* DENV infection of wild-type mice causes little disease; in contrast, in mice lacking of type I IFN receptors (IFANR), DENV infection causes mortality [126].

Secreted type I IFNs trigger autocrine and paracrine induction of cellular antiviral responses and warning signals to noninfected adjacent cells, such as the expression of the interferon stimulated genes (ISGs) [205, 206]. ISGs have been shown to exert numerous antiviral effector functions, many of which are still not fully described [207]. Upon DENV infection, RLRs are activated to trigger antiviral responses based on the induction of type I IFN and pro-inflammatory cytokines [208]. The binding of type I IFN with its receptor activates multi-subsets of ISGs through JAK-STAT signaling which amplifies and sustains the initial antiviral responses [207, 209, 210]. However, ISGs can also be activated in IFN-independent pathways during DENV infection [211]. DENV infection has been shown to trigger the transcriptional activation of ISGs *in vivo* and *in vitro* [208, 212–215]. For instance, a tripartite motif (TRIM) protein encoding gene, *TRIM69*, is induced during DENV infection as an ISG. TRIM69 restricts DENV replication by direct interaction with DENV NS3, which mediates its polyubiquitination and degradation in a process called ISGylation [216]. In addition to ISGs, activation of the transcription factors IRF-3, IRF-7, and NF-κB through either the TLR or RIG-I/MDA5 pathways results in the production of type I IFN which contributes to anti-DENV immunity [217, 218]. IRF-3 and IRF-7 are part of the interferon regulatory factors (IRFs) considered the master regulators of the type I IFN production that contribute to the suppression of viruses [219]. Due to the central importance in viral defense, many pathogenic viruses, including DENV, have evolved mechanisms to suppress IRF signaling. In the case of DENV, the nonstructural proteins restrict IRF3 and IFN response which facilitate DENV replication and virulence [220].

In recent years, considerable advances have been made toward understanding of the specific IFN antagonistic mechanisms evolved by DENV to subvert these intracellular antiviral mechanisms and directly inhibiting these cellular signaling cascades, which results in enhanced virus infection, pathogenesis, and disease [167, 221]. This is supported by the increased susceptibility of mice deficient in IFN-α/β and IFN-γ receptors (AG129) to DENV infection as compared to wild-type mice [124, 126, 127]. Although IFN response is antagonized in mouse, human cells still induce high levels of IFN production in response to DENV, so this pathway is not entirely abrogated in humans during infection [203, 222]. Accordingly, humans infected with DENV have high levels of circulating of type I and type II IFNs [223–225]. Strong IFN-α responses have shown to correlate with milder dengue clinical conditions [226]. Similarly, the levels of the dengue-related gene expression of ISGs have been reported to be lower in patients with more severe disease [227–229] suggesting that DENV may abrogate IFN responses to facilitate viral infection which results in severe manifestations.

From the viral perspective, DENV uses its nonstructural (NS) proteins to block and inhibit the antiviral sensing pathways in infected cells. NS2a, NS3, NS4a, NS4b, and NS5 prevent the virus from being sensed by RIG-I, inhibiting IFNβ induction [230–233]. NS2a, NS4a, and NS4b complex inhibits STAT1 signaling after IFNAR activation *in vitro* [233, 234]. NS5 induces proteasomal degradation of STAT2 which inhibits IFN-mediated response [230]. NS2b induces degradation of cGAS, which prevents DNA sensing resulting from mitochondrial damage [170, 171, 235]. The NS2b/3 protease complex cleaves STING which inhibits IFN production [236]. This phenomenon has been shown to occur in human but not nonhuman primates, suggesting that DENV may have evolved to increase viral titers in human populations, while maintaining decreased titers and pathogenicity in rare animals would serve as a sustainable reservoir in nature [237].

In addition to NS proteins, flavivirus sfRNAs have been described to regulate the innate immune responses via binding and inactivating RNA-binding proteins which are crucial for innate immunity [180, 238]. DENV 3′UTRs possess RNA structures necessary for viral genome cyclization, viral RNA synthesis, translation, and replication [239]. sfRNAs regulate the pathogenicity in both mammalian and mosquito cells after interacting with proteins such as TRIM25 to inhibit RIG-I signaling and translation of ISGs [73, 240, 241]. Interestingly, reduced IFN responses have been found during DENV outbreaks where the infecting DENV serotype produced greater levels of sfRNA than the less pathogenic strains [100, 240]. Thus, high levels of sfRNAs may cause an epidemiological fitness of DENV, which results in lower stimulation of RIG-IMDA5 RNA sensors and reduced production of IFN, causing higher viremia levels that could be translated in more infections and severe diseases.

On the other hand, DENV utilizes the endoplasmic reticulum (ER) of host cells for replication and assembly. In this process, the ER undergoes extensive rearrangements and expansion that requires *de novo* synthesis of viral proteins [71]. Accumulation of unfolded proteins in the ER lumen leads to an unfolded protein response (UPR), a pro-survival cellular reaction induced in response to DENV-mediated ER stress [242, 243]. DENV has evolved to manipulate the UPR to cope with ER stress which hijacks the host cell machinery to evade the host immunity, facilitating viral replication [112]. Distinct *in vitro* and *in vivo* studies have shown that DENV induced ER stress and manipulates the host metabolism and protein production by increasing the autophagy (lipophagy) activity, viral replication, and pathogenesis through UPR signaling pathways [244–247]. Autophagy is the lysosomal degradation of cytoplasmic contents, which results in the recycling of cellular macromolecules as well as the activation of cellular host responses to starvation or stress [248]. Autophagy has been implicated as an innate immune response that would engulf and destroy pathogens by degrading cytosolic contents [249, 250]. In DENV infection, functional autophagy components have been shown to either promote or restrict viral RNA replication and virus production [251–253]. However, DENV has found ways of preventing autophagic processing and degradation of viral components [254, 255]. Several studies have linked DENV induction of autophagy to the regulation of lipid metabolism, leading to increased degradation of lipid droplets that produces more fatty acid material important for viral replication [247]. In this process, the NS3, NS1, and C proteins of DENV have been found to increase fatty acid biosynthesis and recruitment of lipid droplets to the DENV replication complex, facilitating viral particle assembly [256, 257].

Furthermore, several studies have shown that lipids and lipoproteins play a role in modifying DENV infectivity in both mammal and insect cells *in vitro* [258, 259]. Modulation of cholesterol levels in the host cells facilitates viral entry, replication, virus assembly, and control type I IFN response [260, 261]. This modulation involves the regulation of cholesterol levels, expression of cholesterol receptors as well as changes in cholesterol synthesis related to important modifications in the cellular metabolism [114, 262, 263]. Interestingly, clinical studies have found that levels of total serum cholesterol and LDL-C levels are modulated over the course of dengue illness, with generally lower levels associated with increased dengue severity [264–266]. In general, low cholesterol levels have been associated with critical illness related to sepsis and vascular disorders [267]. Thus, the association of cholesterol with severe dengue outcome may be an important indicator of the pathophysiology of DHF/DSS.

About the complement pathway, DENV has evolved strategies to limit recognition and activation of the complement cascade [108, 165]. NS1 is the only flavivirus protein that is secreted by infected cells and has been shown to modulate the complement pathway [14, 268]. NS1 promotes efficient degradation of C4 to C4b to protect DENV from complement-dependent neutralization [13, 269]. The NS1 protein of DENV and other flaviviruses such as WNV NS1 interacts with some components of the alternative complement pathway such as the C3bBb convertase, which limits the formation of C5b-9 membrane attack complex (MAC) [268, 270]. Additional studies have found that NS1 proteins from DENV, WNV, and YFV all attenuate classical and lectin pathway activation by directly interacting with C4, which reduces C4b deposition and C3 convertase (C4b2a) activity [13, 271]. Also, anti-NS1 antibodies have been shown to induce complement consumption and C5b-9 generation [272]. Overall, through protein-to-protein interactions between the viral and host factors involved in antiviral responses and careful manipulation of cellular processes, such as ER expansion, autophagy and lipid metabolism, and complement pathways, DENV hijacks many host antiviral responses to facilitate virus replication leading to pathogenesis.

5. Concluding remarks (Part I)

Dengue is the most prevalent arboviral disease transmitted by mosquitoes, which poses an enormous burden to the public health systems worldwide as more than 40% of the world population is at risk of infection. The infection with any of the four DENV serotypes (DENV1–4) can lead to a wide spectrum of clinical manifestations that range from the asymptomatic or inapparent to moderate flu-like symptoms, known as dengue fever (DF), and life-threatening manifestations identified by the WHO, known as the dengue hemorrhagic fever and dengue shock syndrome (DHF/DSS), also known as severe dengue, with or without warning signs. In endemic areas where multiple DENV serotypes can seasonally circulate, distinct epidemiological studies have demonstrated that an individual human being can be exposed to sequential infections with distinct DENV serotypes, which poses a risk of developing severe manifestations such as DHF/DSS. This phenomenon has been attributed to the potential enhancement activity that the preexisting antibody response elicited from a previous infection with one serotype (e.g., DENV-1) may have on the infection with a different serotype (e.g., DENV-2). This process leads to an increased viral burden that triggers a series of immunological and cellular events (e.g., ADE, cytokine storm, skewed T cell responses, and complement pathways), which despite being intended to prevent the invasion and infection of the infecting viral pathogens, can induce host tissue damage leading to pathology and disease. The cellular and molecular mechanisms involved in this phenomenon will be explained in more detail in the Part II of this chapter entitled "Adaptive immune response and NS1 pathogenesis."

As an arthropod-transmitted virus (arbovirus), DENV is initially transmitted by an infected vector mosquito in which the virus has already been amplified after replication in its distinct tissues, starting at the midgut to finalize in the salivary glands, where a new transmission cycle begins after blood feeding from a new host (**Figure 2**). Following inoculation from the bite of an infected mosquito, viruses undergo replication in the local tissues such as the skin. In the skin, infectious virus particles along with mosquito saliva components including proteases and immunomodulatory proteins among others are sown in the epidermis and dermis, leading to an activation of a cascade of events including the recruitment of skin resident cells (e.g., Langerhans cells, mast cells, and keratinocytes) and new cells (e.g., T cells and neutrophils) into the site of the infection that later serve as viral targets for viral replication. After infection of target cells, sensing of viral products (e.g., PAMPs and DAMPs) results in the activation of innate immune responses (e.g., type I IFN chemokines), the first line of defense, which establishes inflammatory and antiviral states intended to prevent the virus to colonize and to replicate in the skin; however, DENV has elaborated several pathogenic mechanisms to hijack these responses and escape from the normal immune system processing, which results in its dissemination and seeds into the lymph nodes. There, DENV further replicates in monocyte lineage cells, resulting in a primary viremia after its systemic dissemination through the circulatory bloodstream, which results in the subsequent infection of peripheral tissues such as the liver, spleen, and kidney. Overall, the skin represents not only the first line of defense against arboviruses but also the main place where viruses have learned to evade the host immune responses leading to invasion and dissemination toward the establishment of systemic host infection, which will potentially assure subsequent virus transmission into a new host. In this *Part I* of the chapter entitled "Dengue virus tropism, host innate immune responses, and subversion of antiviral responses," we discussed the distinct features of DENV as well as the biological and molecular mechanisms that can tilt the balance to either a local viral infection and dissemination through the skin or to the control and prevention of viral infection by the innate and adaptive immune responses at the site of the infection. Thus, the immunopathogenesis of arboviruses such as DENV in the skin is a critical step and must be a focus of future studies intended to reduce/block arthropod-borne transmission into humans.

Acknowledgements

The authors would like to acknowledge to the Canadian Institutes of Health Research and the International Development Research Centre (Projects 108412 and 109071-002) and the Fondo Mixto CONACYT-Gobierno del Estado de Yucatan (Project YUC-2017-03-01-556).

Author details

Henry Puerta-Guardo[1]*, Scott B. Biering[2], Eva Harris[2], Norma Pavia-Ruz[3], Gonzalo Vázquez-Prokopec[4], Guadalupe Ayora-Talavera[3] and Pablo Manrique-Saide[1]

1 Collaborative Unit for Entomological Bioassays and Laboratory for Biological Control of *Aedes aegypti*, Campus of Biological and Agricultural Sciences, Universidad Autonoma de Yucatan, Merida, Yucatan, Mexico

2 Division of Infectious Diseases and Vaccinology, School of Public Health, University of California, Berkeley, USA

3 Centro de Investigaciones Regionales Dr. Hideyo Noguchi, Universidad Autonoma de Yucatan, Merida Yucatan, Mexico

4 Department of Environmental Sciences, Emory University, Atlanta, Georgia, USA

*Address all correspondence to: hpuertaguardo@gmail.com

References

[1] Bhatt S, Gething PW, Brady OJ, Messina JP, Farlow AW, Moyes CL, et al. The global distribution and burden of dengue. Nature. 2013;**496**(7446):504-507

[2] World Health Organization. Global Strategy for Dengue Prevention and Control 2012-2020. Geneva: World Health Organization; 2012

[3] Guo C, Zhou Z, Wen Z, Liu Y, Zeng C, Xiao D, et al. Global epidemiology of dengue outbreaks in 1990-2015: A systematic review and meta-analysis. Frontiers in Cellular and Infection Microbiology. 2017;**7**:317

[4] Halstead SB. Dengue. Lancet. 2007;**370**(9599):1644-1652

[5] Katzelnick LC, Gresh L, Halloran ME, Mercado JC, Kuan G, Gordon A, et al. Antibody-dependent enhancement of severe dengue disease in humans. Science (New York, N.Y.). 2017;**358**(6365):929-932

[6] Rivino L. Understanding the human T cell response to dengue virus. Advances in Experimental Medicine and Biology. 2018;**1062**:241-250

[7] Mongkolsapaya J, Dejnirattisai W, Xu XN, Vasanawathana S, Tangthawornchaikul N, Chairunsri A, et al. Original antigenic sin and apoptosis in the pathogenesis of dengue hemorrhagic fever. Nature Medicine. 2003;**9**(7):921-927

[8] Rothman AL. Immunity to dengue virus: A tale of original antigenic sin and tropical cytokine storms. Nature Reviews. Immunology. 2011;**11**(8):532-543

[9] Green S, Rothman A. Immunopathological mechanisms in dengue and dengue hemorrhagic fever. Current Opinion in Infectious Diseases. 2006;**19**(5):429-436

[10] Kuczera D, Assolini JP, Tomiotto-Pellissier F, Pavanelli WR, Silveira GF. Highlights for dengue Immunopathogenesis: Antibody-dependent enhancement, cytokine storm, and beyond. Journal of Interferon & Cytokine Research. 2018;**38**(2):69-80

[11] Scaturro P, Cortese M, Chatel-Chaix L, Fischl W, Bartenschlager R. Dengue virus non-structural protein 1 modulates infectious particle production via interaction with the structural proteins. PLOS Pathogens. 2015;**11**(11):e1005277

[12] Muller DA, Young PR. The flavivirus NS1 protein: Molecular and structural biology, immunology, role in pathogenesis and application as a diagnostic biomarker. Antiviral Research. 2013;**98**(2):192-208

[13] Avirutnan P, Fuchs A, Hauhart RE, Somnuke P, Youn S, Diamond MS, et al. Antagonism of the complement component C4 by flavivirus nonstructural protein NS1. The Journal of Experimental Medicine. 2010;**207**(4):793-806

[14] Avirutnan P, Hauhart RE, Somnuke P, Blom AM, Diamond MS, Atkinson JP. Binding of flavivirus nonstructural protein NS1 to C4b binding protein modulates complement activation. Journal of Immunology. 2011;**187**(1):424-433

[15] Avirutnan P, Punyadee N, Noisakran S, Komoltri C, Thiemmeca S, Auethavornanan K, et al. Vascular leakage in severe dengue virus infections: A potential role for the nonstructural viral protein NS1 and complement. The Journal of Infectious Diseases. 2006;**193**(8):1078-1088

[16] Glasner DR, Puerta-Guardo H, Beatty PR, Harris E. The good, the bad,

and the shocking: The multiple roles of dengue virus nonstructural protein 1 in protection and pathogenesis. Annual Review of Virology. 2018;**5**(1):227-253

[17] Puerta-Guardo H, Tabata T, Petitt M, Dimitrova M, Glasner DR, Pereira L, et al. Zika virus nonstructural protein 1 disrupts glycosaminoglycans and causes permeability in developing human placentas. The Journal of Infectious Diseases. 2020;**221**(2):313-324

[18] Glasner DR, Ratnasiri K, Puerta-Guardo H, Espinosa DA, Beatty PR, Harris E. Dengue virus NS1 cytokine-independent vascular leak is dependent on endothelial glycocalyx components. PLOS Pathogens. 2017;**13**(11):e1006673

[19] Chen HR, Chao CH, Liu CC, Ho TS, Tsai HP, Perng GC, et al. Macrophage migration inhibitory factor is critical for dengue NS1-induced endothelial glycocalyx degradation and hyperpermeability. PLOS Pathogens. 2018;**14**(4):e1007033

[20] Chen HR, Chuang YC, Lin YS, Liu HS, Liu CC, Perng GC, et al. Dengue virus nonstructural protein 1 induces vascular leakage through macrophage migration inhibitory factor and autophagy. PLOS Neglected Tropical Diseases. 2016;**10**(7):e0004828

[21] Avirutnan P, Zhang L, Punyadee N, Manuyakorn A, Puttikhunt C, Kasinrerk W, et al. Secreted NS1 of dengue virus attaches to the surface of cells via interactions with heparan sulfate and chondroitin sulfate E. PLOS Pathogens. 2007;**3**(11):e183

[22] Chao CH, Wu WC, Lai YC, Tsai PJ, Perng GC, Lin YS, et al. Dengue virus nonstructural protein 1 activates platelets via Toll-like receptor 4, leading to thrombocytopenia and hemorrhage. PLOS Pathogens. 2019;**15**(4):e1007625

[23] Puerta-Guardo H, Glasner DR, Espinosa DA, Biering SB, Patana M, Ratnasiri K, et al. Flavivirus NS1 triggers tissue-specific vascular endothelial dysfunction reflecting disease tropism. Cell Reports. 2019;**26**(6):1598, 613.e8

[24] Wang C, Puerta-Guardo H, Biering SB, Glasner DR, Tran EB, Patana M, et al. Endocytosis of flavivirus NS1 is required for NS1-mediated endothelial hyperpermeability and is abolished by a single N-glycosylation site mutation. PLOS Pathogens. 2019;**15**(7):e1007938

[25] Xu X, Vaughan K, Weiskopf D, Grifoni A, Diamond MS, Sette A, et al. Identifying candidate targets of immune responses in Zika virus based on homology to epitopes in other Flavivirus species. PLOS Currents. 2016;**8**

[26] Li A, Yu J, Lu M, Ma Y, Attia Z, Shan C, et al. A Zika virus vaccine expressing premembrane-envelope-NS1 polyprotein. Nature Communications. 2018;**9**(1):3067

[27] Wan SW, Chen PW, Chen CY, Lai YC, Chu YT, Hung CY, et al. Therapeutic effects of monoclonal antibody against dengue virus NS1 in a STAT1 knockout mouse model of dengue infection. Journal of Immunology. 2017;**199**(8):2834-2844

[28] Henchal EA, Henchal LS, Schlesinger JJ. Synergistic interactions of anti-NS1 monoclonal antibodies protect passively immunized mice from lethal challenge with dengue 2 virus. The Journal of General Virology. 1988;**69**(Pt 8):2101-2107

[29] Edeling MA, Diamond MS, Fremont DH. Structural basis of flavivirus NS1 assembly and antibody recognition. Proceedings of the National Academy of Sciences of the United States of America. 2014;**111**(11):4285-4290

[30] Shriver-Lake LC, Liu JL, Zabetakis D, Sugiharto VA, Lee CR,

Defang GN, et al. Selection and characterization of anti-dengue NS1 single domain antibodies. Scientific Reports. 2018;**8**(1):18086

[31] Jayathilaka D, Gomes L, Jeewandara C, Jayarathna GSB, Herath D, Perera PA, et al. Role of NS1 antibodies in the pathogenesis of acute secondary dengue infection. Nature Communications. 2018;**9**(1):5242

[32] Amorim JH, Diniz MO, Cariri FA, Rodrigues JF, Bizerra RS, Goncalves AJ, et al. Protective immunity to DENV2 after immunization with a recombinant NS1 protein using a genetically detoxified heat-labile toxin as an adjuvant. Vaccine. 2012;**30**(5):837-845

[33] Wan SW, Lu YT, Huang CH, Lin CF, Anderson R, Liu HS, et al. Protection against dengue virus infection in mice by administration of antibodies against modified nonstructural protein 1. PLOS One. 2014;**9**(3):e92495

[34] Lin YL, Chen LK, Liao CL, Yeh CT, Ma SH, Chen JL, et al. DNA immunization with Japanese encephalitis virus nonstructural protein NS1 elicits protective immunity in mice. Journal of Virology. 1998;**72**(1):191-200

[35] Beatty PR, Puerta-Guardo H, Killingbeck SS, Glasner DR, Hopkins K, Harris E. Dengue virus NS1 triggers endothelial permeability and vascular leak that is prevented by NS1 vaccination. Science Translational Medicine. 2015;7(304):304ra141

[36] Falconar AK. The dengue virus nonstructural-1 protein (NS1) generates antibodies to common epitopes on human blood clotting, integrin/adhesin proteins and binds to human endothelial cells: Potential implications in haemorrhagic fever pathogenesis. Archives of Virology. 1997;**142**(5):897-916

[37] Chen MC, Lin CF, Lei HY, Lin SC, Liu HS, Yeh TM, et al. Deletion of the C-terminal region of dengue virus nonstructural protein 1 (NS1) abolishes anti-NS1-mediated platelet dysfunction and bleeding tendency. Journal of Immunology. 2009;**183**(3):1797-1803

[38] Espinosa DA, Beatty PR, Reiner GL, Sivick KE, Hix Glickman L, Dubensky TW Jr, et al. Cyclic dinucleotide-adjuvanted dengue virus nonstructural protein 1 induces protective antibody and T cell responses. Journal of Immunology. 2019;**202**(4):1153-1162

[39] Lin CF, Lei HY, Shiau AL, Liu CC, Liu HS, Yeh TM, et al. Antibodies from dengue patient sera cross-react with endothelial cells and induce damage. Journal of Medical Virology. 2003;**69**(1):82-90

[40] Bailey MJ, Broecker F, Duehr J, Arumemi F, Krammer F, Palese P, et al. Antibodies elicited by an NS1-based vaccine protect mice against Zika virus. mBio. 2019;**10**(2):e02861-18

[41] Lai YC, Chuang YC, Liu CC, Ho TS, Lin YS, Anderson R, et al. Antibodies against modified NS1 wing domain peptide protect against dengue virus infection. Scientific Reports. 2017;7(1):6975

[42] Reyes-Sandoval A, Ludert JE. The dual role of the antibody response against the flavivirus non-structural protein 1 (NS1) in protection and immuno-pathogenesis. Frontiers in Immunology. 2019;**10**:1651

[43] Kuhn RJ, Zhang W, Rossmann MG, Pletnev SV, Corver J, Lenches E, et al. Structure of dengue virus: Implications for flavivirus organization, maturation, and fusion. Cell. 2002;**108**(5):717-725

[44] Katzelnick LC, Fonville JM, Gromowski GD, Bustos Arriaga J, Green A, James SL, et al. Dengue viruses cluster antigenically but not as discrete serotypes. Science. 2015;**349**(6254):1338-1343

[45] Weaver SC, Vasilakis N. Molecular evolution of dengue viruses: Contributions of phylogenetics to understanding the history and epidemiology of the preeminent arboviral disease. Infection, Genetics and Evolution, Journal of Molecular Epidemiology and Evolutionary Genetics of Infectious Diseases. 2009;**9**(4):523-540

[46] Holmes EC, Twiddy SS. The origin, emergence and evolutionary genetics of dengue virus. Infection, Genetics and Evolution. 2003;**3**(1):19-28

[47] Khan AM, Heiny AT, Lee KX, Srinivasan KN, Tan TW, August JT, et al. Large-scale analysis of antigenic diversity of T-cell epitopes in dengue virus. BMC Bioinformatics. 2006;7(Suppl 5):S4

[48] Lwande OW, Obanda V, Lindström A, Ahlm C, Evander M, Näslund J, et al. Globe-trotting *Aedes aegypti* and *Aedes albopictus*: Risk factors for arbovirus pandemics. Vector Borne and Zoonotic Diseases. 2020;**20**(2):71-81

[49] Gubler DJ. Dengue, urbanization and globalization: The unholy trinity of the 21(st) century. Tropical Medicine and Health. 2011;**39**(4 Suppl):3-11

[50] Paupy C, Delatte H, Bagny L, Corbel V, Fontenille D. Aedes albopictus, an arbovirus vector: From the darkness to the light. Microbes and Infection. 2009;**11**(14-15):1177-1185

[51] Carrington LB, Simmons CP. Human to mosquito transmission of dengue viruses. Frontiers in Immunology. 2014;**5**:290

[52] Chan M, Johansson MA. The incubation periods of dengue viruses. PLOS One. 2012;7(11):e50972

[53] Kuno G, Chang GJ. Biological transmission of arboviruses: Reexamination of and new insights into components, mechanisms, and unique traits as well as their evolutionary trends. Clinical Microbiology Reviews. 2005;**18**(4):608-637

[54] Rathore APS, St John AL. Immune responses to dengue virus in the skin. Open Biology. 2018;**8**(8):180087

[55] Limon-Flores AY, Perez-Tapia M, Estrada-Garcia I, Vaughan G, Escobar-Gutierrez A, Calderon-Amador J, et al. Dengue virus inoculation to human skin explants: An effective approach to assess in situ the early infection and the effects on cutaneous dendritic cells. International Journal of Experimental Pathology. 2005;**86**(5):323-334

[56] Wu SJ, Grouard-Vogel G, Sun W, Mascola JR, Brachtel E, Putvatana R, et al. Human skin Langerhans cells are targets of dengue virus infection. Nature Medicine. 2000;**6**(7):816-820

[57] Schmid MA, Diamond MS, Harris E. Dendritic cells in dengue virus infection: Targets of virus replication and mediators of immunity. Frontiers in Immunology. 2014;**5**:647

[58] Wichit S, Ferraris P, Choumet V, Misse D. The effects of mosquito saliva on dengue virus infectivity in humans. Current Opinion in Virology. 2016;**21**:139-145

[59] Conway MJ, Watson AM, Colpitts TM, Dragovic SM, Li Z, Wang P, et al. Mosquito saliva serine protease enhances dissemination of dengue virus into the mammalian host. Journal of Virology. 2014;**88**(1):164

[60] Schmid MA, Glasner DR, Shah S, Michlmayr D, Kramer LD, Harris E. Mosquito saliva increases endothelial permeability in the skin, immune cell migration, and dengue pathogenesis during antibody-dependent enhancement. PLOS Pathogens. 2016;**12**(6):e1005676-e

[61] Cox J, Mota J, Sukupolvi-Petty S, Diamond MS, Rico-Hesse R. Mosquito bite delivery of dengue virus enhances immunogenicity and pathogenesis in humanized mice. Journal of Virology. 2012;**86**(14):7637-7649

[62] Pingen M, Schmid MA, Harris E, McKimmie CS. Mosquito biting modulates skin response to virus infection. Trends in Parasitology. 2017;**33**(8):645-657

[63] Reyes-del Valle J, Salas-Benito J, Soto-Acosta R, del Angel RM. Dengue virus cellular receptors and tropism. Current Tropical Medicine Reports. 2014;**1**(1):36-43

[64] Perera-Lecoin M, Meertens L, Carnec X, Amara A. Flavivirus entry receptors: An update. Viruses. 2013;**6**(1):69-88

[65] Cruz-Oliveira C, Freire JM, Conceicao TM, Higa LM, Castanho MA, Da Poian AT. Receptors and routes of dengue virus entry into the host cells. FEMS Microbiology Reviews. 2015;**39**(2):155-170

[66] Laureti M, Narayanan D, Rodriguez-Andres J, Fazakerley JK, Kedzierski L. Flavivirus receptors: Diversity, identity, and cell entry. Frontiers in Immunology. 2018;**9**:2180

[67] Begum F, Das S, Mukherjee D, Mal S, Ray U. Insight into the tropism of dengue virus in humans. Viruses. 2019;**11**(12):1136

[68] Clyde K, Kyle JL, Harris E. Recent advances in deciphering viral and host determinants of dengue virus replication and pathogenesis. Journal of Virology. 2006;**80**(23):11418-11431

[69] Stiasny K, Fritz R, Pangerl K, Heinz FX. Molecular mechanisms of flavivirus membrane fusion. Amino Acids. 2011;**41**(5):1159-1163

[70] Heinz FX, Stiasny K. Flaviviruses and their antigenic structure. Journal of Clinical Virology. 2012;**55**(4):289-295

[71] Welsch S, Miller S, Romero-Brey I, Merz A, Bleck CK, Walther P, et al. Composition and three-dimensional architecture of the dengue virus replication and assembly sites. Cell Host & Microbe. 2009;**5**(4):365-375

[72] Lescar J, Soh S, Lee LT, Vasudevan SG, Kang C, Lim SP. The dengue virus replication complex: From RNA replication to protein-protein interactions to evasion of innate immunity. Advances in Experimental Medicine and Biology. 2018;**1062**:115-129

[73] Villordo SM, Carballeda JM, Filomatori CV, Gamarnik AV. RNA structure duplications and flavivirus host adaptation. Trends in Microbiology. 2016;**24**(4):270-283

[74] Villordo SM, Filomatori CV, Sanchez-Vargas I, Blair CD, Gamarnik AV. Dengue virus RNA structure specialization facilitates host adaptation. PLOS Pathogens. 2015;**11**(1):e1004604

[75] El Sahili A, Lescar J. Dengue virus non-structural protein 5. Viruses. 2017;**9**(4):91

[76] Gebhard LG, Incicco JJ, Smal C, Gallo M, Gamarnik AV, Kaufman SB. Monomeric nature of dengue virus NS3 helicase and thermodynamic analysis of the interaction with single-stranded RNA. Nucleic Acids Research. 2014;**42**(18):11668-11686

[77] Liu L, Dong H, Chen H, Zhang J, Ling H, Li Z, et al. Flavivirus RNA cap methyltransferase: Structure, function, and inhibition. Frontiers in Biology (Beijing). 2010;**5**(4):286-303

[78] Xie X, Zou J, Zhang X, Zhou Y, Routh AL, Kang C, et al. Dengue NS2A

protein orchestrates virus assembly. Cell Host & Microbe. 2019;**26**(5):606-22.e8

[79] Plaszczyca A, Scaturro P, Neufeldt CJ, Cortese M, Cerikan B, Ferla S, et al. A novel interaction between dengue virus nonstructural protein 1 and the NS4A-2K-4B precursor is required for viral RNA replication but not for formation of the membranous replication organelle. PLOS Pathogens. 2019;**15**(5):e1007736

[80] Norazharuddin H, Lai NS. Roles and prospects of dengue virus non-structural proteins as antiviral targets: An easy digest. Malaysian Journal of Medical Sciences. 2018;**25**(5):6-15

[81] Xie Q, Zhang B, Yu J, Wu Q, Yang F, Cao H, et al. Structure and function of the non-structural protein of dengue virus and its applications in antiviral therapy. Current Topics in Medicinal Chemistry. 2017;**17**(3):371-380

[82] Wang Q-Y, Dong H, Zou B, Karuna R, Wan KF, Zou J, et al. Discovery of dengue virus NS4B inhibitors. Journal of Virology. 2015;**89**(16):8233

[83] Wu H, Bock S, Snitko M, Berger T, Weidner T, Holloway S, et al. Novel dengue virus NS2B/NS3 protease inhibitors. Antimicrobial Agents and Chemotherapy. 2015;**59**(2):1100

[84] Apte-Sengupta S, Sirohi D, Kuhn RJ. Coupling of replication and assembly in flaviviruses. Current Opinion in Virology. 2014;**9**:134-142

[85] Brady OJ, Gething PW, Bhatt S, Messina JP, Brownstein JS, Hoen AG, et al. Refining the global spatial limits of dengue virus transmission by evidence-based consensus. PLOS Neglected Tropical Diseases. 2012;**6**(8):e1760

[86] Messina JP, Brady OJ, Scott TW, Zou C, Pigott DM, Duda KA, et al. Global spread of dengue virus types: Mapping the 70 year history. Trends in Microbiology. 2014;**22**(3):138-146

[87] Rezza G. Aedes albopictus and the reemergence of dengue. BMC Public Health. 2012;**12**:72

[88] Gubler DJ. Dengue, urbanization and globalization: The unholy trinity of the 21(st) century. Tropical Medicine and Health. 2011;**39**(4 Suppl):3-11

[89] World Health Organization. Dengue Guidelines for Diagnosis, Treatment, Prevention and Control: New Edition. Geneva: World Health Organization; 2009

[90] World Health Organization. Dengue Haemorrhagic Fever: Diagnosis, Treatment, Prevention and Control. 2nd ed. Geneva: World Health Organization; 1997

[91] Hung NT. Fluid management for dengue in children. Paediatrics and International Child Health. 2012;**32**(s1):39-42

[92] Hladish TJ, Pearson CAB, Toh KB, Rojas DP, Manrique-Saide P, Vazquez-Prokopec GM, et al. Designing effective control of dengue with combined interventions. Proceedings of the National Academy of Sciences of the United States of America. 2020;**117**(6):3319-3325

[93] Trung DT, Wills B. Systemic vascular leakage associated with dengue infections—The clinical perspective. Current Topics in Microbiology and Immunology. 2010;**338**:57-66

[94] Yacoub S, Wertheim H, Simmons CP, Screaton G, Wills B. Cardiovascular manifestations of the emerging dengue pandemic. Nature Reviews. Cardiology. 2014;**11**(6):335-345

[95] Yacoub S, Lam PK, Vu le HM, Le TL, Ha NT, Toan TT, et al. Association of microvascular function

and endothelial biomarkers with clinical outcome in dengue: An observational study. The Journal of Infectious Diseases 2016;214(5):697-706

[96] Srikiatkhachorn A. Plasma leakage in dengue haemorrhagic fever. Thrombosis and Haemostasis. 2009;**102**(6):1042-1049

[97] Halstead SB. Controversies in dengue pathogenesis. Paediatrics and International Child Health. 2012;**32**(Suppl 1):5-9

[98] Simmons CP, Farrar JJ, Nguyen VV, Wills B. Dengue. The New England Journal of Medicine. 2012;**366**(15):1423-1432

[99] Vaughn DW, Green S, Kalayanarooj S, Innis BL, Nimmannitya S, Suntayakorn S, et al. Dengue viremia titer, antibody response pattern, and virus serotype correlate with disease severity. The Journal of Infectious Diseases. 2000;**181**(1):2-9

[100] OhAinle M, Balmaseda A, Macalalad AR, Tellez Y, Zody MC, Saborío S, et al. Dynamics of dengue disease severity determined by the interplay between viral genetics and serotype-specific immunity. Science Translational Medicine. 2011;**3**(114):114ra28-114ra28

[101] Malavige GN, Ogg GS. T cell responses in dengue viral infections. Journal of Clinical Virology. 2013;**58**(4):605-611

[102] Srikiatkhachorn A, Mathew A, Rothman AL. Immune-mediated cytokine storm and its role in severe dengue. Seminars in Immunopathology. 2017;**39**(5):563-574

[103] Libraty DH, Young PR, Pickering D, Endy TP, Kalayanarooj S, Green S, et al. High circulating levels of the dengue virus nonstructural protein NS1 early in dengue illness correlate with the development of dengue hemorrhagic fever. The Journal of Infectious Diseases. 2002;**186**(8):1165-1168

[104] Rothman AL. Dengue: Defining protective versus pathologic immunity. The Journal of Clinical Investigation. 2004;**113**(7):946-951

[105] Mangada MM, Rothman AL. Altered cytokine responses of dengue-specific CD4+ T cells to heterologous serotypes. Journal of Immunology. 2005;**175**(4):2676-2683

[106] Guzman MG, Alvarez M, Halstead SB. Secondary infection as a risk factor for dengue hemorrhagic fever/dengue shock syndrome: An historical perspective and role of antibody-dependent enhancement of infection. Archives of Virology. 2013;**158**(7):1445-1459

[107] Sangkawibha N, Rojanasuphot S, Ahandrik S, Viriyapongse S, Jatanasen S, Salitul V, et al. Risk factors in dengue shock syndrome: A prospective epidemiologic study in Rayong, Thailand. I. The 1980 outbreak. American Journal of Epidemiology. 1984;**120**(5):653-669

[108] Conde JN, Silva EM, Barbosa AS, Mohana-Borges R. The complement system in flavivirus infections. Frontiers in Microbiology. 2017;**8**:213

[109] Malasit P. Complement and dengue haemorrhagic fever/shock syndrome. The Southeast Asian Journal of Tropical Medicine and Public Health. 1987;**18**(3):316-320

[110] Rico-Hesse R. Dengue virus markers of virulence and pathogenicity. Future Virology. 2009;**4**(6):581

[111] Diamond MS, Edgil D, Roberts TG, Lu B, Harris E. Infection of human cells by dengue virus is modulated by

different cell types and viral strains. Journal of Virology. 2000;**74**(17):7814

[112] Begum F, Das S, Mukherjee D, Ray U. Hijacking the host immune cells by dengue virus: Molecular interplay of receptors and dengue virus envelope. Microorganisms. 2019;7(9):323

[113] Phoolcharoen W, Smith DR. Internalization of the dengue virus is cell cycle modulated in HepG2, but not vero cells. Journal of Medical Virology. 2004;**74**(3):434-441

[114] Soto-Acosta R, Mosso C, Cervantes-Salazar M, Puerta-Guardo H, Medina F, Favari L, et al. The increase in cholesterol levels at early stages after dengue virus infection correlates with an augment in LDL particle uptake and HMG-CoA reductase activity. Virology. 2013;**442**(2):132-147

[115] King CA, Anderson R, Marshall JS. Dengue virus selectively induces human mast cell chemokine production. Journal of Virology. 2002;**76**(16):8408-8419

[116] King AD, Nisalak A, Kalayanrooj S, Myint KS, Pattanapanyasat K, Nimmannitya S, et al. B cells are the principal circulating mononuclear cells infected by dengue virus. The Southeast Asian Journal of Tropical Medicine and Public Health. 1999;**30**(4):718-728

[117] Salgado DM, Eltit JM, Mansfield K, Panqueba C, Castro D, Vega MR, et al. Heart and skeletal muscle are targets of dengue virus infection. The Pediatric Infectious Disease Journal. 2010;**29**(3):238-242

[118] Jessie K, Fong MY, Devi S, Lam SK, Wong KT. Localization of dengue virus in naturally infected human tissues, by immunohistochemistry and in situ hybridization. The Journal of Infectious Diseases. 2004;**189**(8):1411-1418

[119] Win MM, Charngkaew K, Punyadee N, Aye KS, Win N, Chaisri U, et al. Ultrastructural features of human liver specimens from patients who died of dengue hemorrhagic fever. Tropical Medicine and Infectious Disease. 2019;**4**(2):63

[120] Aye KS, Charngkaew K, Win N, Wai KZ, Moe K, Punyadee N, et al. Pathologic highlights of dengue hemorrhagic fever in 13 autopsy cases from Myanmar. Human Pathology. 2014;**45**(6):1221-1233

[121] Kangwanpong D, Bhamarapravati N, Lucia HL. Diagnosing dengue virus infection in archived autopsy tissues by means of the in situ PCR method: A case report. Clinical and Diagnostic Virology. 1995;**3**(2):165-172

[122] Balsitis SJ, Coloma J, Castro G, Alava A, Flores D, McKerrow JH, et al. Tropism of dengue virus in mice and humans defined by viral nonstructural protein 3-specific immunostaining. The American Journal of Tropical Medicine and Hygiene. 2009;**80**(3):416-424

[123] Balsitis SJ, Williams KL, Lachica R, Flores D, Kyle JL, Mehlhop E, et al. Lethal antibody enhancement of dengue disease in mice is prevented by Fc modification. PLOS Pathogens. 2010;**6**(2):e1000790

[124] Shresta S, Kyle JL, Snider HM, Basavapatna M, Beatty PR, Harris E. Interferon-dependent immunity is essential for resistance to primary dengue virus infection in mice, whereas T- and B-cell-dependent immunity are less critical. Journal of Virology. 2004;**78**(6):2701-2710

[125] Zellweger RM, Prestwood TR, Shresta S. Enhanced infection of liver sinusoidal endothelial cells in a mouse model of antibody-induced severe dengue disease. Cell Host & Microbe. 2010;**7**(2):128-139

[126] Orozco S, Schmid MA, Parameswaran P, Lachica R, Henn MR,

Beatty R, et al. Characterization of a model of lethal dengue virus 2 infection in C57BL/6 mice deficient in the alpha/beta interferon receptor. The Journal of General Virology. 2012;**93**(Pt 10): 2152-2157

[127] Shresta S, Sharar KL, Prigozhin DM, Beatty PR, Harris E. Murine model for dengue virus-induced lethal disease with increased vascular permeability. Journal of Virology. 2006;**80**(20):10208-10217

[128] Zellweger RM, Shresta S. Mouse models to study dengue virus immunology and pathogenesis. Frontiers in Immunology. 2014;**5**:151

[129] Tassaneetrithep B, Burgess TH, Granelli-Piperno A, Trumpfheller C, Finke J, Sun W, et al. DC-SIGN (CD209) mediates dengue virus infection of human dendritic cells. The Journal of Experimental Medicine. 2003;**197**(7):823-829

[130] Navarro-Sanchez E, Altmeyer R, Amara A, Schwartz O, Fieschi F, Virelizier JL, et al. Dendritic-cell-specific ICAM3-grabbing non-integrin is essential for the productive infection of human dendritic cells by mosquito-cell-derived dengue viruses. EMBO Reports. 2003;**4**(7):723-728

[131] Chen ST, Lin YL, Huang MT, Wu MF, Cheng SC, Lei HY, et al. CLEC5A is critical for dengue-virus-induced lethal disease. Nature. 2008;**453**(7195):672-676

[132] Miller JL, de Wet BJ, Martinez-Pomares L, Radcliffe CM, Dwek RA, Rudd PM, et al. The mannose receptor mediates dengue virus infection of macrophages. PLOS Pathogens. 2008;**4**(2):e17

[133] Boonnak K, Dambach KM, Donofrio GC, Tassaneetrithep B, Marovich MA. Cell type specificity and host genetic polymorphisms influence antibody-dependent enhancement of dengue virus infection. Journal of Virology. 2011;**85**(4):1671-1683

[134] Wu MF, Chen ST, Yang AH, Lin WW, Lin YL, Chen NJ, et al. CLEC5A is critical for dengue virus-induced inflammasome activation in human macrophages. Blood. 2013;**121**(1):95-106

[135] Luplertlop N, Misse D, Bray D, Deleuze V, Gonzalez JP, Leardkamolkarn V, et al. Dengue-virus-infected dendritic cells trigger vascular leakage through metalloproteinase overproduction. EMBO Reports. 2006;**7**(11):1176-1181

[136] Avirutnan P, Matangkasombut P. Unmasking the role of mast cells in dengue. eLife. 2013;**2**:e00767

[137] Sherif NA, Zayan AH, Elkady AH, Ghozy S, Ahmed AR, Omran ES, et al. Mast cell mediators in relation to dengue severity: A systematic review and meta-analysis. Reviews in Medical Virology. 2020;**30**(1):e2084

[138] Rathore APS, St John AL. Immune responses to dengue virus in the skin. Open Biology. 2018;**8**(8):180087

[139] Brown MG, Hermann LL, Issekutz AC, Marshall JS, Rowter D, Al-Afif A, et al. Dengue virus infection of mast cells triggers endothelial cell activation. Journal of Virology. 2011;**85**(2):1145

[140] St John AL, Rathore AP, Raghavan B, Ng ML, Abraham SN. Contributions of mast cells and vasoactive products, leukotrienes and chymase, to dengue virus-induced vascular leakage. eLife. 2013;**2**:e00481

[141] Zimmer CL, Cornillet M, Sola-Riera C, Cheung KW, Ivarsson MA, Lim MQ, et al. NK cells are activated and primed for skin-homing during acute dengue virus infection in

humans. Nature Communications. 2019;**10**(1):3897

[142] Durbin AP, Vargas MJ, Wanionek K, Hammond SN, Gordon A, Rocha C, et al. Phenotyping of peripheral blood mononuclear cells during acute dengue illness demonstrates infection and increased activation of monocytes in severe cases compared to classic dengue fever. Virology. 2008;**376**(2):429-435

[143] Castillo JA, Naranjo JS, Rojas M, Castano D, Velilla PA. Role of monocytes in the pathogenesis of dengue. Archivum Immunologiae et Therapiae Experimentalis (Warsz). 2019;**67**(1):27-40

[144] Schmid MA, Harris E. Monocyte recruitment to the dermis and differentiation to dendritic cells increases the targets for dengue virus replication. PLOS Pathogens. 2014;**10**(12):e1004541

[145] Kyle JL, Beatty PR, Harris E. Dengue virus infects macrophages and dendritic cells in a mouse model of infection. The Journal of Infectious Diseases. 2007;**195**(12):1808-1817

[146] Marianneau P, Steffan AM, Royer C, Drouet MT, Jaeck D, Kirn A, et al. Infection of primary cultures of human Kupffer cells by dengue virus: No viral progeny synthesis, but cytokine production is evident. Journal of Virology. 1999;**73**(6):5201-5206

[147] Povoa TF, Alves AM, Oliveira CA, Nuovo GJ, Chagas VL, Paes MV. The pathology of severe dengue in multiple organs of human fatal cases: Histopathology, ultrastructure and virus replication. PLOS One. 2014;**9**(4):e83386

[148] Moi ML, Lim CK, Takasaki T, Kurane I. Involvement of the Fc gamma receptor IIA cytoplasmic domain in antibody-dependent enhancement of dengue virus infection. The Journal of General Virology. 2010;**91**(Pt 1):103-111

[149] Littaua R, Kurane I, Ennis FA. Human IgG Fc receptor II mediates antibody-dependent enhancement of dengue virus infection. Journal of Immunology. 1990;**144**(8):3183-3186

[150] Kontny U, Kurane I, Ennis FA. Gamma interferon augments Fc gamma receptor-mediated dengue virus infection of human monocytic cells. Journal of Virology. 1988;**62**(11):3928-3933

[151] Rodrigo WW, Jin X, Blackley SD, Rose RC, Schlesinger JJ. Differential enhancement of dengue virus immune complex infectivity mediated by signaling-competent and signaling-incompetent human Fcgamma RIA (CD64) or FcgammaRIIA (CD32). Journal of Virology. 2006;**80**(20):10128-10138

[152] Homchampa P, Sarasombath S, Suvatte V, Vongskul M. Natural killer cells in dengue hemorrhagic fever/ dengue shock syndrome. Asian Pacific Journal of Allergy and Immunology. 1988;**6**(2):95-102

[153] Azeredo EL, De Oliveira-Pinto LM, Zagne SM, Cerqueira DI, Nogueira RM, Kubelka CF. NK cells, displaying early activation, cytotoxicity and adhesion molecules, are associated with mild dengue disease. Clinical and Experimental Immunology. 2006;**143**(2):345-356

[154] Kou Z, Quinn M, Chen H, Rodrigo WW, Rose RC, Schlesinger JJ, et al. Monocytes, but not T or B cells, are the principal target cells for dengue virus (DV) infection among human peripheral blood mononuclear cells. Journal of Medical Virology. 2008;**80**(1):134-146

[155] Lin YW, Wang KJ, Lei HY, Lin YS, Yeh TM, Liu HS, et al. Virus

replication and cytokine production in dengue virus-infected human B lymphocytes. Journal of Virology. 2002;**76**(23):12242-12249

[156] Silveira GF, Wowk PF, Cataneo AHD, Dos Santos PF, Delgobo M, Stimamiglio MA, et al. Human T lymphocytes are permissive for dengue virus replication. Journal of Virology. 2018;**92**(10):e02181-17

[157] Kurane I, Kontny U, Janus J, Ennis FA. Dengue-2 virus infection of human mononuclear cell lines and establishment of persistent infections. Archives of Virology. 1990;**110**(1-2):91-101

[158] Boonpucknavig S, Bhamarapravati N, Nimmannitya S, Phalavadhtana A, Siripont J. Immunofluorescent staining of the surfaces of lymphocytes in suspension from patients with dengue hemorrhagic fever. The American Journal of Pathology. 1976;**85**(1):37-48

[159] Mentor NA, Kurane I. Dengue virus infection of human T lymphocytes. Acta Virologica. 1997;**41**(3):175-176

[160] Mota J, Rico-Hesse R. Dengue virus tropism in humanized mice recapitulates human dengue fever. PLOS One. 2011;**6**(6):e20762-e

[161] Takeuchi O, Akira S. Pattern recognition receptors and inflammation. Cell. 2010;**140**(6):805-820

[162] Kawamura T, Ogawa Y, Aoki R, Shimada S. Innate and intrinsic antiviral immunity in skin. Journal of Dermatological Science. 2014;**75**(3):159-166

[163] Thompson MR, Kaminski JJ, Kurt-Jones EA, Fitzgerald KA. Pattern recognition receptors and the innate immune response to viral infection. Viruses. 2011;**3**(6):920-940

[164] Morrison J, Aguirre S, Fernandez-Sesma A. Innate immunity evasion by dengue virus. Viruses. 2012;**4**(3):397-413

[165] Uno N, Ross TM. Dengue virus and the host innate immune response. Emerging Microbes & Infections. 2018;**7**(1):167

[166] Nasirudeen AM, Wong HH, Thien P, Xu S, Lam KP, Liu DX. RIG-I, MDA5 and TLR3 synergistically play an important role in restriction of dengue virus infection. PLOS Neglected Tropical Diseases. 2011;**5**(1):e926

[167] Green AM, Beatty PR, Hadjilaou A, Harris E. Innate immunity to dengue virus infection and subversion of antiviral responses. Journal of Molecular Biology. 2014;**426**(6):1148-1160

[168] Tsai YT, Chang SY, Lee CN, Kao CL. Human TLR3 recognizes dengue virus and modulates viral replication in vitro. Cellular Microbiology. 2009;**11**(4):604-615

[169] Sariol CA, Martínez MI, Rivera F, Rodríguez IV, Pantoja P, Abel K, et al. Decreased dengue replication and an increased anti-viral Humoral response with the use of combined toll-like receptor 3 and 7/8 agonists in macaques. PLOS One. 2011;**6**(4):e19323

[170] Sun B, Sundström KB, Chew JJ, Bist P, Gan ES, Tan HC, et al. Dengue virus activates cGAS through the release of mitochondrial DNA. Scientific Reports. 2017;**7**(1):3594

[171] Aguirre S, Fernandez-Sesma A. Collateral damage during dengue virus infection: Making sense of DNA by cGAS. Journal of Virology. 2017;**91**(14):e01081-e01016

[172] Cai X, Chiu YH, Chen ZJ. The cGAS-cGAMP-STING pathway of cytosolic DNA sensing and signaling. Molecular Cell. 2014;**54**(2):289-296

[173] Gebert LFR, MacRae IJ. Regulation of microRNA function in animals. Nature Reviews. Molecular Cell Biology. 2019;**20**(1):21-37

[174] Stoermer KA, Morrison TE. Complement and viral pathogenesis. Virology. 2011;**411**(2):362-373

[175] O'Brien J, Hayder H, Zayed Y, Peng C. Overview of microRNA biogenesis, mechanisms of actions, and circulation. Frontiers in Endocrinology (Lausanne). 2018;**9**:402

[176] Ding SW, Voinnet O. Antiviral immunity directed by small RNAs. Cell. 2007;**130**(3):413-426

[177] Wong RR, Abd-Aziz N, Affendi S, Poh CL. Role of microRNAs in antiviral responses to dengue infection. Journal of Biomedical Science. 2020;**27**(1):4

[178] Ang F, Wong AP, Ng MM, Chu JJ. Small interference RNA profiling reveals the essential role of human membrane trafficking genes in mediating the infectious entry of dengue virus. Virology Journal. 2010;7:24

[179] Kakumani PK, Ponia SS, Rajgokul SK, Sood V, Chinnappan M, Banerjea AC, et al. Role of RNA interference (RNAi) in dengue virus replication and identification of NS4B as an RNAi suppressor. Journal of Virology. 2013;**87**(16):8870-8883

[180] Mazeaud C, Freppel W, Chatel-Chaix L. The multiples fates of the Flavivirus RNA genome during pathogenesis. Frontiers in Genetics. 2018;**9**:595

[181] Pijlman GP, Funk A, Kondratieva N, Leung J, Torres S, van der Aa L, et al. A highly structured, nuclease-resistant, noncoding RNA produced by flaviviruses is required for pathogenicity. Cell Host & Microbe. 2008;**4**(6):579-591

[182] Schnettler E, Sterken MG, Leung JY, Metz SW, Geertsema C, Goldbach RW, et al. Noncoding flavivirus RNA displays RNA interference suppressor activity in insect and mammalian cells. Journal of Virology. 2012;**86**(24):13486-13500

[183] Moon SL, Anderson JR, Kumagai Y, Wilusz CJ, Akira S, Khromykh AA, et al. A noncoding RNA produced by arthropod-borne flaviviruses inhibits the cellular exoribonuclease XRN1 and alters host mRNA stability. RNA. 2012;**18**(11):2029-2040

[184] Urcuqui-Inchima S, Cabrera J, Haenni AL. Interplay between dengue virus and toll-like receptors, RIG-I/MDA5 and microRNAs: Implications for pathogenesis. Antiviral Research. 2017;**147**:47-57

[185] Jiang L, Sun Q. The expression profile of human peripheral blood mononuclear cell miRNA is altered by antibody-dependent enhancement of infection with dengue virus serotype 3. Virology Journal. 2018;**15**(1):50

[186] Zhu X, He Z, Hu Y, Wen W, Lin C, Yu J, et al. MicroRNA-30e* suppresses dengue virus replication by promoting NF-κB–dependent IFN production. PLOS Neglected Tropical Diseases. 2014;**8**(8):e3088

[187] Castillo JA, Castrillón JC, Diosa-Toro M, Betancur JG, St Laurent G 3rd, Smit JM, et al. Complex interaction between dengue virus replication and expression of miRNA-133a. BMC Infectious Diseases. 2016;**16**:29

[188] Diosa-Toro M, Echavarria-Consuegra L, Flipse J, Fernandez GJ, Kluiver J, van den Berg A, et al. MicroRNA profiling of human primary macrophages exposed to dengue virus identifies miRNA-3614-5p as antiviral and regulator of ADAR1 expression. PLOS Neglected Tropical Diseases. 2017;**11**(10):e0005981

[189] Ouyang X, Jiang X, Gu D, Zhang Y, Kong SK, Jiang C, et al. Dysregulated serum MiRNA profile and promising biomarkers in dengue-infected patients. International Journal of Medical Sciences. 2016;**13**(3):195-205

[190] Shahen M, Guo Z, Shar AH, Ebaid R, Tao Q, Zhang W, et al. Dengue virus causes changes of microRNA-genes regulatory network revealing potential targets for antiviral drugs. BMC Systems Biology. 2018;**12**(1):2

[191] Feng X, Zhou S, Wang J, Hu W. microRNA profiles and functions in mosquitoes. PLOS Neglected Tropical Diseases. 2018;**12**(5):e0006463-e

[192] Su J, Wang G, Li C, Xing D, Yan T, Zhu X, et al. Screening for differentially expressed miRNAs in Aedes albopictus (Diptera: Culicidae) exposed to DENV-2 and their effect on replication of DENV-2 in C6/36 cells. Parasites & Vectors. 2019;**12**(1):44

[193] Su J, Li C, Zhang Y, Yan T, Zhu X, Zhao M, et al. Identification of microRNAs expressed in the midgut of *Aedes albopictus* during dengue infection. Parasites & Vectors. 2017;**10**(1):63

[194] Lee W-S, Webster JA, Madzokere ET, Stephenson EB, Herrero LJ. Mosquito antiviral defense mechanisms: A delicate balance between innate immunity and persistent viral infection. Parasites & Vectors. 2019;**12**(1):165

[195] Blair CD. Mosquito RNAi is the major innate immune pathway controlling arbovirus infection and transmission. Future Microbiology. 2011;**6**(3):265-277

[196] Shahid I. RNA association, RNA interference, and microRNA pathways in dengue fever virus-host interaction. Current Topics in Tropical Emerging Diseases and Travel Medicine. 2018;**6**:93-114

[197] Shresta S. Role of complement in dengue virus infection: Protection or pathogenesis? mBio. 2012;**3**(1):e00003-12

[198] Cabezas S, Bracho G, Aloia AL, Adamson PJ, Bonder CS, Smith JR, et al. Dengue virus induces increased activity of the complement alternative pathway in infected cells. Journal of Virology. 2018;**92**(14):e00633-e00618

[199] Carr JM, Cabezas-Falcon S, Dubowsky JG, Hulme-Jones J, Gordon DL. Dengue virus and the complement alternative pathway. FEBS Letters. 2020;**594**:2543-2555

[200] Bokisch VA, Top FH Jr, Russell PK, Dixon FJ, Muller-Eberhard HJ. The potential pathogenic role of complement in dengue hemorrhagic shock syndrome. The New England Journal of Medicine. 1973;**289**(19):996-1000

[201] Koyama S, Ishii KJ, Coban C, Akira S. Innate immune response to viral infection. Cytokine. 2008;**43**(3):336-341

[202] Takeuchi O, Akira S. Innate immunity to virus infection. Immunological Reviews. 2009;**227**(1):75-86

[203] Munoz-Jordan JL, Sanchez-Burgos GG, Laurent-Rolle M, Garcia-Sastre A. Inhibition of interferon signaling by dengue virus. Proceedings of the National Academy of Sciences of the United States of America. 2003;**100**(24):14333-14338

[204] Diamond MS, Roberts TG, Edgil D, Lu B, Ernst J, Harris E. Modulation of dengue virus infection in human cells by alpha, beta, and gamma interferons. Journal of Virology. 2000;**74**(11):4957-4966

[205] Perry AK, Chen G, Zheng D, Tang H, Cheng G. The host type I interferon response to viral and

bacterial infections. Cell Research. 2005;**15**(6):407-422

[206] Baum A, García-Sastre A. Induction of type I interferon by RNA viruses: Cellular receptors and their substrates. Amino Acids. 2010;**38**(5):1283-1299

[207] Schoggins JW, Rice CM. Interferon-stimulated genes and their antiviral effector functions. Current Opinion in Virology. 2011;**1**(6):519-525

[208] Huang X, Yue Y, Li D, Zhao Y, Qiu L, Chen J, et al. Antibody-dependent enhancement of dengue virus infection inhibits RLR-mediated type-I IFN-independent signalling through upregulation of cellular autophagy. Scientific Reports. 2016;**6**:22303

[209] Schoggins JW, Wilson SJ, Panis M, Murphy MY, Jones CT, Bieniasz P, et al. A diverse range of gene products are effectors of the type I interferon antiviral response. Nature. 2011;**472**(7344):481-485

[210] Liu SY, Sanchez DJ, Aliyari R, Lu S, Cheng G. Systematic identification of type I and type II interferon-induced antiviral factors. Proceedings of the National Academy of Sciences of the United States of America. 2012;**109**(11):4239-4244

[211] Pulit-Penaloza JA, Scherbik SV, Brinton MA. Type 1 IFN-independent activation of a subset of interferon stimulated genes in West Nile virus Eg101-infected mouse cells. Virology. 2012;**425**(2):82-94

[212] Sariol CA, Muñoz-Jordán JL, Abel K, Rosado LC, Pantoja P, Giavedoni L, et al. Transcriptional activation of interferon-stimulated genes but not of cytokine genes after primary infection of rhesus macaques with dengue virus type 1. Clinical and Vaccine Immunology. 2007;**14**(6):756

[213] Wu X, Dao Thi VL, Huang Y, Billerbeck E, Saha D, Hoffmann H-H, et al. Intrinsic immunity shapes viral resistance of stem cells. Cell. 2018;**172**(3):423-438.e25

[214] Dai J, Pan W, Wang P. ISG15 facilitates cellular antiviral response to dengue and west nile virus infection in vitro. Virology Journal. 2011;**8**(1):468

[215] Jiang D, Weidner JM, Qing M, Pan X-B, Guo H, Xu C, et al. Identification of five interferon-induced cellular proteins that inhibit West Nile virus and dengue virus infections. Journal of Virology. 2010;**84**(16):8332

[216] Wang K, Zou C, Wang X, Huang C, Feng T, Pan W, et al. Interferon-stimulated TRIM69 interrupts dengue virus replication by ubiquitinating viral nonstructural protein 3. PLOS Pathogens. 2018;**14**(8):e1007287-e

[217] Hertzog PJ, O'Neill LA, Hamilton JA. The interferon in TLR signaling: More than just antiviral. Trends in Immunology. 2003;**24**(10):534-539

[218] Chen H-W, King K, Tu J, Sanchez M, Luster AD, Shresta S. The roles of IRF-3 and IRF-7 in innate antiviral immunity against dengue virus. Journal of Immunology (Baltimore, Md. : 1950). 2013;**191**(8):4194-4201

[219] Carlin AF, Plummer EM, Vizcarra EA, Sheets N, Joo Y, Tang W, et al. An IRF-3-, IRF-5-, and IRF-7-independent pathway of dengue viral resistance utilizes IRF-1 to stimulate type I and II interferon responses. Cell Reports. 2017;**21**(6):1600-1612

[220] Dalrymple NA, Cimica V, Mackow ER. Dengue virus NS proteins inhibit RIG-I/MAVS Signaling by blocking TBK1/IRF3 phosphorylation: Dengue virus serotype 1 NS4A is a unique interferon-regulating

virulence determinant. MBio. 2015;**6**(3):e00553-15

[221] Modhiran N, Kalayanarooj S, Ubol S. Subversion of innate defenses by the interplay between DENV and pre-existing enhancing antibodies: TLRs signaling collapse. PLOS Neglected Tropical Diseases. 2010;**4**(12):e924

[222] Munoz-Jordan JL. Subversion of interferon by dengue virus. Current Topics in Microbiology and Immunology. 2010;**338**:35-44

[223] Kurane I, Innis BL, Nimmannitya S, Nisalak A, Meager A, Ennis FA. High levels of interferon alpha in the sera of children with dengue virus infection. The American Journal of Tropical Medicine and Hygiene. 1993;**48**(2):222-229

[224] Chakravarti A, Kumaria R. Circulating levels of tumour necrosis factor-alpha & interferon-gamma in patients with dengue & dengue haemorrhagic fever during an outbreak. The Indian Journal of Medical Research. 2006;**123**(1):25-30

[225] Nguyen TH, Lei HY, Nguyen TL, Lin YS, Huang KJ, Le BL, et al. Dengue hemorrhagic fever in infants: A study of clinical and cytokine profiles. The Journal of Infectious Diseases. 2004;**189**(2):221-232

[226] De La Cruz Hernandez SI, Puerta-Guardo H, Flores-Aguilar H, Gonzalez-Mateos S, Lopez-Martinez I, Ortiz-Navarrete V, et al. A strong interferon response correlates with a milder dengue clinical condition. Journal of Clinical Virology. 2014;**60**(3):196-199

[227] Fink J, Gu F, Ling L, Tolfvenstam T, Olfat F, Chin KC, et al. Host gene expression profiling of dengue virus infection in cell lines and patients. PLOS Neglected Tropical Diseases. 2007;**1**(2):e86

[228] Simmons CP, Popper S, Dolocek C, Chau TN, Griffiths M, Dung NT, et al. Patterns of host genome-wide gene transcript abundance in the peripheral blood of patients with acute dengue hemorrhagic fever. The Journal of Infectious Diseases. 2007;**195**(8):1097-1107

[229] Nascimento EJ, Braga-Neto U, Calzavara-Silva CE, Gomes AL, Abath FG, Brito CA, et al. Gene expression profiling during early acute febrile stage of dengue infection can predict the disease outcome. PLOS One. 2009;**4**(11):e7892

[230] Ashour J, Laurent-Rolle M, Shi PY, Garcia-Sastre A. NS5 of dengue virus mediates STAT2 binding and degradation. Journal of Virology. 2009;**83**(11):5408-5418

[231] Rodriguez-Madoz JR, Belicha-Villanueva A, Bernal-Rubio D, Ashour J, Ayllon J, Fernandez-Sesma A. Inhibition of the type I interferon response in human dendritic cells by dengue virus infection requires a catalytically active NS2B3 complex. Journal of Virology. 2010;**84**(19):9760-9774

[232] Muñoz-Jordán JL, Laurent-Rolle M, Ashour J, Martínez-Sobrido L, Ashok M, Lipkin WI, et al. Inhibition of alpha/beta interferon signaling by the NS4B protein of flaviviruses. Journal of Virology. 2005;**79**(13):8004

[233] Mazzon M, Jones M, Davidson A, Chain B, Jacobs M. Dengue virus NS5 inhibits interferon-alpha signaling by blocking signal transducer and activator of transcription 2 phosphorylation. The Journal of Infectious Diseases. 2009;**200**(8):1261-1270

[234] Shresta S, Sharar KL, Prigozhin DM, Snider HM, Beatty PR, Harris E. Critical roles for both STAT1-dependent and STAT1-independent pathways in the control of primary dengue virus infection in mice. Journal of Immunology. 2005;**175**(6):3946-3954

[235] Aguirre S, Luthra P, Sanchez-Aparicio MT, Maestre AM, Patel J, Lamothe F, et al. Dengue virus NS2B protein targets cGAS for degradation and prevents mitochondrial DNA sensing during infection. Nature Microbiology. 2017;**2**:17037

[236] Aguirre S, Maestre AM, Pagni S, Patel JR, Savage T, Gutman D, et al. DENV inhibits type I IFN production in infected cells by cleaving human STING. PLOS Pathogens. 2012;**8**(10):e1002934

[237] Stabell AC, Meyerson NR, Gullberg RC, Gilchrist AR, Webb KJ, Old WM, et al. Dengue viruses cleave STING in humans but not in nonhuman primates, their presumed natural reservoir. eLife. 2018;**7**:e31919

[238] Diosa-Toro M, Prasanth KR, Bradrick SS, Garcia Blanco MA. Role of RNA-binding proteins during the late stages of flavivirus replication cycle. Virology Journal. 2020;**17**(1):60

[239] Alvarez DE, De Lella Ezcurra AL, Fucito S, Gamarnik AV. Role of RNA structures present at the 3'UTR of dengue virus on translation, RNA synthesis, and viral replication. Virology. 2005;**339**(2):200-212

[240] Manokaran G, Finol E, Wang C, Gunaratne J, Bahl J, Ong EZ, et al. Dengue subgenomic RNA binds TRIM25 to inhibit interferon expression for epidemiological fitness. Science. 2015;**350**(6257):217-221

[241] Pompon J, Manuel M, Ng GK, Wong B, Shan C, Manokaran G, et al. Dengue subgenomic flaviviral RNA disrupts immunity in mosquito salivary glands to increase virus transmission. PLOS Pathogens. 2017;**13**(7):e1006535

[242] Pena J, Harris E. Early dengue virus protein synthesis induces extensive rearrangement of the endoplasmic reticulum independent of the UPR and SREBP-2 pathway. PLOS One. 2012;**7**(6):e38202

[243] Umareddy I, Pluquet O, Wang QY, Vasudevan SG, Chevet E, Gu F. Dengue virus serotype infection specifies the activation of the unfolded protein response. Virology Journal. 2007;**4**:91

[244] Perera N, Miller JL, Zitzmann N. The role of the unfolded protein response in dengue virus pathogenesis. Cellular Microbiology. 2017;**19**(5):e12734

[245] Lee YR, Kuo SH, Lin CY, Fu PJ, Lin YS, Yeh TM, et al. Dengue virus-induced ER stress is required for autophagy activation, viral replication, and pathogenesis both in vitro and in vivo. Scientific Reports. 2018;**8**(1):489

[246] Ke PY. The multifaceted roles of autophagy in Flavivirus-host interactions. International Journal of Molecular Sciences. 2018;**19**(12):3940

[247] Heaton NS, Randall G. Dengue virus-induced autophagy regulates lipid metabolism. Cell Host & Microbe. 2010;**8**(5):422-432

[248] Mizushima N. Autophagy: Process and function. Genes & Development. 2007;**21**(22):2861-2873

[249] Dong X, Levine B. Autophagy and viruses: Adversaries or allies? Journal of Innate Immunity. 2013;**5**(5):480-493

[250] Kuballa P, Nolte WM, Castoreno AB, Xavier RJ. Autophagy and the immune system. Annual Review of Immunology. 2012;**30**:611-646

[251] Mateo R, Nagamine CM, Spagnolo J, Méndez E, Rahe M, Gale M, et al. Inhibition of cellular autophagy deranges dengue virion maturation. Journal of Virology. 2013;**87**(3):1312

[252] Heaton NS, Randall G. Dengue virus and autophagy. Viruses. 2011;**3**(8):1332-1341

[253] Panyasrivanit M, Khakpoor A, Wikan N, Smith DR. Linking dengue virus entry and translation/replication through amphisomes. Autophagy. 2009;**5**(3):434-435

[254] Metz P, Chiramel A, Chatel-Chaix L, Alvisi G, Bankhead P, Mora-Rodríguez R, et al. Dengue virus inhibition of autophagic flux and dependency of viral replication on proteasomal degradation of the autophagy receptor p62. Journal of Virology. 2015;**89**(15):8026

[255] Acharya B, Gyeltshen S, Chaijaroenkul W, Na-Bangchang K. Significance of autophagy in dengue virus infection: A brief review. The American Journal of Tropical Medicine and Hygiene. 2019;**100**(4):783-790

[256] Heaton NS, Perera R, Berger KL, Khadka S, Lacount DJ, Kuhn RJ, et al. Dengue virus nonstructural protein 3 redistributes fatty acid synthase to sites of viral replication and increases cellular fatty acid synthesis. Proceedings of the National Academy of Sciences of the United States of America. 2010;**107**(40):17345-17350

[257] Samsa MM, Mondotte JA, Iglesias NG, Assuncao-Miranda I, Barbosa-Lima G, Da Poian AT, et al. Dengue virus capsid protein usurps lipid droplets for viral particle formation. PLOS Pathogens. 2009;**5**(10):e1000632

[258] Melo CFOR, Delafiori J, Dabaja MZ, de Oliveira DN, Guerreiro TM, Colombo TE, et al. The role of lipids in the inception, maintenance and complications of dengue virus infection. Scientific Reports. 2018;**8**(1):11826

[259] Perera R, Riley C, Isaac G, Hopf-Jannasch AS, Moore RJ, Weitz KW, et al. Dengue virus infection perturbs lipid homeostasis in infected mosquito cells. PLOS Pathogens. 2012;**8**(3):e1002584-e

[260] Leier HC, Messer WB, Tafesse FG. Lipids and pathogenic flaviviruses: An intimate union. PLOS Pathogens. 2018;**14**(5):e1006952

[261] Randall G. Lipid droplet metabolism during dengue virus infection. Trends in Microbiology. 2018;**26**(8):640-642

[262] Osuna-Ramos JF, Reyes-Ruiz JM, Del Angel RM. The role of host cholesterol during Flavivirus infection. Frontiers in Cellular and Infection Microbiology. 2018;**8**:388

[263] Soto-Acosta R, Bautista-Carbajal P, Cervantes-Salazar M, Angel-Ambrocio AH, del Angel RM. DENV up-regulates the HMG-CoA reductase activity through the impairment of AMPK phosphorylation: A potential antiviral target. PLOS Pathogens. 2017;**13**(4):e1006257

[264] Duran A, Carrero R, Parra B, Gonzalez A, Delgado L, Mosquera J, et al. Association of lipid profile alterations with severe forms of dengue in humans. Archives of Virology. 2015;**160**(7):1687-1692

[265] Lima WG, Souza NA, Fernandes SOA, Cardoso VN, Godoi IP. Serum lipid profile as a predictor of dengue severity: A systematic review and meta-analysis. Reviews in Medical Virology. 2019;**29**(5):e2056

[266] van Gorp EC, Suharti C, Mairuhu AT, Dolmans WM, van Der Ven J, Demacker PN, et al. Changes in the plasma lipid profile as a potential predictor of clinical outcome in dengue hemorrhagic fever. Clinical Infectious Diseases. 2002;**34**(8):1150-1153

[267] Biswas HH, Gordon A, Nuñez A, Perez MA, Balmaseda A, Harris E. Lower low-density lipoprotein cholesterol levels are associated with severe dengue outcome. PLOS Neglected Tropical Diseases. 2015;**9**(9):e0003904-e

[268] Conde JN, da Silva EM, Allonso D, Coelho DR, Andrade IDS, de Medeiros LN, et al. Inhibition of the membrane attack complex by dengue virus NS1 through interaction with vitronectin and terminal complement proteins. Journal of Virology. 2016;**90**(21):9570-9581

[269] Avirutnan P, Hauhart RE, Somnuke P, Blom AM, Diamond MS, Atkinson JP. Binding of Flavivirus nonstructural protein NS1 to C4b binding protein modulates complement activation. The Journal of Immunology. 2011;**187**(1):424

[270] Chung KM, Liszewski MK, Nybakken G, Davis AE, Townsend RR, Fremont DH, et al. West Nile virus nonstructural protein NS1 inhibits complement activation by binding the regulatory protein factor H. Proceedings of the National Academy of Sciences of the United States of America. 2006;**103**(50):19111-19116

[271] Schlesinger JJ. Flavivirus nonstructural protein NS1: Complementary surprises. Proceedings of the National Academy of Sciences. 2006;**103**(50):18879

[272] Thiemmeca S, Tamdet C, Punyadee N, Prommool T, Songjaeng A, Noisakran S, et al. Secreted NS1 protects dengue virus from mannose-binding Lectin–mediated neutralization. The Journal of Immunology. 2016;**197**(10):4053

Chapter 5

Dengue Immunopathogenesis: A Crosstalk between Host and Viral Factors Leading to Disease: PART II - DENV Infection, Adaptive Immune Responses, and NS1 Pathogenesis

Henry Puerta-Guardo, Scott B. Biering, Eva Harris, Norma Pavia-Ruz, Gonzalo Vázquez-Prokopec, Guadalupe Ayora-Talavera and Pablo Manrique-Saide

Abstract

Severe disease is associated with serial infection with DENV of different serotypes. Thus, primary DENV infections normally cause asymptomatic infections, and secondary heterotypic infections with a new DENV serotype potentially increase the risks of developing severe disease. Despite many proposed hypotheses trying to explain it, the exact immunological mechanism leading to severe dengue disease is unknown. In turn, severe manifestations are believed to be a consequence of the combinations of many immunopathogenic mechanisms involving viral and host factors leading to increased pathogenesis and disease. Of these mechanisms, the adaptive immune response has been proposed to play a critical role in the development of severe dengue manifestations. This includes the effect of non-neutralizing but enhancing antibodies produced during primary infections, which results in enhanced-DENV infection of Fc-γ-receptor-expressing cells (e.g. monocytes and macrophages) during DENV heterotypic exposure in a phenomenon called *antibody-dependent enhancement* (ADE); the increased activation of memory T cells during secondary infections, which has low affinity for the current infecting serotype and high affinity for a past infection with a different serotype known as *the original antigenic sin*; the unbalanced production of pro-inflammatory cytokines that have a direct effect on vascular endothelial cells resulting in plasma leak in a phenomenon known as *cytokine storm*; and the excessive activation of the *complement system* that causes exacerbated inflammatory responses, increasing disease severity. In addition to the adaptive immune responses, a secreted viral factor known as the *nonstructural protein 1* (NS1) has been recently proposed as the missing corner piece of the DENV pathogenesis influencing disease. This *Part II* of the chapter will discuss the interplay between the distinct host adaptive immune responses and viral factors that together contribute to the development of DENV pathogenesis and severe disease.

Keywords: dengue, immunopathogenesis, dengue shock syndrome, severe dengue, adaptive immune response, antibody response, ADE, *cytokine storm*, T cells, complement system, *viral toxin*, NS1, endothelial dysfunction, vascular leak

1. Dengue immunopathogenesis and severe disease: host and viral factors

As discussed in *Part I* of this chapter, severe dengue is mainly characterized by the altered endothelial function in blood vessels and the disruption of the coagulation cascade that results in hypotension, shock, and severe hemorrhage manifestations [1, 2]. As the epidemiology of dengue indicates that appearance of severe manifestations occurs when the peak of viremia has passed, the key biological mechanisms leading to the pathogenesis of clinical complications during DENV infection, are believed to involve the activity of short-lived biological mediators closely linked to host innate and adaptive immune responses [3–6].

This *Part II* of the dengue immunopathogenesis section will address the multifactorial immunopathogenic process of DENV infection from the perspective of the pre-existing serotype cross-reactive antibodies, the hyperactivation of DENV-infected immune cells (e.g. monocytes, mast cells) leading to increased cytokine production, the role of T cell responses, the activation of complement pathways, and the new pathogenic roles of the secreted NS1 of DENV that may act together to occasionally cause severe dengue manifestations followed by shock and potentially death [1, 6–21].

1.1 Antibody response to DENV infection

The DENV complex refers to a group of four evolutionarily distinct, but antigenically and genetically related DENV serotypes (DENV-1 to DENV-4) [22]. During dengue disease, the humoral immune response is vital for controlling DENV virus infection and for the development of acquired immunity [10]. Neutralizing antibodies against the four serotypes are critical components of the protective immune response [23]. In this sense, during primary DENV infection, it is expected that a neutralizing type-specific antibody response should provide long-term protection against the primary DENV infecting serotype, but only transient protection against other DENV serotypes (cross-reactive antibodies) (See Figure 1 *Part I*). Infection with a primary serotype is thought to induce lifelong immunity that protects against re-infection with the same serotype (homotypic) [7, 23]. However, homotypic DENV infections have been found in symptomatic dengue cases in a community-based prospective cohort study suggesting that recurrent DENV infections, particularly in endemic areas can occurs in patients over time [24]. After subsequent infection with a different serotype (secondary infection), the neutralizing antibody response becomes broadly neutralizing and is thought to reduce the incidence of severe disease [25] (See Figure 1C, *Part I*). In fact, individuals with higher cross-reactive neutralizing antibody titers originated from pre-infection correlates with reduced likelihood of symptomatic secondary infection [23]. However, numerous studies worldwide involving human infections during dengue epidemics (e.g. hospitalized cases) or multiple epidemiological studies from prospective cohorts strongly support the heterotypic secondary DENV infection, defined as two or more sequential infections by different serotypes, as the epidemiologic greatest risk factor for developing severe dengue disease [17, 26–29].

Antibody responses during DENV infection are mainly directed against the envelope protein (E), the major structural protein of the virion, and the dominant antigenic target for DENV neutralizing antibodies during natural infection, thus the focus of vaccine candidates design [30–32]. Antibodies specific for DENV proteins can mediate a wide range of functions *in vitro* [10]. They can neutralize DENV infection by direct hindering of virus-receptor interactions, blocking viral fusion with the endosomal membrane within host cells, viral clearance in a Fc-receptor dependent manner, lysis of virus infected cells via complement activation, and antibody dependent cell cytotoxicity (ADCC) of infected cells [33] (**Figure 1**). The E glycoprotein is composed of three structural domains (DI, DII, DIII), and the most extensive characterization of B cell epitopes has been conducted against them [34]. Neutralizing antibodies against the E protein of DENV include antibodies to nearly all the epitopes [35]. However, during the natural course of infection, the serological response to the E glycoprotein is highly serotype cross-reactive and predominantly targets epitopes containing highly conserved residues, for instance, the fusion loop of the domain II [31]. In addition, high-avidity and highly neutralizing antibodies against DENV, bind to domain III (DIII) of the E glycoprotein, which is implicated in DENV binding to its cognate receptor [36, 37]. These antibodies appear to be most effective at providing protection from infection and/or disease [38–40]. However, with an ~60% amino acid divergence between the E glycoproteins of all four DENV serotypes, immunity to one serotype usually does not confer long-lasting cross-protective immunity to the other serotypes [41]. A mature DENV particle contains 180 copies of the E protein covering the surface of the virion in either dimeric or trimeric (pre-fusion) conformations [42]. Neutralization is estimated to require a minimum occupancy of ~30 epitope sites per virion [34]. This may be attributed to the dense arrangement of E glycoproteins on the virion surface which has shown to be important for antigenicity, as many potently neutralizing human antibodies against flaviviruses that target either hidden cryptic or quaternary epitopes extent through multiple E proteins [43–47].

On the other hand, the adaptive immune response during DENV infection can also generate antibodies against pre-M proteins which are highly serotype cross-reactive [48]. Despite this high cross-reactivity, anti-pre-M antibodies rarely neutralize DENV infection even at high concentrations [48]. The pre-M protein forms a heterodimer with the E protein, and it gets cleaved by host cell-expressed furin during the final stage of virion maturation before egress [42]. The cleavage of pre-M is required for the activation of flavivirus infectivity, including DENV [49]. In the mature virion, the remaining M protein fragment is completely hidden by the E protein dimers which makes it inaccessible to antibody binding [34]. Therefore, maturation state of the virion matters and may influence the interaction between immature virus particles and anti-pre-M antibodies leading to neutralization or enhancement of the infection (**Figure 1**). The potential role of anti-E or pre-M antibodies in increasing DENV infection and pathogenesis will be further discussed later in this chapter.

Antibody responses in DENV infection can be also directed against several non-structural proteins such as NS1, NS3, and NS5 as found in sera collected from DENV infected patients [50, 51]. These antibody responses have been mainly detected during secondary cases which open the possibility of implementing it in early diagnostic assays of DENV infection [51, 52]. NS3 (viral helicase/protease) and NS5 (virus RNA dependent polymerase) localize exclusively within virus-infected cells, but cell lysis owing to viral cytopathic effect or immune cell-mediated lysis may make these proteins accessible for binding to B cell receptors, inducing an antibody response [40, 52]. In this same line of interest, T cells may play an important role in the immune response against DENV nonstructural proteins. This topic will be later discussed in this chapter. On the other hand, the NS1 protein is the only flavivirus glycoprotein secreted by infected cells [53]. NS1 forms a multimeric structures either expressed on the surface of infected cells (dimer) or released as a soluble

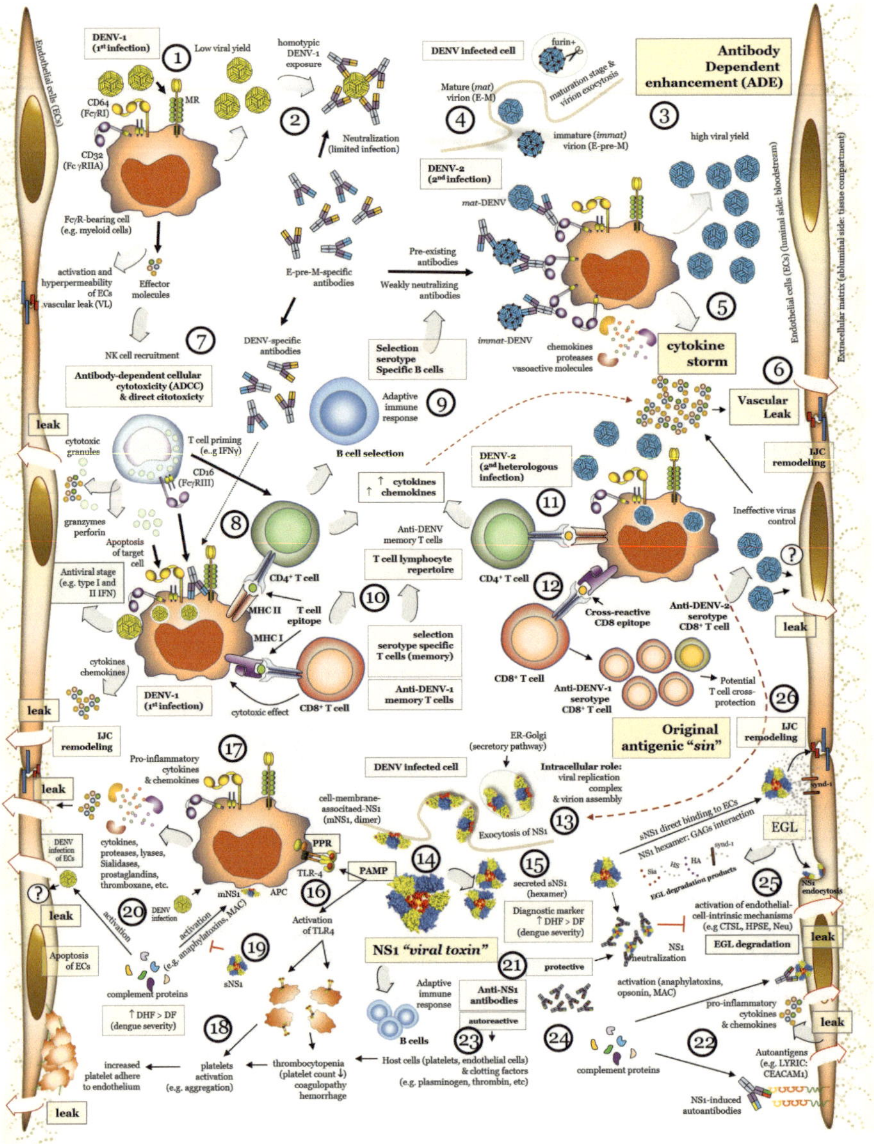

Figure 1.

The supercomplex interplay of the immunopathogenic mechanisms triggered by systemic DENV infection leading to disease. The DENV complex is composed by four serotypes [1–4], and a primary infection with any of these serotypes triggers an adaptive immune response that results in the generation of neutralizing antibodies mainly directed against the infecting serotype, for instance, DENV-1 (here in yellow) [1, 2] (see also Figure 1c, Part I). When the host is re-exposed to the same DENV serotype as the one from the primary infection (homotypic infection), the neutralizing antibodies generated during the first encounter, prevent APCs to be infected [2]. However, during a sequential DENV infection with a different serotype, here DENV-2 (in blue) [3], the pre-existing antibody response (1st DENV infection) do not neutralize but increases the infection of APCs via a mechanism called antibody-dependent-enhancement (ADE). This ADE phenomenon relies on the cell surface expression of Fcγ-receptors (FcγRs) including FcγRI (CD64) and FcγRII (CD32) mainly found in monocytes/macrophages and dendritic cells [1, 3], also Fc εR found in mast cells resident of the skin (see also Figure 2, Part I). Importantly, ADE can be also modulated by the structural heterogeneity of the DENV particles (maturation state) [4]. During the DENV replication cycle, right before virus exocytosis of the infected cell, the newly assembled virus particles suffer a final processing step known as the 'maturation state' of the virion, in which the pre-M protein is cleaved by the cellular protease, furin. Inefficient furin activity leads to the release of viral particles containing a wide variety of pre-M/E protein complex known as partially mature virions [4]. Although immature and partially mature DENV viral particles are unable to infect cells via its cognate receptor, they can use the ADE mechanisms as a way to infect FcR-bearing cells which results in increased viral production (high virus yield) and increased secretion of cytokines and chemokines and other soluble components with vasoactive and pro-inflammatory activities in a process known as the 'cytokine storm'. [5] The term "cytokine storm" is referred to the exacerbated and unbalanced production of cytokines and chemokines which exert many effector functions including antiviral response and inflammation. Many of these components pose some vasoactive activities which alter the homeostasis of mostly all biological barriers including the microvascular endothelium, leading to a phenomenon called vascular leak (hereafter, 'leak'), a consequence of the increased endothelial cell (EC) permeability, and a hallmark of severe dengue disease [6]. The homeostasis of the endothelial barrier is mainly maintained by two structures: a) the endothelial glycocalyx layer (EGL), a network of membrane-bound glycosaminoglycans (e.g heparan sulfate [HS], hyaluronic acid [HA], chondroitin sulfate [CS]) and proteoglycans (e.g syndecan-1, perlecan, glypicans), covering the endothelium luminally and playing critical roles in vascular physiology and pathology, including mechanotransduction, hemostasis, signaling, and blood cell-vessel wall interactions; and b) the intercellular junction complex (IJC), mainly composed of the tight (e.g. ZO-1, occluding, claudins) and adherens (e.g. VE-cadherin, beta-catenin) junction proteins that maintain the cell-to-cell contacts to control fluids and small molecules exchange between the luminal side (bloodstream) and the abluminal side (tissues compartment) of blood vessels. The disruption of any of these two main components under pathological conditions leads to increased inflammatory responses with pathogenic consequences involving barrier dysfunction and vascular disorders that result in excessive extravasation of fluids and proteins into the tissues, hypotension, shock, and sometimes, death. In addition to modulating the endothelial barrier function, cytokine and chemokines secreted by DENV infected cells pose important effector functions that promote the recruitment and activation of other immune cells such as NK cells with the ability to induce apoptosis of susceptible target cells (e.g. DENV infected cells) via NK cell-mediated cytotoxicity, and antibody (Ab)-dependent NK cell-mediated cytotoxicity (ADCC) [7]. Activation of NK cells also lead to the secretion of an array of immunoregulatory cytokines which conditioned a bidirectional crosstalk between NK cells and other immune cells such as dendritic cells (DC), macrophages, mast cells, and T cells. The release of cytotoxic granules and cytokines by NK cells may also contribute to a cytokine storm, and the tissue damage associated with infection clearance may exacerbate the pro-inflammatory environment. On the other hand, during DENV infection of immunes cells, viral clearance of DENV results from a coordinated action of multiple cell types and mechanisms including innate immune responses such as the production of type I and type II interferons, cell killing by cytotoxic lymphocytes and production of neutralizing antibodies by B cells [7, 8, 9]. Intracellular expression of newly synthesized DENV proteins (e.g. NS3, NS1, NS5 proteins) enter the MHC class I and II presentation pathways in which viral peptide epitopes are presented on the cell surface either through MHC class II molecules for CD4+ T cells, and MHC class I molecules for CD8+ T cells, which principally lyse infected cells but also produce cytokines with effector functions on the endothelial biology. Like with the antibody response, after primary DENV infection, T cell responses are mainly characterized by higher homotypic than heterotypic responses [8, 10]. However, during DENV secondary infections, this pattern breaks down as B and T cells induced by the prior exposure to a different DENV serotype rapidly turn into highly serotype cross-reactive responses mainly directed against the previously encountered DENV serotype [11]. This phenomenon results in the consistent preferential expansion of pre-existing cross-reactive heterologous memory T cells with higher avidity for the previous DENV serotype and weak-affinity for the new infecting DENV, that may lead to an inefficient in clearing DENV infection, while producing excessive cytokines, leading to the onset of immune pathology such as vascular leak which results in severe disease. This alteration in the T cell immune responses, skewed by the 'memory' of the previous infection, is referred to as 'original antigenic sin' [12]. In addition to these host factors, the non-structural protein 1 (NS1) of DENV is a multifaceted viral factor that has been also demonstrated to play many roles in DENV pathogenesis. In DENV infected cells, NS1 can be found intracellularly expressed as a monomer in the ER where it forms dimers that play critical roles in the viral replication cycle, particularly the assembly of new viral particles [13]. Secreted NS1 protein from DENV infected cells is a hexameric protein with a barrel-like shape that contains a hydrophobic lipid core (cholesterol and triglycerides), and three domains known as the "wing domain"(here in yellow), the β-ladder domain (in blue), and the β-roll domain (in red) ([14], see also Figure 1B). Plasma circulating levels of soluble NS1 (sNS1) have been described to correlate with the appearance of severe disease manifestations such as dengue hemorrhagic fever (DHF) in DENV-infected patients [15]. sNS1 from DENV has been shown to act as a potential pathogen associated-molecular pattern (PAMP) that on immune cells and platelets interacts with Toll-like receptor 4 (TLR4), a pattern-recognition-receptor (PPR) [16] resulting in the production of pro-inflammatory cytokines from human PBMCs and monocytes [17] and the activation of human platelets which results in their aggregation and increase adherent onto the ECs lining the blood vessels, which hampers the homeostasis of the EC-barrier and the microvasculature [18]. Due to its ability to trigger the production of cytokines via TLR4, the term 'viral toxin' is now used to describe this pathogenic function of sNS1 during systemic DENV infection [14]. Furthermore, sNS1 can activate and block the antiviral activity of the complement pathway, an important component of the innate immune response against many human pathogen infections [19]. NS1 can either lead to pathogenesis by increasing the deposition of active complement components on the surface of ECs and human tissues [20], or by directly interacting with the component itself blocking its function or getting rid of some of the critical components involved in complement activation cascade [19]. An additional route for NS1 to cause virus pathogenesis or protection is related to the adaptive immune response generated against the secreted NS1 protein during DENV infection [21]. First, NS1-induced autoantibodies (anti-NS1 antibodies that recognize antigens on the host components) increase the activation of ECs causing barrier dysfunction by increasing the production of proinflammatory cytokines and the action of the complement pathway or binds to autoantigens encoded in proteins of the clotting cascade such as plasminogen, thrombin, and fibrinogen inducing coagulation disorders that along with the thrombocytopenia leads to bleeding manifestations [22, 23]. Second, anti-NS1 antibodies have been reported to prevent the direct interaction of sNS1 with the surface of ECs which blocks the NS1-induced activation of endothelial-intrinsic pathways leading to the disruption of the EGL and the remodeling the cell-to-cell contacts which disrupts the integrity of the intercellular junction complex formed by tight and adherens junction proteins (TJ/AJ) [24–26]. Overall, this summary figure represents the complex crosstalk between distinct host and viral factors that together trigger a diverse cascade of effector functions leading to protection or pathogenesis, the latter sometimes associated to the development of life-threatening disease manifestations that can result in death.

hexameric during DENV infection *in vitro* and *in vivo* (See Figure 1B, *Part I*) [12, 54–56]. Specific antibodies for NS1 proteins have been also found circulating in DENV infected patients, particularly in secondary cases and are highly serotype cross-reactive [57–59].

In vivo experiments using mouse models for DENV infection, the adoptive transfer of immune serum or monoclonal antibodies specific for pre-M, E or NS1 proteins prevented mortality from lethal challenge with DENV [9, 38, 60–63]. Similarly, passive transfer of anti-E antibodies can protect against infection with DENV in nonhuman primate models [64, 65]. Dengue virus-specific antibodies of the appropriate subclasses can also bind to complement proteins and promote their activation. Fixation of complement to virions by antibodies specific for the pre-M and/or E proteins can inhibit viral infection [66]. NS1-specific antibodies mediate complement-dependent lysis of infected cells; however, this may not fully explain their protective effects *in vivo* [67]. Additionally, NS1-specific antibodies may also contribute to antibody-dependent cellular cytotoxicity [67, 68]. Recently, the role of the antibody immune response against the soluble DENV NS1 has become more relevant in the development of future dengue vaccines [9, 62, 69] as NS1 was described to play a key role in the development of DENV pathogenesis. Further evidences from a candidate dengue vaccine has demonstrated the functionality of anti-NS1-specific IgG responses against NS1 pathogenesis *in vitro* [70]. The phenomenon of NS1 being directly involved in modulating DENV pathogenesis will be discussed in more detail in a different section of this chapter.

1.2 Antibody-dependent enhancement of DENV infection and the cytokine storm

DENV has four distinct serotypes, and infection with one serotype results in the development of homotypic immunity which has been suggested to confer a durable and possible life-long protection against the infecting DENV serotype, but only short-term cross-reactive protection against other serotypes (heterotypic immunity) [13]. This cross-serotype–reactive antibody response is thought to wane to subneutralizing levels, where antibodies still bind, but do not neutralize the infecting virion. In turn, these antibodies contribute to enhanced infection of Fc receptors (FcRs) bearing cells during heterologous DENV encounters (**Figure 1**) [71, 72]. This phenomenon called "*antibody dependent enhancement*" or ADE, potentially increases the risk of developing severe disease by virtue of increasing the number of virus infected cells and therefore the viral biomass *in vivo* accompanied by hyperactivation of infected-immune cells and increased release of vasoactive mediators that resembles some pathologic features of what occurs in patients suffering severe dengue disease including capillary permeability and vascular leak (**Figure 1**) [73–78].

Multiple prospective cohort studies in Asia and Latin America have identified secondary infection as an epidemiological risk factor for severe dengue [17, 28, 79, 80]. Classical epidemiologic and observational studies have suggested that pre-existing sub-neutralizing antibodies in closely association with immunologic markers and clinical events supports the hypothesis of ADE and the risk of severe dengue during secondary infections [16, 26, 27, 78, 81–83]. Maternally derived subneutralizing levels of DENV-reactive IgGs have been also postulated to be a critical risk factor for severe dengue during infancy [26, 27, 84–86]. Numerous studies performed in animal models have reiterated that ADE results in higher viral load in patients at specific concentration of antibodies (*a peak of enhancement*), especially at early stages of infection, thereby increasing the risk of developing DHF/DSS [14, 87]. Studies performed in rhesus monkeys confirmed that passive transfer of immune serum or monoclonal antibodies resulted in increased viremia; however, no apparent signs of severe disease was observed, indicating that severe dengue manifestations may not only be a main consequence of increased viremia [65, 88].

Despite all these evidences, yet no conclusive evidence exist that a risk of severe dengue disease and ADE occur in humans. A recent study using samples from a well-characterized DENV cohort study in children showed that the risk of developing severe dengue disease during secondary dengue infections existed within a narrow range of preexisting anti-DENV antibody titers, *a peak of enhancement*, detected in humans [29]. Recently, a phase 3 clinical trial of the only dengue vaccine licensed, Dengvaxia [89] showed an increased risk of hospitalization for severe dengue in children not exposed to DENV before vaccination [90], raising concerns about the need to assess dengue vaccine safety at the earliest development stages prior to human vaccination, and confirming that vaccination of DENV-naïve individuals may induce poorly neutralizing anti-DENV antibodies that increase the risk of severe dengue disease [91]. All these observations indicate that ADE may occur in humans and should be an obligate consideration for future designing, implementation, and evaluation of vaccine trials, especially those in the flavivirus field.

DENV-ADE can be mediated by E protein-specific antibodies either at low antibody concentrations or low antibody avidity, when the number of antibody molecules bound per virion is below the threshold necessary for neutralization of the virus (*a peak of enhancement*) [92]. As DENV E protein binds to cellular receptors and mediates viral fusion during entry, it is thought to be the major target of neutralizing antibodies [33, 41, 93]. However, a substantial proportion of antibodies generated in response to natural DENV infection are directed toward the pre-M protein which represents an important part of the adaptive immune response in DENV infected patients [40, 94].

During DENV infection, the cleavage of pre-M protein represents a critical step for the virus maturation process [49, 95, 96]. As the cleavage of pre-M is not complete in all dengue virions, a proportion of secreted viral particles from infected cells are partially mature dengue virions that contain a varying amount of cleaved and uncleaved pre-M proteins [42, 96, 97]. Immature dengue viral particles contains regular trimeric E-pre-M protein complexes and are noninfectious [49, 98]. In contrast, some partially mature forms, containing some pre-M protein–E protein trimers, are partially infectious. In both cases, uncleaved pre-M protein on immature or partially mature virions can be targeted by the host anti-pre-M antibody response which despite being highly cross-reactive among all four DENV serotypes, can rarely neutralize virus infection even at high concentrations, but promote ADE (**Figure 1**) [48, 75, 76, 98, 99].

Historically, the DENV-ADE phenomenon has been recapitulated by numerous *in vitro* studies where FcR-bearing immunes cells including human monocyte/macrophages-like cell lines [48, 73, 74, 77, 98–103], human pre-basophil-like and immature mast cell-like cells [104, 105], human primary derived-monocytes/macrophages, dendritic cells, mast cells [75, 76, 106–110], and human derived-PBMCs [111, 112] have been infected with distinct DENV serotype strains in the presence of monoclonal antibodies or human derived-serum/plasma obtained from DENV infected cases [59, 72, 75, 76, 104, 105, 113–115]. Controversially, DENV-ADE for other considered immune cells such as endothelial cells [116, 117] have been also described *in vitro* and *in vivo* [118–121]. However, histochemistry of autopsy samples from fatal dengue cases and *in vitro* assays using peripheral blood cells revealed that macrophages/monocytes are primary targets for DENV infection and not endothelial cells [122–127].

In vitro, the increased infection of these target cells results in augmented expression/production of cytokines and vasoactive mediators and their release into the extracellular milieu where provoke an exacerbated activation of neighboring immune cells and endothelial cells which leads to another critical phenomenon that may frequently occur during severe dengue infections known as the "*cytokine storm*" [10, 11, 73, 107, 128–130]. This phenomenon has been described for several other virus infections (such as influenza viruses, hantaviruses, and potentially coronaviruses), where the scenario envisioned is that this excessive immune activation creates a cascade of cytokine production or "*cytokine storm*" resulting in increased vascular permeability [131–134]. *In vivo*, experimental DENV infection in AG129 [135], showed that sub-neutralizing concentrations of anti-E or anti-pre-M antibodies increased DENV pathogenesis and mortality in mice mainly associated with increased circulation of pro-inflammatory cytokines and increased vascular leakage [40, 48, 87, 118, 136].

Mechanistically, it is thought that ADE-DENV infection of Fc receptor-bearing cells, particularly through the Fc-gamma-receptor IIA (FcγRIIA or CD32) [75, 102, 137, 138], not only results in a large virus-infected cell mass, rather the activation of intracellular signaling pathways [109, 139–142] which leads to the increased secretion of vasoactive immune products by infected cells, such as TNF-α, a cytokine produced by activated monocytes, which in elevated levels has been found in serum of DHF/DSS patients [71, 86, 143–145]. In addition to TNF- α, an important number of immune modulators have been described to be implicated in DENV pathogenesis acting upon a complicated network of events to provoke the severe dengue outcomes mainly related to increased vascular leakage. In DENV-infected primary monocytes or monocytic cell lines, the production of IL-6, IL-8, and interferon gamma-induced protein 10 (IP-10), IL-12p70, IL-1β, IL-10 and the prostaglandin E2 (PGE2) have been found upregulated [73, 74, 76, 77, 109, 112, 137, 142, 146]. In DENV-infected dendritic cells, the production of inflammatory cytokines TNF-α, IFN-α, IL-6, IL-10; the chemokines IFN-γ-inducible chemokines CXCL9, CXCL10, and CXCL11, PGE2, and also matrix metalloproteinases (MMPs) such as MMP-2 and MMP-9 were found increasingly produced [75, 76, 147–149]. On the other hand, DENV infection of mast cells has showed to elicit the release of potent vasoactive cytokines such as IL-1β and IL-6; chemokines, such as CCL3, CCL4, CCL5 and CXCL10, and other mast cell-derived mediators including proteases such as chymase and tryptase, leukotrienes, prostaglandins, histamine, and vascular endothelial growth factor (VEGF) which shows the significant influence of mast cells in immunity and pathogenesis during DENV infection [104, 107, 150, 151].

In humans, increased levels of many of these soluble factors including IFN-γ, TNF-α, IL-1β, IL-4, IL-6, IL-7, IL-10, IL-13, IL-15, IL-17, IL-18, macrophage migration inhibitory factor (MIF), chemokines such as IL-8, CCL2, CCL4, CCL5, CXCL10 (IP-10) and the monocyte chemoattractant protein-1 (MCP-1) have been reported in patients with DHF when compared to DF [1, 10, 152–154]. Studies show that elevated levels of IL-6, IL-10, IFN-γ, MIF, and CCL-4 could be used as potential biomarkers of severe dengue [155, 156]. Additional biological markers such as serum lipids [157, 158], prostaglandins, leukotrienes and thromboxane [151, 159], free radical compounds such as reactive oxygen and nitrogen oxide species [160, 161], MPPs [162–164], and several components of the endothelium in the microvasculature such as the vascular cell adhesion molecule 1 (VCAM-1), Angiopoietin-1 and -2 (Ang-1, -2), endothelial-1, [5, 163, 165–167] or carbohydrates including glycosaminoglycans (GAGs) and proteoglycans (e.g. HSPG) [168–171] have been suggested to play important roles in the pathogenesis of different viral infections, including DENV. Changes in the plasma or urine levels of these molecules have been shown to act as potential predictors for clinical outcome between patients with different stages of DHF disease severity and predictors of disease severity in animal models *in vivo* [168, 170–174].

1.3 T cell responses and "the antigenic sin" of DENV infection

During DENV replication cycle, the viral genomic RNA encodes for a single polyprotein that after being cleaved by cellular and viral proteases yield three structural proteins and seven nonstructural proteins [42, 175] (See Figure 1A, *Part I*). Numerous studies have demonstrated that DENV infection leads to potent T cell responses, and many DENV-T cell epitopes have been found throughout the DENV polyprotein *ex vivo* using human leukocytes and *in vivo* using murine models [176–179]. These T cell epitopes appear to follow the general principles of T cell epitope immunogenicity, as they show similar MHC molecule binding kinetics to those of other immunodominant viral epitopes. Several studies indicate that nonstructural proteins are more frequently recognized by CD8+ T cells, while structural proteins are better recognized by CD4+ T cells. [180, 181]. However, most of the identified CD8+ and/or CD4+ T cells epitopes predominantly reside in the nonstructural proteins 3 (NS3) suggesting that NS3 protein is immunodominantly recognized by T cell epitopes in humans infected with DENV [8, 177, 182–184]. On the other hand, CD8+ and CD4+ T cell responses have been also identified, to a lesser extent, against other viral proteins such as the viral capsid, Ns1, NS2A/B, NS4A/B, and NS5 proteins [177, 178, 185, 186]. The recognition pattern of T cell receptors (TCRs) to these proteins expressed in the context of MHC differs according to the type of HLA which confers either susceptibility or protection to severe dengue infections [187, 188]. HLA class I and class II alleles have been shown to be associated with the development of DHF/DSS in different populations [182, 187, 189–192]. However, some specific HLA alleles are found to be more significantly common among patients with dengue fever than those undergoing severe dengue manifestations suggesting a protective effect of DENV-specific T cells [191]. Overall, the T cell immunodominance of DENV is quite complex and widely focused on different epitopes identified across the whole virus proteome [177, 183, 192]. Given that around 70% of amino acid identity exist between all four DENV serotypes, T cell epitopes are also highly cross-reactive and this has been suggested to play important roles in protective immunity not only against DENV but also other related flavivirus such as Zika virus (ZIKV) [193–195].

The protective role of T cells in viral infections is well established [196]. Dengue virus-specific T cells recognize virus-infected cells and respond with a diverse set of effector functions, including proliferation, target cell lysis and the production of a range of cytokines [197]. *In vivo*, CD8+ T cells control viral infection via direct cytotoxicity, and production of pro-inflammatory cytokines such as IFN-γ and TNF-α; in turn, CD4+ T cells induce enhancement of B and CD8+ T cell responses, production of inflammatory and anti-viral cytokines, cytotoxicity, and promotion of memory responses to defeat viral infections [178, 179, 198–200]. T cell activity requires the presentation of viral peptides on the surface of infected cells in the context of MHC molecules and, unlike B cells, T cells do not recognize intact virions [196]. *In vitro*, DENV specific CD8+ memory T-cells can lyse MHC-matched virus-infected cells as an antiviral mechanism leading to protection [199, 201]. Activation of cytotoxic CD8+ T cells after presentation of viral peptides by infected antigen presenting cells (APCs) can generate immediate effector functions by expressing cytotoxic molecules such as granzyme B and perforin to kill virus-infected cells via MHC I- and MHC II-dependent mechanisms [10]. *In vivo* studies have shown that adoptive transfer of DENV-specific CD8+ T cell can partially protect mice from lethal challenge with DENV [202]. Other studies involving immunization with antigens that induce DENV-specific T cells but not neutralizing antibodies, have also shown that T cells are enough to protect mice from lethal infection [179, 203, 204]. These studies suggest that CD4+ or CD8+ T cells may have beneficial roles in controlling virus replication during DENV infections.

Although T cells have important functions in combating viral pathogens, both pathological and protective effects of T cells have been reported in the context of DENV infection [177, 178]. The association of severe dengue symptoms with a rapid decline in viral loads and a peak of pro-inflammatory cytokine secretion have led to the proposal of a role for a T cell mediated immune response in driving immunopathology in severe dengue [205]. T cell responses after primary DENV infections are characterized by higher homotypic than heterotypic responses [194]. However, in secondary DENV infections, T cell responses are highly serotype cross-reactive [206] with higher responses maintained to the previously encountered DENV serotype [207]. This alteration in the T cell immune responses, skewed by the 'memory' of the previous infection, is referred to as '*original antigenic sin*" [10, 207] (**Figure 1**). According to this hypothesis, secondary DENV infection is dominated by the expansion of pre-existing nonprotective, cross-reactive and low affinity T cells to the new infecting serotype that results in ineffective viral control and elicit an aberrant immune response that contribute to immunopathology and severe dengue disease through an excessive production of inflammatory cytokines [10, 177, 178, 205, 207, 208]. Distinct studies *in vitro* using tetramers containing peptides from either the primary or secondary infecting viruses, have provided evidences for the original antigenic sin occurring in secondary T cell responses to DENV [207, 209].

The magnitude of the T cell response positively correlates with disease severity [183, 207]. Studies of the function of dengue-specific T cells has revealed an interesting difference between mild and severe infections [183]. Profound activation of naïve T cells into effector T cells and increased cytokine production have been reported in patients with DHF during both primary and secondary DENV infections [1]. T cell responses in severe dengue patients mainly produce IFN-γ and TNF-α [183]. Additionally, a broad spectrum of cytokines has been shown to be produced by DENV-specific T cells in responses to the recognition of peptide–MHC complexes on target cells. This array of cytokines follows a T helper 1 (TH1)- or TH0-like profile including the production of IFN-γ, TNF-α, IL-2, and MIP1β, also known as CCL4, and less commonly, the TH2-type cytokines, IL-4 [15, 193]. Many of these T cell-derived cytokines have pleiotropic effects, including the induction or enhancement of inflammation and the alteration of vascular permeability that may contribute to the systemic disturbances leading to DHF [1, 10, 208].

Despite all this evidence, the relative contribution of DENV activated T cells in dengue pathogenesis and control of viral infection is still controversial. Severe dengue can occur during a primary dengue infection in which cross-reactive T cells and original antigenic sin would not be operative [210]. In addition, the relatively low numbers of circulating T cells seen during acute DENV infection and the temporal mismatch between the appearance of DENV NS3-specific CD8+ T cells, and the appearance of vascular leakage manifestations, suggests that other mechanisms independent of CD8+ T cells are responsible for early triggering of capillary leakage in children with DHF [207, 211]. A recent study found that numbers of DENV-specific T cells were augmented in the skin of DENV-infected patients compared to those circulating in the peripheral blood, suggesting that during the acute phase, DENV-specific T cells may migrate to the skin and return the bloodstream upon viral clearance [212, 213]. During secondary infections, the expansion of the low-avidity T cells specific for the primary DENV infection may delay viral clearance and thereby lead to higher viral loads. These results may explain the asynchronies timing between T cells circulating in the blood and the beginning of capillary permeability that occurs in DENV infection. However, in the absence of a good animal model of disease, it remains controversial whether the expansion of low-avidity cross-reactive T cells in secondary dengue infection contributes to disease pathogenesis. In summary, during DENV infection, the generation of an early T cell response may be protective, whereas the late generation of T cell populations that have a proportion of low-avidity T cells and are skewed to inflammatory cytokine production in the absence of degranulation may predispose to immunopathology in the presence of high viral antigen loads that contributes to the cytokine storm and vascular leak.

1.4 DENV infection, NS1 pathogenesis, and vascular leak

The hallmark and critical feature of severe dengue disease is the increased capillary permeability, causing plasma leakage, which can lead to hemodynamic compromise and dengue shock syndrome (DSS) [2–4]. The plasma leakage syndrome, is defined as the extensive extravasation and accumulation of fluids out of blood vessels into the surrounding tissues and serous cavities, causing serositis which includes pleural effusion, and pericardial and peritoneal ascites, leading to hemoconcentration, hypotension, organ disfunction, and life-threatening shock [6, 214]. In DENV infection, the transient nature of plasma leakage, its association with the late febrile phase and the paucity of structural damage to the vasculature identified by autopsy studies initially suggested that circulating factors were primarily responsible for this phenomenon [5, 125, 126, 205].

Although a major risk factor for developing severe dengue disease is related to the DENV-ADE phenomenon that correlates with increased plasma levels of pro-inflammatory cytokines found in the acute phase of patients undergoing severe dengue manifestations [1, 83], ADE alone seems not to be sufficient to explain the vascular pathology associated with DHF since not all secondary heterotypic infections results in severe disease, and many individuals also experience DHF during primary infection [16]. The association of severe dengue symptoms with a rapid decline in viral loads and a peak of pro-inflammatory cytokine secretion suggests that although subneutralizing antibodies can increase dengue disease severity via ADE, other factors may also influence disease outcome, driving the immunopathology in severe dengue [10, 205].

Very recently, a new piece in DENV pathogenesis puzzle, known as the nonstructural protein 1 or NS1, was reported to directly be involved in inducing endothelial dysfunction *in vitro* and vascular leakage *in vivo* via alteration of the endothelial barrier function and activation of immune cells and platelets, the latter resulting in induction of pro-inflammatory signaling pathways leading to increased secretion of vasoactive molecules and vascular leakage [9, 215, 216]. Initially recognized as a soluble complement-fixing (SCF) antigen detected in the blood of DENV-infected patients [217], NS1 of the flavivirus genus including DENV, is the only flaviviral protein described to be secreted by infected mammalian and insect cells [218–221], which circulates in the bloodstream of DENV-infected patients for up to 14 days since the onset of symptoms [222]. This bioavailability feature of NS1 launched it as a diagnostic marker for acute primary and secondary DENV infections and potentially other flavivirus diseases [54, 223–225]. NS1 antigenemia can reach as high as 50 μg/mL during the acute phase of dengue illness correlating with the development of DHF and sometimes fatality cases [12, 14, 54, 170, 223, 226–228]. These observations suggest that circulating levels of NS1 in the bloodstream of patients during the clinical phase of the disease may contribute to DENV pathogenesis.

In infected cells, NS1 is found as a membrane-associated dimer in both cellular compartments and on the cell surface. NS1 is intracellularly generated as a monomeric glycoprotein in the ER of DENV infected cells, where it has been demonstrated to play essential roles as cofactor in virus replication and virus assembly by recruiting cellular proteins as well as viral proteins such as the envelope protein during virus morphogenesis which results in the biogenesis of the membranous DENV RC organelle [229–233]. NS1 is also secreted by infected cells and recent structural analyses showed that secreted NS1 circulates as a soluble hexamer glycoprotein with an atypical open barrel-shape that contains a prominent central lipid-enriched core of triglycerides, cholesteryl esters, and phospholipids that evocates a plasma high-density lipoprotein [53, 234] (**Figure 1**). Elucidation of the crystal structures of the NS1 hexamers reveal an amphipathic molecule with a hydrophobic inner face and a hydrophilic outer face containing three structural domains known as the hydrophobic "β-roll", the "wing" domain, and the c-terminal "β-ladder" domain that likely have distinct roles in membrane association, replication complex assembly, and interactions with the immune system and are the basis for elucidating the molecular mechanism of NS1 function [235, 236] (See Figure 1B, *Part I*). These same structural domains were also identified by cryo-EM reconstruction studies of other related flavivirus NS1 proteins such as West Nile virus (WNV), Zika virus (ZIKV), and yellow fever virus (YFV) [237–239].

In addition to the role played in viral replication, NS1 participates in dengue immunopathogenesis by inhibiting platelet aggregation and prothrombin activation, directing complement against endothelial cells, inducing endothelial cell apoptosis, and facilitating the evasion of DENV particles from complement system–dependent neutralization [229, 240]. Regarding the complement pathways, NS1 mediates complement inactivation through multiple interactions with the complement proteins including factor H, C1s and C4, and the C4 binding protein [241–244]. These interactions result in attenuation of complement classical, lectin, and alternative pathways suggesting that extracellular NS1 protein may function to minimize immune system responses by decreasing complement recognition of DENV infected cells [19]. However, in flavivirus infections, the complement system has been described to play an important role in protecting the host but also influencing disease pathogenesis [19]. In DENV infected patients with DSS, accelerated complement consumption and a marked reduction in plasma complement components has been observed, which led to the proposal that complement activation plays an important role in disease pathogenesis [20, 245]. Recent studies from human autopsies have identified more evidences of increased deposition of complement components from both classical and alternative pathways associated with increased liver damage [126].

In the context of DENV NS1, both soluble NS1 and cell membrane-associated NS1 have been identified to triggers complement activation and anaphylatoxin formation in the presence of polyclonal or monoclonal anti-NS1 antibodies [246] (**Figure 1**). *In vitro* and *in vivo* experiments using anti-NS1 specific antibodies as well as antiserum obtained from DENV immunized mice and rabbits have reported their cross-reactivity with various epitopes found on human plasma proteins involved in coagulation pathways such as fibrinogen, plasminogen, and thrombin as well as integrin/adhesion proteins, endothelial cells and platelets leading to inflammation, apoptosis, and dysfunction of endothelial cells and platelets which sometimes results in bleeding issues [247–252]. Based on these evidences, autoimmune mechanisms mediated by anti-NS1 antibodies have been also proposed to lead to symptoms of DHF related to increasing vascular permeability maybe in a complement dependent manner. However, numerous past and new growing evidence describing the role of anti-NS1 antibody responses in NS1-immunized mouse models, DENV infected patients or DENV vaccine trails suggest an important protective effect of anti-NS1 immune responses as prophylactic or therapeutic options against DENV infection and other related flavivirus infections [9, 57, 62, 63, 70, 186, 253–260]. Therefore, the dual role of anti-NS1 antibodies in protection and disease still represents a critical challenge that needs to be overcome to develop an effective and safe NS1-based vaccine against flavivirus infections.

As mentioned previously, endothelial barrier dysfunction leading to vascular leakage and shock are the major causes of death in patients with dengue hemorrhagic fever (DHF) and dengue shock syndrome (DSS) [2]. The vascular alterations observed in dengue cases have been described to be a consequence of the imbalance of the host immune system, specially cytokine storm, cytotoxic T cell and complement activations [1, 10, 11], in addition to endothelium injuries caused by the direct infection of the virus of endothelial cells, as reported by several *in vitro* studies [261, 262]. Endothelial cells, lining the inner side of blood vessels, constitute a critical component of the vascular endothelium which are in direct contact with the plasma proteins and all cellular components circulating in the bloodstream [263]. Under homeostatic conditions, this layer of endothelial cells crucially conducts several essential processes such as maintenance of vessel integrity, supply of oxygen and nutrients to underlying tissues and patrolling immune cell trafficking [264, 265]. Thus, alterations on its integrity under pathologic circumstances result in malfunction which contributes to inflammation and disease [265] (**Figure 1**).

Secreted hexameric DENV NS1 protein has been described to attaches to the surface of uninfected cells, primarily human endothelial cells *in vitro* and *in vivo* via interactions with heparan sulfate and chondroitin sulfate E [266]. In 2015, a new role for soluble NS1 in eliciting direct pathogenic effects in DENV disease was described [9]. In this study, the barrier function of human pulmonary microvascular endothelial cells (HPMEC) cultured under polarized conditions on semipermeable membrane filters (*e.g.* Transwells inserts) was compromised after being exposed to physiological concentrations (0.5–5 ug/mL) of recombinant soluble and hexameric NS1 proteins from all four DENV serotypes (DENV 1–4) *in vitro*. Interestingly, this pathogenic effect was recapitulated *in vivo* when inoculation of mice (e.g. *Ifnar*$^{-/-}$) with only DENV NS1 in the absence of DENV infection results in increased mice morbidity. More interesting, a combination of DENV NS1 with a sublethal dose of DENV2 made mice succumbed. These NS1-induced morbidity/mortality effects *in vivo* was significantly related to the increased vascular leak observed in these mice, phenomenon that was shown to be prevented by NS1 immunization or prophylactic treatment of mice using NS1-derived mouse antiserum or anti-NS1 monoclonal antibodies that also blocked NS1-increased permeability of HPMEC cultures *in vitro*. This study demonstrate how NS1 alone was able to mediate DENV pathogenesis by triggering endothelial dysfunction *in vitro* which was linked to increased vascular leak and mortality *in vivo* [9]. Interestingly, an additional study showed that the secreted form of NS1 may act as a pathogen associated-molecular pattern (PAMP) as purified NS1 protein was able to directly activate mouse macrophages and human PBMCs via Toll-like receptor 4 (TLR4), which leads to the induction and release of pro-inflammatory cytokines and chemokines *in vitro* (*e.g.* TNF-α, IL-6, IFN-β, IL-1β, and IL-12); later, this effect was prevented by TLR4 antagonists and anti-TLR4 antibody treatment in a mouse model of DENV infection [215]. These evidences strongly support the important contribution of NS1 in modulating the endothelial cell biology and the inflammatory responses of immune cells as two of the main mechanisms described to influence DENV pathogenesis and therefore severe disease.

On the endothelium, two main structures work together to maintain the homeostasis of the microvasculature: a network of glycosaminoglycans, glycoproteins, and proteoglycans known as the endothelial glycocalyx layer (EGL) and an array of protein-to-protein interactions that integrates the intercellular junction complex (IJC), mainly composed by tight and adherens junction proteins, and other structures such as gaps and desmosomes [257–259]. Based on the first set of evidence showing a direct role of NS1 on the endothelial cell barrier, subsequent studies have identified distinct mechanisms triggered by DENV NS1 to cause endothelial hyperpermeability and vascular leak such as disruption of EGL (*e.g.* sialic acid, heparan sulfate, syndecan-1) expressed on the surface of HPMEC and the microvasculature *in vivo* via activation/expression of endothelial enzymes including sialidases, heparanase, and cathepsin L, a lysosomal cysteine proteinase, all of these occurring in a cytokine-independent manner [267, 268] (**Figure 1**). An additional study corroborates these findings showing that NS1 induces the increased secretion of vasoactive molecules such as the macrophage migration inhibitory factor (MIF) and the angiopoietin-1 and 2 (Ang-1/Ang-2) from human endothelial cells (e.g. HMEC-1 from dermis) and DENV infected patients. These molecules were shown to activate autophagy pathways, phosphorylation cascades, and actin cytoskeleton rearrangements leading to disarrangement and internalization of VE-cadherin, an adherens junction protein of endothelial cell-to-cell contacts, inflammation, and also secretion of heparanase, shedding of sydencan-1 (CD138), and expression of MMP-9 from immune cells, resulting in degradation of EGL and hyperpermeability *in vitro* [269–272]. Follow up studies in human primary monocytes, monocytic cell lines, and human platelets stimulated with exogenous NS1 *in vitro* have additionally demonstrated the NS1-mediated activation and stimulation of pro-inflammatory cytokines and proteases (*e.g.* MMPs) via TLR4 signaling supporting previous reports of NS1 protein acting as a PAMP leading to inflammation, thrombocytopenia, hemorrhage and disease in DENV infection [273–275].

Besides DENV, the flavivirus genus includes other human medically important mosquito-borne pathogens such as ZIKV, WNV, Japanese encephalitis virus (JEV), and YFV [276]. In humans, flaviviruses can cause a wide spectrum of systemic or neurotropic-encephalitic pathologies ranging from clinically inapparent infections to severe, sometimes fatal disease, characterized by hemorrhagic manifestations and vascular leakage with organ failure (DENV and YFV), encephalitic manifestations (JEV and WNV), and congenital Zika syndrome in pregnancy and Guillain-Barré syndrome in adults associated with ZIKV infection [277, 278]. In recent studies, NS1 proteins from other DENV-closely related flavivirus including ZIKV, WNV, JEV, and YFV also demonstrated to cause endothelial hyperpermeability and vascular leak [172, 173, 279]. Interestingly, NS1 proteins selectively bind to and alters permeability of human endothelial cells from distinct tissues including lung, dermis, umbilical vein, brain, and liver *in vitro* and causes tissue-specific vascular leakage in mice, reflecting the pathophysiology of each flavivirus. Mechanistically, flaviviruses NS1 trigger the disruption of EGL components to cause endothelial hyperpermeability [172, 173, 253, 279]. On the vascular endothelium, the EGL constitutes a network of GAGs such as heparan sulfate, chondroitin sulfate, and hyaluronic acid, and proteoglycans (e.g., syndecans, glypicans, and perlecan) that contributes to maintain the homeostasis of the endothelial barrier function [280]. Degradation of the EGL and the detection of its degradation products in cell supernatants and human plasma have been linked to virus pathogenesis and disease severity in several viral hemorrhagic fever diseases [281], including dengue, where increased levels of heparan sulfate, hyaluronic acid, sialic acid, and syndecan-1 have been found to correlate with severe dengue disease in humans and lethality in animal models [3, 168–170, 172].

This NS1 pathogenic effect on the endothelium requires the internalization of the soluble NS1 protein inside human endothelial cells [279] (**Figure 1**). This process occurs via clathrin-mediated endocytosis and relies on one of the glycosylation sites (Asparigine-207) located in the *Wing* domain of NS1 [279]. DENV NS1 contains two conserved N-linked glycans at the asparagine-130 (N130) and the asparagine-207 (N207) which have been implicated in NS1 hexamer secretion, stability, and function [234, 236, 282, 283]. Previous studies investigating the importance of the N-glycans on NS1 have found that deglycosylated flaviviral NS1 proteins at either site, exhibited significant attenuation of neurovirulence in mice compared to the wild-type virus [284–286]. Additional *in vitro* studies have shown that endocytosis of DENV NS1 occur in human hepatocytes which may potentialize subsequent DENV infection [221].

Flavivirus infection has been shown to compromise the integrity of many biological barriers, including the lung microvascular endothelium and the blood–brain barrier, which are usually able to protect against virus infection [287, 288]. Numerous studies of flavivirus infection in different animal models as well as human autopsies have shown a selective tropism of distinct groups of flaviviruses that target different tissues, leading to systemic versus neurotropic-encephalitic pathology [277]. The fact that NS1 internalization is required to induce endothelial hyperpermeability and increased vascular leak through a flaviviral-conserved endothelial cell-intrinsic pathways, and the finding that the flaviviral virulence depends on the expression of N-glycans on soluble NS1, suggest the possibility that NS1 may favor virus propagation and pathogenesis *in vivo*. During the acute phase of DENV infection high NS1 antigenemia have been correlated with increased risk of developing severe dengue disease, including vascular leakage [12, 14]; however, little is known about circulating levels of NS1 from other flavivirus infections. Future studies intended to investigate the kinetics and dynamics of NS1 circulation in flavivirus-infected patients different than DENV, will help to better understand the role of NS1 in flavivirus pathogenesis and disease. NS1 is well conserved among flaviviruses (20–40% identity, 60–80% similarity) [289], therefore, these findings reveal the capacity of a secreted viral protein from related flaviviruses named as NS1 flaviviral toxin as critical for pan-flavivirus pathogenesis through modulation of the endothelial barrier function in a tissue-specific manner, potentially influencing virus dissemination and pathogenesis of target organs and representing a novel target for anti-flaviviral therapy and potential vaccine candidates against flavivirus infections.

2. Concluding remarks (*PART II*)

Systemic vascular leakage associated with DENV infection is the most serious complication and the most important contributor to severe clinical outcomes during severe dengue disease that result in life-threatening complications such as hypotension, organ failure, and shock. Epidemiological data strongly associate severe dengue disease with secondary heterotypic DENV infections occurring in the presence of pre-existing antibody responses, widely attributed to the phenomenon of *antibody-dependent enhancement* (ADE). Numerous studies *in vivo* and *in vitro* have tightened DENV-ADE to the increased activation of immune cells such as monocytes, macrophages, dendritic cells, and mast cells leading to the generation of the pro-inflammatory environment found in many patients undergoing severe dengue, known as "*cytokine storm*". Along with DENV-ADE, heterotypic immunity originated during primary DENV infection may also lead to alterations in immune responses of T cells, skewed by the 'memory' of the previous infection, referred to as '*original antigenic sin*'. These DENV cross-reactive T cell responses produce only inflammatory cytokines and might be inherently inefficient in killing DENV-infected cells, resulting in enhanced infection, which may predispose to the immunopathology of DENV.

Along with this evidence, in the last decades, several other immunologic mechanisms such as activation of complement pathways and autoimmune responses (e.g. mimetic anti-DENV antibodies) have been also linked to ensure severe dengue manifestations leading to the activation and apoptosis of immune cells and endothelial cells, aggregation of platelets, and inactivation of plasma proteins involved in coagulation cascades. On the other hand, viral biomarkers such as NS1, which high circulating levels correlated with the appearance of severe dengue disease, was reported to modulate complement pathways, facilitating virus infection via immune evasion strategies. NS1 has demonstrated to exert an amazing array of different functions. More recently, NS1 was demonstrated to be a multitasking protein of the flavivirus genus which could directly cause disruption of the EGL and endothelial cell-to-cell contacts, two main components of the homeostasis balance in the microvasculature, and to induce the production of soluble immunoregulators resulting in increased endothelial barrier dysfunction and vascular leakage. This evidence provides new insights into the biology of the multifaceted NS1 protein of flavivirus that may improve the understanding of the flavivirus pathogenesis, strongly supporting the inclusion of NS1 protein in flavivirus vaccine development and the generation of new targets for future therapies against flavivirus infections.

In conclusion, the immunopathogenesis of DENV infection represents an extraordinarily complex interplay between several viral and host factors that together contribute intimately to the activation of distinct immunopathological processes that although were intended to control the viral infection and replication, instead unleash an unbalanced host immune response leading to increased endothelial dysfunction and vascular leakage, reflected in the appearance of dengue severe manifestations. As no effective vaccine or antiviral therapy are available to treat either prophylactically or therapeutically the DENV infection, the incidence of dengue disease is expanding globally and continues to threat the public health services worldwide, particularly in endemic areas. An increased understanding of DENV immunopathogenesis mechanisms involved in the development of severe disease, their components, biological triggers, and their potential connections will assist not only the development of potentially more effective novel therapeutic interventions but also the understanding of dengue vaccine efficacy or vaccine adverse events that can be considered during vaccine trial interventions.

Acknowledgements

To the Canadian Institutes of Health Research and the International Development Research Centre (Projects 108,412 & 109,071–002) and the Fondo Mixto CONACYT-Gobierno del Estado de Yucatan (Project YUC-2017-2103-01-556).

Author details

Henry Puerta-Guardo[1*], Scott B. Biering[2], Eva Harris[2],
Norma Pavia-Ruz[3], Gonzalo Vázquez-Prokopec[4], Guadalupe Ayora-Talavera[3]
and Pablo Manrique-Saide[1]

1 Collaborative Unit for Entomological Bioassays and Laboratory for Biological Control of *Aedes aegypti*, Campus of Biological and Agricultural Sciences, Universidad Autonoma de Yucatan, Merida, Yucatan, Mexico

2 Division of Infectious Diseases and Vaccinology, School of Public Health, University of California, Berkeley, USA

3 Centro de Investigaciones Regionales, Dr. Hideyo Noguchi, Universidad Autonoma de Yucatan, Merida, Yucatan, Mexico

4 Department of Environmental Sciences, Emory University, Atlanta, Georgia, USA

*Address all correspondence to: hpuertaguardo@gmail.com

References

[1] Green S, Rothman A. Immunopathological mechanisms in dengue and dengue hemorrhagic fever. Current Opinion in Infectious Diseases. 2006;**19**(5):429-436

[2] World Health O. Dengue Guidelines for Diagnosis, Treatment, Prevention and Control: New Edition. Geneva: World Health Organization; 2009

[3] Trung DT, Wills B. Systemic vascular leakage associated with dengue infections—the clinical perspective. Current Topics in Microbiology and Immunology. 2010;**338**:57-66

[4] Yacoub S, Wertheim H, Simmons CP, Screaton G, Wills B. Cardiovascular manifestations of the emerging dengue pandemic. Nature Reviews. Cardiology. 2014;**11**(6):335-345

[5] Yacoub S, Lam PK, Vu le HM, Le TL, Ha NT, Toan TT, et al. Association of microvascular function and endothelial biomarkers with clinical outcome in dengue: An observational study. The Journal of Infectious Diseases. 2016;**214**(5):697-706

[6] Srikiatkhachorn A. Plasma leakage in dengue haemorrhagic fever. Thrombosis and Haemostasis. 2009;**102**(6):1042-1049

[7] OhAinle M, Balmaseda A, Macalalad AR, Tellez Y, Zody MC, Saborío S, et al. Dynamics of dengue disease severity determined by the interplay between viral genetics and serotype-specific immunity. Science Translational Medicine. 2011;**3**(114):114ra28-114ra28

[8] Malavige GN, Ogg GS. T cell responses in dengue viral infections. Journal of Clinical Virology. 2013;**58**(4):605-611

[9] Beatty PR, Puerta-Guardo H, Killingbeck SS, Glasner DR, Hopkins K, Harris E. Dengue virus NS1 triggers endothelial permeability and vascular leak that is prevented by NS1 vaccination. Science Translational Medicine. 2015;**7**(304):304ra141

[10] Rothman AL. Immunity to dengue virus: A tale of original antigenic sin and tropical cytokine storms. Nature Reviews. Immunology. 2011;**11**(8):532-543

[11] Srikiatkhachorn A, Mathew A, Rothman AL. Immune-mediated cytokine storm and its role in severe dengue. Seminars in Immunopathology. 2017;**39**(5):563-574

[12] Libraty DH, Young PR, Pickering D, Endy TP, Kalayanarooj S, Green S, et al. High circulating levels of the dengue virus nonstructural protein NS1 early in dengue illness correlate with the development of dengue hemorrhagic fever. The Journal of Infectious Diseases. 2002;**186**(8):1165-1168

[13] Rothman AL. Dengue: Defining protective versus pathologic immunity. The Journal of Clinical Investigation. 2004;**113**(7):946-951

[14] Vaughn DW, Green S, Kalayanarooj S, Innis BL, Nimmannitya S, Suntayakorn S, et al. Dengue viremia titer, antibody response pattern, and virus serotype correlate with disease severity. The Journal of Infectious Diseases. 2000;**181**(1):2-9

[15] Mangada MM, Rothman AL. Altered cytokine responses of dengue-specific CD4+ T cells to heterologous serotypes. Journal of Immunology. 2005;**175**(4):2676-2683

[16] Guzman MG, Alvarez M, Halstead SB. Secondary infection as a risk factor for dengue hemorrhagic fever/dengue shock syndrome: An historical perspective and role of

antibody-dependent enhancement of infection. Archives of Virology. 2013;**158**(7):1445-1459

[17] Sangkawibha N, Rojanasuphot S, Ahandrik S, Viriyapongse S, Jatanasen S, Salitul V, et al. Risk factors in dengue shock syndrome: A prospective epidemiologic study in Rayong, Thailand. I. The 1980 outbreak. American Journal of Epidemiology. 1984;**120**(5):653-669

[18] Wang WH, Urbina AN, Chang MR, Assavalapsakul W, Lu PL, Chen YH, et al. Dengue hemorrhagic fever—a systemic literature review of current perspectives on pathogenesis, prevention and control. Journal of Microbiology, Immunology, and Infection. 2020;**20**:30067

[19] Conde JN, Silva EM, Barbosa AS, Mohana-Borges R. The complement system in Flavivirus infections. Frontiers in Microbiology. 2017;**8**:213

[20] Malasit P. Complement and dengue haemorrhagic fever/shock syndrome. The Southeast Asian Journal of Tropical Medicine and Public Health. 1987;**18**(3):316-320

[21] Rico-Hesse R. Dengue virus markers of virulence and pathogenicity. Future Virology. 2009;**4**(6):581

[22] Katzelnick LC, Fonville JM, Gromowski GD, Bustos Arriaga J, Green A, James SL, et al. Dengue viruses cluster antigenically but not as discrete serotypes. Science. 2015;**349**(6254):1338-1343

[23] Katzelnick LC, Montoya M, Gresh L, Balmaseda A, Harris E. Neutralizing antibody titers against dengue virus correlate with protection from symptomatic infection in a longitudinal cohort. Proceedings of the National Academy of Sciences of the United States of America. 2016;**113**(3):728-733

[24] Waggoner JJ, Balmaseda A, Gresh L, Sahoo MK, Montoya M, Wang C, et al. Homotypic dengue virus reinfections in Nicaraguan children. The Journal of Infectious Diseases. 2016;**214**(7):986-993

[25] Olkowski S, Forshey BM, Morrison AC, Rocha C, Vilcarromero S, Halsey ES, et al. Reduced risk of disease during postsecondary dengue virus infections. The Journal of Infectious Diseases. 2013;**208**(6):1026-1033

[26] Simmons CP, Chau TN, Thuy TT, Tuan NM, Hoang DM, Thien NT, et al. Maternal antibody and viral factors in the pathogenesis of dengue virus in infants. The Journal of Infectious Diseases. 2007;**196**(3):416-424

[27] Kliks SC, Nimmanitya S, Nisalak A, Burke DS. Evidence that maternal dengue antibodies are important in the development of dengue hemorrhagic fever in infants. The American Journal of Tropical Medicine and Hygiene. 1988;**38**(2):411-419

[28] Kouri GP, Guzman MG, Bravo JR, Triana C. Dengue haemorrhagic fever/dengue shock syndrome: Lessons from the Cuban epidemic, 1981. Bulletin of the World Health Organization. 1989;**67**(4):375-380

[29] Katzelnick LC, Gresh L, Halloran ME, Mercado JC, Kuan G, Gordon A, et al. Antibody-dependent enhancement of severe dengue disease in humans. Science. 2017;**358**(6365):929-932

[30] Tsai WY, Chen HL, Tsai JJ, Dejnirattisai W, Jumnainsong A, Mongkolsapaya J, et al. Potent neutralizing human monoclonal antibodies preferentially target mature dengue virus particles: Implication for novel strategy for dengue vaccine. Journal of Virology. 2018;**92**(23)

[31] Lai CY, Tsai WY, Lin SR, Kao CL, Hu HP, King CC, et al. Antibodies to

envelope glycoprotein of dengue virus during the natural course of infection are predominantly cross-reactive and recognize epitopes containing highly conserved residues at the fusion loop of domain II. Journal of Virology. 2008;**82**(13):6631-6643

[32] Schieffelin JS, Costin JM, Nicholson CO, Orgeron NM, Fontaine KA, Isern S, et al. Neutralizing and non-neutralizing monoclonal antibodies against dengue virus E protein derived from a naturally infected patient. Virology Journal. 2010;**7**(1):28

[33] Pierson TC, Fremont DH, Kuhn RJ, Diamond MS. Structural insights into the mechanisms of antibody-mediated neutralization of flavivirus infection: Implications for vaccine development. Cell Host & Microbe. 2008;**4**(3):229-238

[34] Heinz FX, Stiasny K. Flaviviruses and their antigenic structure. Journal of Clinical Virology. 2012;**55**(4):289-295

[35] Sun H, Chen Q, Lai H. Development of antibody therapeutics against Flaviviruses. International Journal of Molecular Sciences. 2017;**19**(1):54

[36] Hu D, Zhu Z, Li S, Deng Y, Wu Y, Zhang N, et al. A broadly neutralizing germline-like human monoclonal antibody against dengue virus envelope domain III. PLoS Pathogens. 2019;**15**(6):e1007836

[37] Durham ND, Agrawal A, Waltari E, Croote D, Zanini F, Fouch M, et al. Broadly neutralizing human antibodies against dengue virus identified by single B cell transcriptomics. eLife. 2019;**8**:e52384

[38] Sukupolvi-Petty S, Austin SK, Engle M, Brien JD, Dowd KA, Williams KL, et al. Structure and function analysis of therapeutic monoclonal antibodies against dengue virus type 2. Journal of Virology. 2010;**84**(18):9227-9239

[39] Guzman MG, Hermida L, Bernardo L, Ramirez R, Guillen G. Domain III of the envelope protein as a dengue vaccine target. Expert Review of Vaccines. 2010;**9**(2):137-147

[40] Beltramello M, Williams KL, Simmons CP, Macagno A, Simonelli L, Quyen NT, et al. The human immune response to dengue virus is dominated by highly cross-reactive antibodies endowed with neutralizing and enhancing activity. Cell Host & Microbe. 2010;**8**(3):271-283

[41] Heinz FX, Stiasny K. Flaviviruses and flavivirus vaccines. Vaccine. 2012;**30**(29):4301-4306

[42] Kuhn RJ, Zhang W, Rossmann MG, Pletnev SV, Corver J, Lenches E, et al. Structure of dengue virus: Implications for flavivirus organization, maturation, and fusion. Cell. 2002;**108**(5):717-725

[43] Gallichotte EN, Widman DG, Yount BL, Wahala WM, Durbin A, Whitehead S, et al. A new quaternary structure epitope on dengue virus serotype 2 is the target of durable type-specific neutralizing antibodies. MBio. 2015;**6**(5):e01461-15

[44] Widman DG, Young E, Nivarthi U, Swanstrom JA, Royal SR, Yount BL, et al. Transplantation of a quaternary structure neutralizing antibody epitope from dengue virus serotype 3 into serotype 4. Scientific Reports. 2017;**7**(1):17169

[45] de Alwis R, Smith SA, Olivarez NP, Messer WB, Huynh JP, Wahala WM, et al. Identification of human neutralizing antibodies that bind to complex epitopes on dengue virions. Proceedings of the National Academy of Sciences of the United States of America. 2012;**109**(19):7439-7444

[46] Dejnirattisai W, Wongwiwat W, Supasa S, Zhang X, Dai X, Rouvinsky A, et al. Corrigendum: A new class of highly potent, broadly neutralizing

antibodies isolated from viremic patients infected with dengue virus. Nature Immunology. 2015;**16**(7):785

[47] Li J, Watterson D, Chang CW, Che XY, Li XQ, Ericsson DJ, et al. Structural and functional characterization of a cross-reactive dengue virus neutralizing antibody that recognizes a cryptic epitope. Structure. 2018;**26**(1):51-9.e4

[48] Dejnirattisai W, Jumnainsong A, Onsirisakul N, Fitton P, Vasanawathana S, Limpitikul W, et al. Cross-reacting antibodies enhance dengue virus infection in humans. Science. 2010;**328** (5979):745-748

[49] Zybert IA, van der Ende-Metselaar H, Wilschut J, Smit JM. Functional importance of dengue virus maturation: Infectious properties of immature virions. The Journal of General Virology. 2008;**89** (Pt 12):3047-3051

[50] Dos Santos Franco L, Gushi LT, Luiz WB, Amorim JH. Seeking Flavivirus cross-protective immunity. Frontiers in Immunology. 2019;**10**:2260

[51] Churdboonchart V, Bhamarapravati N, Peampramprecha S, Sirinavin S. Antibodies against dengue viral proteins in primary and secondary dengue hemorrhagic fever. The American Journal of Tropical Medicine and Hygiene. 1991;**44**(5):481-493

[52] Valdes K, Alvarez M, Pupo M, Vazquez S, Rodriguez R, Guzman MG. Human dengue antibodies against structural and nonstructural proteins. Clinical and Diagnostic Laboratory Immunology. 2000;**7**(5):856-857

[53] Gutsche I, Coulibaly F, Voss JE, Salmon J, d'Alayer J, Ermonval M, et al. Secreted dengue virus nonstructural protein NS1 is an atypical barrel-shaped high-density lipoprotein. Proceedings of the National Academy of Sciences of the United States of America. 2011;**108**(19):8003-8008

[54] Young PR, Hilditch PA, Bletchly C, Halloran W. An antigen capture enzyme-linked immunosorbent assay reveals high levels of the dengue virus protein NS1 in the sera of infected patients. Journal of Clinical Microbiology. 2000;**38**(3):1053-1057

[55] Thomas L, Najioullah F, Verlaeten O, Martial J, Brichler S, Kaidomar S, et al. Relationship between nonstructural protein 1 detection and plasma virus load in dengue patients. The American Journal of Tropical Medicine and Hygiene. 2010;**83**(3):696-699

[56] Dussart P, Labeau B, Lagathu G, Louis P, Nunes MR, Rodrigues SG, et al. Evaluation of an enzyme immunoassay for detection of dengue virus NS1 antigen in human serum. Clinical and Vaccine Immunology. 2006;**13**(11):1185-1189

[57] Jayathilaka D, Gomes L, Jeewandara C, Jayarathna GSB, Herath D, Perera PA, et al. Role of NS1 antibodies in the pathogenesis of acute secondary dengue infection. Nature Communications. 2018;**9**(1):5242

[58] Shu PY, Chen LK, Chang SF, Yueh YY, Chow L, Chien LJ, et al. Dengue NS1-specific antibody responses: Isotype distribution and serotyping in patients with dengue fever and dengue hemorrhagic fever. Journal of Medical Virology. 2000;**62**(2):224-232

[59] Shriver-Lake LC, Liu JL, Zabetakis D, Sugiharto VA, Lee CR, Defang GN, et al. Selection and characterization of anti-dengue NS1 single domain antibodies. Scientific Reports. 2018;**8**(1):18086

[60] Edeling MA, Austin SK, Shrestha B, Dowd KA, Mukherjee S, Nelson CA, et al. Potent dengue virus neutralization

by a therapeutic antibody with low monovalent affinity requires bivalent engagement. PLoS Pathogens. 2014;**10**(4):e1004072

[61] Kaufman BM, Summers PL, Dubois DR, Cohen WH, Gentry MK, Timchak RL, et al. Monoclonal antibodies for dengue virus prM glycoprotein protect mice against lethal dengue infection. The American Journal of Tropical Medicine and Hygiene. 1989;**41**(5):576-580

[62] Hertz T, Beatty PR, MacMillen Z, Killingbeck SS, Wang C, Harris E. Antibody epitopes identified in critical regions of dengue virus nonstructural 1 protein in mouse vaccination and natural human infections. Journal of Immunology. 2017;**198**(10):4025-4035

[63] Henchal EA, Henchal LS, Schlesinger JJ. Synergistic interactions of anti-NS1 monoclonal antibodies protect passively immunized mice from lethal challenge with dengue 2 virus. The Journal of General Virology 1988;69 (Pt 8):2101-2107

[64] Lai CJ, Goncalvez AP, Men R, Wernly C, Donau O, Engle RE, et al. Epitope determinants of a chimpanzee dengue virus type 4 (DENV-4)-neutralizing antibody and protection against DENV-4 challenge in mice and rhesus monkeys by passively transferred humanized antibody. Journal of Virology. 2007;**81**(23):12766-12774

[65] Goncalvez AP, Engle RE, St Claire M, Purcell RH, Lai CJ. Monoclonal antibody-mediated enhancement of dengue virus infection in vitro and in vivo and strategies for prevention. Proceedings of the National Academy of Sciences of the United States of America. 2007;**104**(22):9422-9427

[66] Mehlhop E, Ansarah-Sobrinho C, Johnson S, Engle M, Fremont DH, Pierson TC, et al. Complement protein C1q inhibits antibody-dependent enhancement of flavivirus infection in an IgG subclass-specific manner. Cell Host & Microbe. 2007;**2**(6):417-426

[67] Falgout B, Bray M, Schlesinger JJ, Lai CJ. Immunization of mice with recombinant vaccinia virus expressing authentic dengue virus nonstructural protein NS1 protects against lethal dengue virus encephalitis. Journal of Virology. 1990;**64**(9):4356-4363

[68] Garcia G, Arango M, Perez AB, Fonte L, Sierra B, Rodriguez-Roche R, et al. Antibodies from patients with dengue viral infection mediate cellular cytotoxicity. Journal of Clinical Virology. 2006;**37**(1):53-57

[69] Reyes-Sandoval A, Ludert JE. The dual role of the antibody response against the Flavivirus non-structural protein 1 (NS1) in protection and Immuno-pathogenesis. Frontiers in Immunology. 2019;**10**:1651

[70] Sharma M, Glasner DR, Watkins H, Puerta-Guardo H, Kassa Y, Egan MA, et al. Magnitude and functionality of the NS1-specific antibody response elicited by a live-attenuated tetravalent dengue vaccine candidate. The Journal of Infectious Diseases. 2020;**221**(6):867-877

[71] Kliks SC, Nisalak A, Brandt WE, Wahl L, Burke DS. Antibody-dependent enhancement of dengue virus growth in human monocytes as a risk factor for dengue hemorrhagic fever. The American Journal of Tropical Medicine and Hygiene. 1989;**40**(4):444-451

[72] Halstead SB, O'Rourke EJ. Antibody-enhanced dengue virus infection in primate leukocytes. Nature. 1977;**265**(5596):739-741

[73] Puerta-Guardo H, Raya-Sandino A, González-Mariscal L, Rosales VH, Ayala-Dávila J, Chávez-Mungía B, et al. The cytokine response of U937-derived

macrophages infected through antibody-dependent enhancement of dengue virus disrupts cell apical-junction complexes and increases vascular permeability. Journal of Virology. 2013;**87**(13):7486-7501

[74] Chareonsirisuthigul T, Kalayanarooj S, Ubol S. Dengue virus (DENV) antibody-dependent enhancement of infection upregulates the production of anti-inflammatory cytokines, but suppresses anti-DENV free radical and pro-inflammatory cytokine production, in THP-1 cells. The Journal of General Virology 2007;**88** (Pt 2):365-375

[75] Boonnak K, Slike BM, Burgess TH, Mason RM, Wu SJ, Sun P, et al. Role of dendritic cells in antibody-dependent enhancement of dengue virus infection. Journal of Virology. 2008;**82**(8):3939-3951

[76] Boonnak K, Dambach KM, Donofrio GC, Tassaneetrithep B, Marovich MA. Cell type specificity and host genetic polymorphisms influence antibody-dependent enhancement of dengue virus infection. Journal of Virology. 2011;**85**(4):1671-1683

[77] Ubol S, Phuklia W, Kalayanarooj S, Modhiran N. Mechanisms of immune evasion induced by a complex of dengue virus and preexisting enhancing antibodies. The Journal of Infectious Diseases. 2010;**201**(6):923-935

[78] Halstead SB, Nimmannitya S, Yamarat C, Russell PK. Hemorrhagic fever in Thailand; recent knowledge regarding etiology. Japanese Journal of Medical Science & Biology. 1967;**20** Suppl:96-103

[79] Endy TP, Nisalak A, Chunsuttiwat S, Libraty DH, Green S, Rothman AL, et al. Spatial and temporal circulation of dengue virus serotypes: A prospective study of primary school children in Kamphaeng Phet, Thailand. American Journal of Epidemiology. 2002;**156**(1):52-59

[80] Gibbons RV, Kalanarooj S, Jarman RG, Nisalak A, Vaughn DW, Endy TP, et al. Analysis of repeat hospital admissions for dengue to estimate the frequency of third or fourth dengue infections resulting in admissions and dengue hemorrhagic fever, and serotype sequences. The American Journal of Tropical Medicine and Hygiene. 2007;**77**(5):910-913

[81] Gan ES, Ting DH, Chan KR. The mechanistic role of antibodies to dengue virus in protection and disease pathogenesis. Expert Review of Anti-Infective Therapy. 2017;**15**(2):111-119

[82] Halstead SB. Observations related to pathogensis of dengue hemorrhagic fever. VI. Hypotheses and discussion. The Yale Journal of Biology and Medicine. 1970;**42**(5):350-362

[83] Halstead SB, Nimmannitya S, Cohen SN. Observations related to pathogenesis of dengue hemorrhagic fever. IV. Relation of disease severity to antibody response and virus recovered. The Yale Journal of Biology and Medicine. 1970;**42**(5):311-328

[84] Chau TN, Hieu NT, Anders KL, Wolbers M, Lien le B, Hieu LT, et al. Dengue virus infections and maternal antibody decay in a prospective birth cohort study of Vietnamese infants. The Journal of Infectious Diseases. 2009;**200**(12):1893-1900

[85] Chau TN, Quyen NT, Thuy TT, Tuan NM, Hoang DM, Dung NT, et al. Dengue in Vietnamese infants—results of infection-enhancement assays correlate with age-related disease epidemiology, and cellular immune responses correlate with disease severity. The Journal of Infectious Diseases. 2008;**198**(4):516-524

[86] Nguyen TH, Lei HY, Nguyen TL, Lin YS, Huang KJ, Le BL, et al. Dengue hemorrhagic fever in infants: A study of clinical and cytokine profiles. The Journal of Infectious Diseases. 2004;**189**(2):221-232

[87] Balsitis SJ, Williams KL, Lachica R, Flores D, Kyle JL, Mehlhop E, et al. Lethal antibody enhancement of dengue disease in mice is prevented by fc modification. PLoS Pathogens. 2010;**6**(2):e1000790

[88] Halstead SB. In vivo enhancement of dengue virus infection in rhesus monkeys by passively transferred antibody. The Journal of Infectious Diseases. 1979;**140**(4):527-533

[89] Hadinegoro SR, Arredondo-Garcia JL, Capeding MR, Deseda C, Chotpitayasunondh T, Dietze R, et al. Efficacy and long-term safety of a dengue vaccine in regions of endemic disease. The New England Journal of Medicine. 2015;**373**(13):1195-1206

[90] Sridhar S, Luedtke A, Langevin E, Zhu M, Bonaparte M, Machabert T, et al. Effect of dengue Serostatus on dengue vaccine safety and efficacy. The New England Journal of Medicine. 2018;**379**(4):327-340

[91] Ferguson NM, Rodriguez-Barraquer I, Dorigatti I, Mier YT-RL, Laydon DJ, Cummings DA. Benefits and risks of the Sanofi-Pasteur dengue vaccine: Modeling optimal deployment. Science. 2016;**353**(6303):1033-1036

[92] Pierson TC, Xu Q, Nelson S, Oliphant T, Nybakken GE, Fremont DH, et al. The stoichiometry of antibody-mediated neutralization and enhancement of West Nile virus infection. Cell Host & Microbe. 2007;**1**(2):135-145

[93] Roehrig JT. Antigenic structure of flavivirus proteins. Advances in Virus Research. 2003;**59**:141-175

[94] Smith SA, Zhou Y, Olivarez NP, Broadwater AH, de Silva AM, Crowe JE Jr. Persistence of circulating memory B cell clones with potential for dengue virus disease enhancement for decades following infection. Journal of Virology. 2012;**86**(5):2665-2675

[95] Kuhn RJ, Dowd KA, Beth Post C, Pierson TC. Shake, rattle, and roll: Impact of the dynamics of flavivirus particles on their interactions with the host. Virology. 2015;**479-480**:508-517

[96] Pierson TC, Diamond MS. Degrees of maturity: The complex structure and biology of flaviviruses. Current Opinion in Virology. 2012;**2**(2):168-175

[97] Junjhon J, Edwards TJ, Utaipat U, Bowman VD, Holdaway HA, Zhang W, et al. Influence of pr-M cleavage on the heterogeneity of extracellular dengue virus particles. Journal of Virology. 2010;**84**(16):8353-8358

[98] Rodenhuis-Zybert IA, van der Schaar HM, da Silva Voorham JM, van der Ende-Metselaar H, Lei HY, Wilschut J, et al. Immature dengue virus: a veiled pathogen? PLoS Pathogens. 2010;**6**(1):e1000718

[99] Rodenhuis-Zybert IA, Wilschut J, Smit JM. Partial maturation: An immune-evasion strategy of dengue virus? Trends in Microbiology. 2011;**19**(5):248-254

[100] Smith SA, Nivarthi UK, de Alwis R, Kose N, Sapparapu G, Bombardi R, et al. Dengue virus prM-specific human monoclonal antibodies with virus replication-enhancing properties recognize a single Immunodominant antigenic site. Journal of Virology. 2016;**90**(2):780-789

[101] Ayala-Nunez NV, Hoornweg TE, van de Pol DP, Sjollema KA, Flipse J, van der Schaar HM, et al. How antibodies alter the cell entry pathway of dengue virus particles in macrophages. Scientific Reports. 2016;**6**:28768

[102] Kontny U, Kurane I, Ennis FA. Gamma interferon augments Fc gamma receptor-mediated dengue virus infection of human monocytic cells. Journal of Virology. 1988;**62**(11):3928-3933

[103] Littaua R, Kurane I, Ennis FA. Human IgG fc receptor II mediates antibody-dependent enhancement of dengue virus infection. Journal of Immunology. 1990;**144**(8):3183-3186

[104] Brown MG, McAlpine SM, Huang YY, Haidl ID, Al-Afif A, Marshall JS, et al. RNA sensors enable human mast cell anti-viral chemokine production and IFN-mediated protection in response to antibody-enhanced dengue virus infection. PLoS One. 2012;**7**(3):e34055-e

[105] Brown MG, Huang YY, Marshall JS, King CA, Hoskin DW, Anderson R. Dramatic caspase-dependent apoptosis in antibody-enhanced dengue virus infection of human mast cells. Journal of Leukocyte Biology. 2009;**85**(1):71-80

[106] Brown MG, King CA, Sherren C, Marshall JS, Anderson R. A dominant role for FcgammaRII in antibody-enhanced dengue virus infection of human mast cells and associated CCL5 release. Journal of Leukocyte Biology. 2006;**80**(6):1242-1250

[107] King CA, Anderson R, Marshall JS. Dengue virus selectively induces human mast cell chemokine production. Journal of Virology. 2002;**76**(16):8408-8419

[108] Diamond MS, Edgil D, Roberts TG, Lu B, Harris E. Infection of human cells by dengue virus is modulated by different cell types and viral strains. Journal of Virology. 2000;**74**(17):7814

[109] Tsai T-T, Chuang Y-J, Lin Y-S, Chang C-P, Wan S-W, Lin S-H, et al. Antibody-dependent enhancement infection facilitates dengue virus-regulated signaling of IL-10 production in monocytes. PLoS Neglected Tropical Diseases. 2014;**8**(11):e3320

[110] Flipse J, Diosa-Toro MA, Hoornweg TE, van de Pol DP, Urcuqui-Inchima S, Smit JM. Antibody-dependent enhancement of dengue virus infection in primary human macrophages; balancing higher fusion against antiviral responses. Scientific Reports. 2016;**6**:29201

[111] Jiang L, Sun Q. The expression profile of human peripheral blood mononuclear cell miRNA is altered by antibody-dependent enhancement of infection with dengue virus serotype 3. Virology Journal. 2018;**15**(1):50

[112] Sun P, Bauza K, Pal S, Liang Z, Wu SJ, Beckett C, et al. Infection and activation of human peripheral blood monocytes by dengue viruses through the mechanism of antibody-dependent enhancement. Virology. 2011;**421**(2):245-252

[113] Morens DM, Halstead SB. Measurement of antibody-dependent infection enhancement of four dengue virus serotypes by monoclonal and polyclonal antibodies. The Journal of General Virology 1990;**71**(Pt 12): 2909-2914

[114] Modhiran N, Kalayanarooj S, Ubol S. Subversion of innate defenses by the interplay between DENV and pre-existing enhancing antibodies: TLRs signaling collapse. PLoS Neglected Tropical Diseases. 2010;**4**(12):e924

[115] Fang YT, Wan SW, Lu YT, Yao JH, Lin CF, Hsu LJ, et al. Autophagy facilitates antibody-enhanced dengue virus infection in human pre-basophil/mast cells. PLoS One. 2014;**9**(10):e110655

[116] Al-Soudi A, Kaaij MH, Tas SW. Endothelial cells: From innocent bystanders to active participants in immune responses. Autoimmunity Reviews. 2017;**16**(9):951-962

[117] Young MR. Endothelial cells in the eyes of an immunologist. Cancer Immunology, Immunotherapy. 2012;**61**(10):1609-1616

[118] Zellweger RM, Prestwood TR, Shresta S. Enhanced infection of liver sinusoidal endothelial cells in a mouse model of antibody-induced severe dengue disease. Cell Host & Microbe. 2010;**7**(2):128-139

[119] Arevalo MT, Simpson-Haidaris PJ, Kou Z, Schlesinger JJ, Jin X. Primary human endothelial cells support direct but not antibody-dependent enhancement of dengue viral infection. Journal of Medical Virology. 2009;**81**(3):519-528

[120] Talavera D, Castillo AM, Dominguez MC, Gutierrez AE, Meza I. IL8 release, tight junction and cytoskeleton dynamic reorganization conducive to permeability increase are induced by dengue virus infection of microvascular endothelial monolayers. The Journal of General Virology. 2004;**85**(Pt 7):1801-1813

[121] Povoa TF, Alves AM, Oliveira CA, Nuovo GJ, Chagas VL, Paes MV. The pathology of severe dengue in multiple organs of human fatal cases: Histopathology, ultrastructure and virus replication. PLoS One. 2014;**9**(4):e83386

[122] Bruggeman CW, Houtzager J, Dierdorp B, Kers J, Pals ST, Lutter R, et al. Tissue-specific expression of IgG receptors by human macrophages ex vivo. PLoS One. 2019;**14**(10):e0223264

[123] Jessie K, Fong MY, Devi S, Lam SK, Wong KT. Localization of dengue virus in naturally infected human tissues, by immunohistochemistry and in situ hybridization. The Journal of Infectious Diseases. 2004;**189**(8):1411-1418

[124] Kangwanpong D, Bhamarapravati N, Lucia HL. Diagnosing dengue virus infection in archived autopsy tissues by means of the in situ PCR method: A case report. Clinical and Diagnostic Virology. 1995;**3**(2):165-172

[125] Win MM, Charngkaew K, Punyadee N, Aye KS, Win N, Chaisri U, et al. Ultrastructural features of human liver specimens from patients who died of dengue hemorrhagic fever. Tropical Medicine and Infectious Diseases. 2019;**4**(2):63

[126] Aye KS, Charngkaew K, Win N, Wai KZ, Moe K, Punyadee N, et al. Pathologic highlights of dengue hemorrhagic fever in 13 autopsy cases from Myanmar. Human Pathology. 2014;**45**(6):1221-1233

[127] Begum F, Das S, Mukherjee D, Mal S, Ray U. Insight into the tropism of dengue virus in humans. Viruses. 2019;**11**(12):1136

[128] Kuczera D, Assolini JP, Tomiotto-Pellissier F, Pavanelli WR, Silveira GF. Highlights for dengue Immunopathogenesis: Antibody-dependent enhancement, cytokine storm, and beyond. Journal of Interferon & Cytokine Research. 2018;**38**(2):69-80

[129] Lin YW, Wang KJ, Lei HY, Lin YS, Yeh TM, Liu HS, et al. Virus replication and cytokine production in dengue virus-infected human B lymphocytes. Journal of Virology. 2002;**76**(23):12242-12249

[130] Anderson R, Wang S, Osiowy C, Issekutz AC. Activation of endothelial cells via antibody-enhanced dengue virus infection of peripheral blood monocytes. Journal of Virology. 1997;**71**(6):4226-4232

[131] Tisoncik JR, Korth MJ, Simmons CP, Farrar J, Martin TR, Katze MG. Into the eye of the cytokine storm. Microbiology and Molecular Biology Reviews. 2012;**76**(1):16-32

[132] Khaiboullina SF, Levis S, Morzunov SP, Martynova EV, Anokhin VA, Gusev OA, et al. Serum cytokine profiles differentiating hemorrhagic fever with renal syndrome and hantavirus pulmonary syndrome. Frontiers in Immunology. 2017;**8**:567

[133] Guo X-ZJ, Thomas PG. New fronts emerge in the influenza cytokine storm. Seminars in Immunopathology. 2017;**39**(5):541-550

[134] Ye Q, Wang B, Mao J. The pathogenesis and treatment of the 'Cytokine Storm' in COVID-19. The Journal of Infection. 2020;**S0163-4453**(20):30165-30161

[135] Shresta S, Kyle JL, Snider HM, Basavapatna M, Beatty PR, Harris E. Interferon-dependent immunity is essential for resistance to primary dengue virus infection in mice, whereas T- and B-cell-dependent immunity are less critical. Journal of Virology. 2004;**78**(6):2701-2710

[136] Ng JKW, Zhang SL, Tan HC, Yan B, Maria Martinez Gomez J, Tan WY, et al. First experimental In vivo model of enhanced dengue disease severity through maternally acquired heterotypic dengue antibodies. PLoS Pathogens. 2014;**10**(4):e1004031

[137] Moi ML, Lim CK, Takasaki T, Kurane I. Involvement of the fc gamma receptor IIA cytoplasmic domain in antibody-dependent enhancement of dengue virus infection. The Journal of General Virology. 2010;**91**(Pt 1):103-111

[138] Rodrigo WW, Jin X, Blackley SD, Rose RC, Schlesinger JJ. Differential enhancement of dengue virus immune complex infectivity mediated by signaling-competent and signaling-incompetent human Fcgamma RIA (CD64) or FcgammaRIIA (CD32). Journal of Virology. 2006;**80**(20):10128-10138

[139] Flipse J, Wilschut J, Smit JM. Molecular mechanisms involved in antibody-dependent enhancement of dengue virus infection in humans. Traffic. 2013;**14**(1):25-35

[140] Chan CYY, Low JZH, Gan ES, Ong EZ, Zhang SL, Tan HC, et al. Antibody-dependent dengue virus entry modulates cell intrinsic responses for enhanced infection. mSphere. 2019;**4**(5):e00528-19

[141] Halstead SB, Mahalingam S, Marovich MA, Ubol S, Mosser DM. Intrinsic antibody-dependent enhancement of microbial infection in macrophages: Disease regulation by immune complexes. The Lancet Infectious Diseases. 2010;**10**(10):712-722

[142] Huang X, Yue Y, Li D, Zhao Y, Qiu L, Chen J, et al. Antibody-dependent enhancement of dengue virus infection inhibits RLR-mediated type-I IFN-independent signalling through upregulation of cellular autophagy. Scientific Reports. 2016;**6**:22303

[143] Hober D, Poli L, Roblin B, Gestas P, Chungue E, Granic G, et al. Serum levels of tumor necrosis factor-alpha (TNF-alpha), interleukin-6 (IL-6), and interleukin-1 beta (IL-1 beta) in dengue-infected patients. The American Journal of Tropical Medicine and Hygiene. 1993;**48**(3):324-331

[144] Vitarana T, de Silva H, Withana N, Gunasekera C. Elevated tumour necrosis factor in dengue fever and dengue haemorrhagic fever. The Ceylon Medical Journal. 1991;**36**(2):63-65

[145] Meena AA, Murugesan A, Sopnajothi S, Yong YK, Ganesh PS, Vimali IJ, et al. Increase of plasma TNF-alpha is associated with decreased levels of blood platelets in clinical dengue infection. Viral Immunology. 2020;**33**(1):54-60

[146] Tan TY, Chu JJH. Dengue virus-infected human monocytes trigger late

activation of caspase-1, which mediates pro-inflammatory IL-1beta secretion and pyroptosis. The Journal of General Virology. 2013;**94**(Pt 10):2215-2220

[147] Libraty DH, Pichyangkul S, Ajariyakhajorn C, Endy TP, Ennis FA. Human dendritic cells are activated by dengue virus infection: Enhancement by gamma interferon and implications for disease pathogenesis. Journal of Virology. 2001;**75**(8):3501-3508

[148] Luplertlop N, Misse D, Bray D, Deleuze V, Gonzalez JP, Leardkamolkarn V, et al. Dengue-virus-infected dendritic cells trigger vascular leakage through metalloproteinase overproduction. EMBO Reports. 2006;**7**(11):1176-1181

[149] Wu WL, Ho LJ, Chang DM, Chen CH, Lai JH. Triggering of DC migration by dengue virus stimulation of COX-2-dependent signaling cascades in vitro highlights the significance of these cascades beyond inflammation. European Journal of Immunology. 2009;**39**(12):3413-3422

[150] King CA, Marshall JS, Alshurafa H, Anderson R. Release of vasoactive cytokines by antibody-enhanced dengue virus infection of a human mast cell/basophil line. Journal of Virology. 2000;**74**(15):7146-7150

[151] Avirutnan P, Matangkasombut P. Unmasking the role of mast cells in dengue. eLife. 2013;**2**:e00767

[152] Patro ARK, Mohanty S, Prusty BK, Singh DK, Gaikwad S, Saswat T, et al. Cytokine signature associated with disease severity in dengue. Viruses. 2019;**11**(1):34

[153] Espada-Murao LA, Morita K. Dengue and soluble mediators of the innate immune system. Tropical Medicine and Health. 2011;**39**(4 Suppl):53-62

[154] Srikiatkhachorn A, Green S. Markers of dengue disease severity. Current Topics in Microbiology and Immunology. 2010;**338**:67-82

[155] John DV, Lin YS, Perng GC. Biomarkers of severe dengue disease - a review. Journal of Biomedical Science. 2015;**22**:83

[156] Robinson M, Einav S. Towards predicting progression to severe dengue. Trends in Microbiology. 2020;**28**(6):478-486

[157] Lima WG, Souza NA, Fernandes SOA, Cardoso VN, Godoi IP. Serum lipid profile as a predictor of dengue severity: A systematic review and meta-analysis. Reviews in Medical Virology. 2019;**29**(5):e2056

[158] van Gorp EC, Suharti C, Mairuhu AT, Dolmans WM, van Der Ven J, Demacker PN, et al. Changes in the plasma lipid profile as a potential predictor of clinical outcome in dengue hemorrhagic fever. Clinical Infectious Diseases. 2002;**34**(8):1150-1153

[159] Malavige GN, Ogg GS. Pathogenesis of vascular leak in dengue virus infection. Immunology. 2017;**151**(3):261-269

[160] Chaturvedi UC, Nagar R. Nitric oxide in dengue and dengue haemorrhagic fever: Necessity or nuisance? FEMS Immunology and Medical Microbiology. 2009;**56**(1):9-24

[161] Cheng YL, Lin YS, Chen CL, Wan SW, Ou YD, Yu CY, et al. Dengue virus infection causes the activation of distinct NF-kappaB pathways for inducible nitric oxide synthase and TNF-alpha expression in RAW264.7 cells. Mediators of Inflammation. 2015;**2015**:274025

[162] Voraphani N, Khong-phatthanayothin A, Srikaew K, Tontulawat P, Poovorawan Y. Matrix metalloproteinase-9 (mmp-9) in children with dengue virus infection.

Japanese Journal of Infectious Diseases. 2010;**63**(5):346-348

[163] Her Z, Kam YW, Gan VC, Lee B, Thein TL, Tan JJ, et al. Severity of plasma leakage is associated with high levels of interferon gamma-inducible protein 10, hepatocyte growth factor, matrix metalloproteinase 2 (MMP-2), and MMP-9 during dengue virus infection. The Journal of Infectious Diseases. 2017;**215**(1):42-51

[164] Kubelka CF, Azeredo EL, Gandini M, Oliveira-Pinto LM, Barbosa LS, Damasco PV, et al. Metalloproteinases are produced during dengue fever and MMP9 is associated with severity. The Journal of Infection. 2010;**61**(6):501-505

[165] Figueroa CL, Gelvez M, Niederbacher J. Regulators of endothelial integrity as severity predictors in dengue. Biomédica. 2016;**36**(0):148-155

[166] van de Weg CA, Pannuti CS, van den Ham HJ, de Araujo ES, Boas LS, Felix AC, et al. Serum angiopoietin-2 and soluble VEGF receptor 2 are surrogate markers for plasma leakage in patients with acute dengue virus infection. Journal of Clinical Virology. 2014;**60**(4):328-335

[167] Mariko R, Darwin E, Yanwirasti Y, Hadinegoro SR. The difference of Angiopoietin-2 levels between dengue hemorrhagic fever patients with shock and without shock. Open Access Macedonian Journal of Medical Sciences. 2019;7(13):2119-2122

[168] Tang TH, Alonso S, Ng LF, Thein TL, Pang VJ, Leo YS, et al. Increased serum hyaluronic acid and Heparan sulfate in dengue fever: Association with plasma leakage and disease severity. Scientific Reports. 2017;7:46191

[169] Suwarto S, Sasmono RT, Sinto R, Ibrahim E, Suryamin M. Association of Endothelial Glycocalyx and Tight and Adherens junctions with severity of plasma leakage in dengue infection. The Journal of Infectious Diseases. 2017;**215**(6):992-999

[170] Lin CY, Kolliopoulos C, Huang CH, Tenhunen J, Heldin CH, Chen YH, et al. High levels of serum hyaluronan is an early predictor of dengue warning signs and perturbs vascular integrity. eBioMedicine. 2019;**48**:425-441

[171] Espinosa DA, Beatty PR, Puerta-Guardo H, Islam MN, Belisle JT, Perera R, et al. Increased serum sialic acid is associated with morbidity and mortality in a murine model of dengue disease. The Journal of General Virology. 2019;**100**(11):1515-1522

[172] Puerta-Guardo H, Tabata T, Petitt M, Dimitrova M, Glasner DR, Pereira L, et al. Zika virus nonstructural protein 1 disrupts Glycosaminoglycans and causes permeability in developing human placentas. The Journal of Infectious Diseases. 2020;**221**(2):313-324

[173] Puerta-Guardo H, Glasner DR, Espinosa DA, Biering SB, Patana M, Ratnasiri K, et al. Flavivirus NS1 triggers tissue-specific vascular endothelial dysfunction reflecting disease tropism. Cell Reports. 2019;**26**(6):1598-613.e8

[174] Wills BA, Oragui EE, Dung NM, Loan HT, Chau NV, Farrar JJ, et al. Size and charge characteristics of the protein leak in dengue shock syndrome. The Journal of Infectious Diseases. 2004;**190**(4):810-818

[175] Apte-Sengupta S, Sirohi D, Kuhn RJ. Coupling of replication and assembly in flaviviruses. Current Opinion in Virology. 2014;**9**:134-142

[176] Vaughan K, Greenbaum J, Blythe M, Peters B, Sette A. Meta-analysis of all immune epitope data

in the Flavivirus genus: Inventory of current immune epitope data status in the context of virus immunity and immunopathology. Viral Immunology. 2010;**23**(3):259-284

[177] Weiskopf D, Sette A. T-cell immunity to infection with dengue virus in humans. Frontiers in Immunology. 2014;**5**:93

[178] Tian Y, Grifoni A, Sette A, Weiskopf D. Human T cell response to dengue virus infection. Frontiers in Immunology. 2019;**10**:2125

[179] Yauch LE, Zellweger RM, Kotturi MF, Qutubuddin A, Sidney J, Peters B, et al. A protective role for dengue virus-specific CD8+ T cells. Journal of Immunology (Baltimore, Md.: 1950). 2009;**182**(8):4865-4873

[180] Rivino L, Kumaran EA, Jovanovic V, Nadua K, Teo EW, Pang SW, et al. Differential targeting of viral components by CD4+ versus CD8+ T lymphocytes in dengue virus infection. Journal of Virology. 2013;**87**(5):2693-2706

[181] Weiskopf D, Cerpas C, Angelo MA, Bangs DJ, Sidney J, Paul S, et al. Human CD8+ T-cell responses against the 4 dengue virus serotypes are associated with distinct patterns of protein targets. The Journal of Infectious Diseases. 2015;**212**(11):1743-1751

[182] Appanna R, Huat TL, See LL, Tan PL, Vadivelu J, Devi S. Cross-reactive T-cell responses to the nonstructural regions of dengue viruses among dengue fever and dengue hemorrhagic fever patients in Malaysia. Clinical and Vaccine Immunology. 2007;**14**(8):969-977

[183] Duangchinda T, Dejnirattisai W, Vasanawathana S, Limpitikul W, Tangthawornchaikul N, Malasit P, et al. Immunodominant T-cell responses to dengue virus NS3 are associated with DHF. Proceedings of the National Academy of Sciences of the United States of America. 2010;**107**(39):16922-16927

[184] Simmons CP, Dong T, Chau NV, Dung NT, Chau TN, Thao le TT, et al. Early T-cell responses to dengue virus epitopes in Vietnamese adults with secondary dengue virus infections. Journal of Virology. 2005;**79**(9):5665-5675

[185] Green S, Kurane I, Pincus S, Paoletti E, Ennis FA. Recognition of dengue virus NS1-NS2a proteins by human CD4+ cytotoxic T lymphocyte clones. Virology. 1997;**234**(2):383-386

[186] Espinosa DA, Beatty PR, Reiner GL, Sivick KE, Hix Glickman L, Dubensky TW Jr, et al. Cyclic dinucleotide-Adjuvanted dengue virus nonstructural protein 1 induces protective antibody and T cell responses. Journal of Immunology. 2019;**202**(4):1153-1162

[187] Loke H, Bethell DB, Phuong CX, Dung M, Schneider J, White NJ, et al. Strong HLA class I--restricted T cell responses in dengue hemorrhagic fever: A double-edged sword? The Journal of Infectious Diseases. 2001;**184**(11):1369-1373

[188] Xavier-Carvalho C, Cardoso CC, de Souza Kehdy F, Pacheco AG, Moraes MO. Host genetics and dengue fever. Infection, Genetics and Evolution. 2017;**56**:99-110

[189] Malavige GN, Rostron T, Rohanachandra LT, Jayaratne SD, Fernando N, De Silva AD, et al. HLA class I and class II associations in dengue viral infections in a Sri Lankan population. PLoS One. 2011;**6**(6):e20581

[190] Nguyen TP, Kikuchi M, Vu TQ, Do QH, Tran TT, Vo DT, et al. Protective and enhancing HLA alleles, HLA-DRB1*0901 and HLA-A*24, for severe

forms of dengue virus infection, dengue hemorrhagic fever and dengue shock syndrome. PLoS Neglected Tropical Diseases. 2008;**2**(10):e304

[191] Stephens HA. HLA and other gene associations with dengue disease severity. Current Topics in Microbiology and Immunology. 2010;**338**:99-114

[192] Weiskopf D, Angelo MA, de Azeredo EL, Sidney J, Greenbaum JA, Fernando AN, et al. Comprehensive analysis of dengue virus-specific responses supports an HLA-linked protective role for CD8+ T cells. Proceedings of the National Academy of Sciences of the United States of America. 2013;**110**(22):E2046-E2053

[193] Bashyam HS, Green S, Rothman AL. Dengue virus-reactive CD8+ T cells display quantitative and qualitative differences in their response to variant epitopes of heterologous viral serotypes. Journal of Immunology. 2006;**176**(5):2817-2824

[194] Imrie A, Meeks J, Gurary A, Sukhbataar M, Kitsutani P, Effler P, et al. Differential functional avidity of dengue virus-specific T-cell clones for variant peptides representing heterologous and previously encountered serotypes. Journal of Virology. 2007;**81**(18):10081-10091

[195] Rivino L, Lim MQ. CD4(+) and CD8(+) T-cell immunity to dengue—lessons for the study of Zika virus. Immunology. 2017;**150**(2):146-154

[196] Rosendahl Huber S, van Beek J, de Jonge J, Luytjes W, van Baarle D. T cell responses to viral infections—opportunities for peptide vaccination. Frontiers in Immunology. 2014;**5**:171

[197] Kurane I, Matsutani T, Suzuki R, Takasaki T, Kalayanarooj S, Green S, et al. T-cell responses to dengue virus in humans. Tropical Medicine and Health. 2011;**39**(4 Suppl):45-51

[198] Gagnon SJ, Ennis FA, Rothman AL. Bystander target cell lysis and cytokine production by dengue virus-specific human CD4(+) cytotoxic T-lymphocyte clones. Journal of Virology. 1999;**73**(5):3623-3629

[199] Kurane I, Meager A, Ennis FA. Dengue virus-specific human T cell clones. Serotype crossreactive proliferation, interferon gamma production, and cytotoxic activity. The Journal of Experimental Medicine. 1989;**170**(3):763-775

[200] Aberle JH, Koblischke M, Stiasny K. CD4 T cell responses to flaviviruses. Journal of Clinical Virology. 2018;**108**:126-131

[201] Bukowski JF, Kurane I, Lai CJ, Bray M, Falgout B, Ennis FA. Dengue virus-specific cross-reactive CD8+ human cytotoxic T lymphocytes. Journal of Virology. 1989;**63**(12):5086-5091

[202] An J, Zhou DS, Zhang JL, Morida H, Wang JL, Yasui K. Dengue-specific CD8+ T cells have both protective and pathogenic roles in dengue virus infection. Immunology Letters. 2004;**95**(2):167-174

[203] Elong Ngono A, Chen HW, Tang WW, Joo Y, King K, Weiskopf D, et al. Protective role of cross-reactive CD8 T cells against dengue virus infection. eBioMedicine. 2016;**13**:284-293

[204] Zellweger RM, Tang WW, Eddy WE, King K, Sanchez MC, Shresta S. CD8+ T cells can mediate short-term protection against heterotypic dengue virus reinfection in mice. Journal of Virology. 2015;**89**(12):6494-6505

[205] Screaton G, Mongkolsapaya J, Yacoub S, Roberts C. New insights into the immunopathology and control of dengue virus infection. Nature Reviews. Immunology. 2015;**15**(12):745-759

[206] Mathew A, Kurane I, Green S, Stephens HA, Vaughn DW, Kalayanarooj S, et al. Predominance of HLA-restricted cytotoxic T-lymphocyte responses to serotype-cross-reactive epitopes on nonstructural proteins following natural secondary dengue virus infection. Journal of Virology. 1998;**72**(5):3999-4004

[207] Mongkolsapaya J, Dejnirattisai W, Xu XN, Vasanawathana S, Tangthawornchaikul N, Chairunsri A, et al. Original antigenic sin and apoptosis in the pathogenesis of dengue hemorrhagic fever. Nature Medicine. 2003;**9**(7):921-927

[208] Dong T, Moran E, Vinh Chau N, Simmons C, Luhn K, Peng Y, et al. High pro-inflammatory cytokine secretion and loss of high avidity cross-reactive cytotoxic T-cells during the course of secondary dengue virus infection. PLoS One. 2007;**2**(12):e1192

[209] Friberg H, Beaumier CM, Park S, Pazoles P, Endy TP, Mathew A, et al. Protective versus pathologic pre-exposure cytokine profiles in dengue virus infection. PLoS Neglected Tropical Diseases. 2018;**12**(12):e0006975

[210] Halstead SB. Controversies in dengue pathogenesis. Paediatrics and International Child Health. 2012;**32**(Suppl 1):5-9

[211] Dung NT, Duyen HT, Thuy NT, Ngoc TV, Chau NV, Hien TT, et al. Timing of CD8+ T cell responses in relation to commencement of capillary leakage in children with dengue. Journal of Immunology. 2010;**184**(12):7281-7287

[212] Rivino L, Kumaran EA, Thein TL, Too CT, Gan VC, Hanson BJ, et al. Virus-specific T lymphocytes home to the skin during natural dengue infection. Science Translational Medicine. 2015;7(278):278ra35

[213] Rivino L. Understanding the human T cell response to dengue virus. Advances in Experimental Medicine and Biology. 2018;**1062**:241-250

[214] Karkhanis VS, Joshi JM. Pleural effusion: diagnosis, treatment, and management. Open Access Emergency Medicine. 2012;**4**:31-52

[215] Modhiran N, Watterson D, Muller DA, Panetta AK, Sester DP, Liu L, et al. Dengue virus NS1 protein activates cells via toll-like receptor 4 and disrupts endothelial cell monolayer integrity. Science Translational Medicine. 2015;**7**(304):304ra142

[216] Thomas SJ. NS1: A corner piece in the dengue pathogenesis puzzle? Science Translational Medicine. 2015;**7**(304):304fs37

[217] Smith TJ, Brandt WE, Swanson JL, McCown JM, Buescher EL. Physical and biological properties of dengue-2 virus and associated antigens. Journal of Virology. 1970;**5**(4):524-532

[218] Alcala AC, Hernandez-Bravo R, Medina F, Coll DS, Zambrano JL, Del Angel RM, et al. The dengue virus non-structural protein 1 (NS1) is secreted from infected mosquito cells via a non-classical caveolin-1-dependent pathway. The Journal of General Virology. 2017;**98**(8):2088-2099

[219] Alcala AC, Medina F, Gonzalez-Robles A, Salazar-Villatoro L, Fragoso-Soriano RJ, Vasquez C, et al. The dengue virus non-structural protein 1 (NS1) is secreted efficiently from infected mosquito cells. Virology. 2016;**488**:278-287

[220] Ludert JE, Mosso C, Ceballos-Olvera I, del Angel RM. Use of a commercial enzyme immunoassay to monitor dengue virus replication in cultured cells. Virology Journal. 2008;**5**:51

[221] Alcon-LePoder S, Drouet M-T, Roux P, Frenkiel M-P, Arborio M, Durand-Schneider A-M, et al. The secreted form of dengue virus nonstructural protein NS1 is endocytosed by hepatocytes and accumulates in late endosomes: Implications for viral infectivity. Journal of Virology. 2005;**79**(17):11403-11411

[222] Hu D, Di B, Ding X, Wang Y, Chen Y, Pan Y, et al. Kinetics of non-structural protein 1, IgM and IgG antibodies in dengue type 1 primary infection. Virology Journal. 2011;**8**:47

[223] Alcon S, Talarmin A, Debruyne M, Falconar A, Deubel V, Flamand M. Enzyme-linked Immunosorbent assay specific to dengue virus type 1 nonstructural protein NS1 reveals circulation of the antigen in the blood during the acute phase of disease in patients experiencing primary or secondary infections. Journal of Clinical Microbiology. 2002;**40**(2):376

[224] Peeling RW, Artsob H, Pelegrino JL, Buchy P, Cardosa MJ, Devi S, et al. Evaluation of diagnostic tests: Dengue. Nature Reviews. Microbiology. 2010;**8**(12 Suppl): S30-S38

[225] Casenghi M, Kosack C, Li R, Bastard M, Ford N. NS1 antigen detecting assays for diagnosing acute dengue infection in people living in or returning from endemic countries. Cochrane Database of Systematic Reviews. 2018;**2018**(5):CD011155

[226] Libraty DH, Endy TP, Houng HS, Green S, Kalayanarooj S, Suntayakorn S, et al. Differing influences of virus burden and immune activation on disease severity in secondary dengue-3 virus infections. The Journal of Infectious Diseases. 2002;**185**(9):1213-1221

[227] Nunes PCG, Nogueira RMR, Heringer M, Chouin-Carneiro T. Damasceno Dos Santos Rodrigues C, de Filippis AMB, et al. NS1 Antigenemia and Viraemia load: Potential markers of progression to dengue fatal outcome? Viruses. 2018;**10**(6)

[228] Martinez-Cuellar C, Lovera D, Galeano F, Gatti L, Arbo A. Non-structural protein 1 (NS1) of dengue virus detection correlates with severity in primary but not in secondary dengue infection. Journal of Clinical Virology. 2020;**124**:104259

[229] Muller DA, Young PR. The flavivirus NS1 protein: Molecular and structural biology, immunology, role in pathogenesis and application as a diagnostic biomarker. Antiviral Research. 2013;**98**(2):192-208

[230] Mackenzie JM, Jones MK, Young PR. Immunolocalization of the dengue virus nonstructural glycoprotein NS1 suggests a role in viral RNA replication. Virology. 1996;**220**(1):232-240

[231] Scaturro P, Cortese M, Chatel-Chaix L, Fischl W, Bartenschlager R. Dengue virus non-structural protein 1 modulates infectious particle production via interaction with the structural proteins. PLoS Pathogens. 2015;**11**(11):e1005277

[232] Plaszczyca A, Scaturro P, Neufeldt CJ, Cortese M, Cerikan B, Ferla S, et al. A novel interaction between dengue virus nonstructural protein 1 and the NS4A-2K-4B precursor is required for viral RNA replication but not for formation of the membranous replication organelle. PLoS Pathogens. 2019;**15**(5):e1007736

[233] Cervantes-Salazar M, Angel-Ambrocio AH, Soto-Acosta R, Bautista-Carbajal P, Hurtado-Monzon AM, Alcaraz-Estrada SL, et al. Dengue virus NS1 protein interacts with the ribosomal protein RPL18: This interaction is required for viral translation and

replication in Huh-7 cells. Virology. 2015;**484**:113-126

[234] Flamand M, Megret F, Mathieu M, Lepault J, Rey FA, Deubel V. Dengue virus type 1 nonstructural glycoprotein NS1 is secreted from mammalian cells as a soluble Hexamer in a glycosylation-dependent fashion. Journal of Virology. 1999;**73**(7):6104

[235] Akey DL, Brown WC, Dutta S, Konwerski J, Jose J, Jurkiw TJ, et al. Flavivirus NS1 structures reveal surfaces for associations with membranes and the immune system. Science. 2014;**343**(6173):881-885

[236] Akey DL, Brown WC, Jose J, Kuhn RJ, Smith JL. Structure-guided insights on the role of NS1 in flavivirus infection. BioEssays. 2015;**37**(5):489-494

[237] Edeling MA, Diamond MS, Fremont DH. Structural basis of Flavivirus NS1 assembly and antibody recognition. Proceedings of the National Academy of Sciences of the United States of America. 2014;**111**(11):4285-4290

[238] Brown WC, Akey DL, Konwerski JR, Tarrasch JT, Skiniotis G, Kuhn RJ, et al. Extended surface for membrane association in Zika virus NS1 structure. Nature Structural & Molecular Biology. 2016;**23**(9):865-867

[239] Wang H, Han M, Qi J, Hilgenfeld R, Luo T, Shi Y, et al. Crystal structure of the C-terminal fragment of NS1 protein from yellow fever virus. Science China. Life Sciences. 2017;**60**(12):1403-1406

[240] Amorim JH, Alves RP, Boscardin SB, Ferreira LC. The dengue virus non-structural 1 protein: Risks and benefits. Virus Research. 2014;**181**:53-60

[241] Avirutnan P, Fuchs A, Hauhart RE, Somnuke P, Youn S, Diamond MS, et al. Antagonism of the complement component C4 by flavivirus nonstructural protein NS1. The Journal of Experimental Medicine. 2010;**207**(4):793-806

[242] Avirutnan P, Hauhart RE, Somnuke P, Blom AM, Diamond MS, Atkinson JP. Binding of flavivirus nonstructural protein NS1 to C4b binding protein modulates complement activation. Journal of Immunology. 2011;**187**(1):424-433

[243] Chung KM, Liszewski MK, Nybakken G, Davis AE, Townsend RR, Fremont DH, et al. West Nile virus nonstructural protein NS1 inhibits complement activation by binding the regulatory protein factor H. Proceedings of the National Academy of Sciences of the United States of America. 2006;**103**(50):19111-19116

[244] Conde JN, da Silva EM, Allonso D, Coelho DR, Andrade IDS, de Medeiros LN, et al. Inhibition of the membrane attack complex by dengue virus NS1 through interaction with Vitronectin and terminal complement proteins. Journal of Virology. 2016;**90**(21):9570-9581

[245] Bokisch VA, Top FH Jr, Russell PK, Dixon FJ, Muller-Eberhard HJ. The potential pathogenic role of complement in dengue hemorrhagic shock syndrome. The New England Journal of Medicine. 1973;**289**(19):996-1000

[246] Avirutnan P, Punyadee N, Noisakran S, Komoltri C, Thiemmeca S, Auethavornanan K, et al. Vascular leakage in severe dengue virus infections: A potential role for the nonstructural viral protein NS1 and complement. The Journal of Infectious Diseases. 2006;**193**(8):1078-1088

[247] Falconar AK. The dengue virus nonstructural-1 protein (NS1) generates antibodies to common epitopes on human blood clotting, integrin/adhesin proteins and binds to human endothelial cells: Potential

implications in haemorrhagic fever pathogenesis. Archives of Virology. 1997;**142**(5):897-916

[248] Chuang YC, Lin YS, Liu HS, Yeh TM. Molecular mimicry between dengue virus and coagulation factors induces antibodies to inhibit thrombin activity and enhance fibrinolysis. Journal of Virology. 2014;**88**(23):13759-13768

[249] Lin CF, Lei HY, Shiau AL, Liu CC, Liu HS, Yeh TM, et al. Antibodies from dengue patient sera cross-react with endothelial cells and induce damage. Journal of Medical Virology. 2003;**69**(1):82-90

[250] Lin CF, Lei HY, Liu CC, Liu HS, Yeh TM, Wang ST, et al. Generation of IgM anti-platelet autoantibody in dengue patients. Journal of Medical Virology. 2001;**63**(2):143-149

[251] Lin CF, Lei HY, Shiau AL, Liu HS, Yeh TM, Chen SH, et al. Endothelial cell apoptosis induced by antibodies against dengue virus nonstructural protein 1 via production of nitric oxide. Journal of Immunology. 2002;**169**(2):657-664

[252] Chen MC, Lin CF, Lei HY, Lin SC, Liu HS, Yeh TM, et al. Deletion of the C-terminal region of dengue virus nonstructural protein 1 (NS1) abolishes anti-NS1-mediated platelet dysfunction and bleeding tendency. Journal of Immunology. 2009;**183**(3):1797-1803

[253] Glasner DR, Puerta-Guardo H, Beatty PR, Harris E. The good, the bad, and the shocking: The multiple roles of dengue virus nonstructural protein 1 in protection and pathogenesis. Annual Review of Virology. 2018;**5**(1):227-253

[254] Wan SW, Chen PW, Chen CY, Lai YC, Chu YT, Hung CY, et al. Therapeutic effects of monoclonal antibody against dengue virus NS1 in a STAT1 knockout mouse model of dengue infection. Journal of Immunology. 2017;**199**(8):2834-2844

[255] Wan SW, Lu YT, Huang CH, Lin CF, Anderson R, Liu HS, et al. Protection against dengue virus infection in mice by administration of antibodies against modified nonstructural protein 1. PLoS One. 2014;**9**(3):e92495

[256] Lin YL, Chen LK, Liao CL, Yeh CT, Ma SH, Chen JL, et al. DNA immunization with Japanese encephalitis virus nonstructural protein NS1 elicits protective immunity in mice. Journal of Virology. 1998;**72**(1):191-200

[257] Amorim JH, Diniz MO, Cariri FA, Rodrigues JF, Bizerra RS, Goncalves AJ, et al. Protective immunity to DENV2 after immunization with a recombinant NS1 protein using a genetically detoxified heat-labile toxin as an adjuvant. Vaccine. 2012;**30**(5):837-845

[258] Bailey MJ, Broecker F, Duehr J, Arumemi F, Krammer F, Palese P, et al. Antibodies elicited by an NS1-based vaccine protect mice against Zika virus. MBio. 2019;**10**(2):e02861-18

[259] Schlesinger JJ, Brandriss MW, Cropp CB, Monath TP. Protection against yellow fever in monkeys by immunization with yellow fever virus nonstructural protein NS1. Journal of Virology. 1986;**60**(3):1153-1155

[260] Li A, Yu J, Lu M, Ma Y, Attia Z, Shan C, et al. A Zika virus vaccine expressing premembrane-envelope-NS1 polyprotein. Nature Communications. 2018;**9**(1):3067

[261] Dalrymple NA, Mackow ER. Roles for endothelial cells in dengue virus infection. Advances in Virology. 2012;**2012**:840654

[262] Avirutnan P, Malasit P, Seliger B, Bhakdi S, Husmann M. Dengue virus infection of human endothelial cells leads to chemokine production,

complement activation, and apoptosis. The Journal of Immunology. 1998;**161**(11):6338

[263] Félétou M. The endothelium: Part 1: Multiple Functions of the Endothelial Cells—Focus on Endothelium-Derived Vasoactive Mediators. San Rafael (CA): Morgan & Claypool Life Sciences; 2011. Available from: https://www.ncbi.nlm.nih.gov/books/NBK57148/

[264] Yuan SYR, Robert R Rigor. Regulation of Endothelial Barrier Function. San Rafael (CA): Morgan & Claypool Life Sciences; 2010. Available from: https://www.ncbi.nlm.nih.gov/books/NBK54117/

[265] Pober JS, Sessa WC. Evolving functions of endothelial cells in inflammation. Nature Reviews. Immunology. 2007;**7**(10):803-815

[266] Avirutnan P, Zhang L, Punyadee N, Manuyakorn A, Puttikhunt C, Kasinrerk W, et al. Secreted NS1 of dengue virus attaches to the surface of cells via interactions with heparan sulfate and chondroitin sulfate E. PLoS Pathogens. 2007;**3**(11):e183

[267] Puerta-Guardo H, Glasner DR, Harris E. Dengue virus NS1 disrupts the endothelial Glycocalyx, leading to Hyperpermeability. PLoS Pathogens. 2016;**12**(7):e1005738

[268] Glasner DR, Ratnasiri K, Puerta-Guardo H, Espinosa DA, Beatty PR, Harris E. Dengue virus NS1 cytokine-independent vascular leak is dependent on endothelial glycocalyx components. PLoS Pathogens. 2017;**13**(11):e1006673

[269] Chen HR, Chuang YC, Lin YS, Liu HS, Liu CC, Perng GC, et al. Dengue virus nonstructural protein 1 induces vascular leakage through macrophage migration inhibitory factor and autophagy. PLoS Neglected Tropical Diseases. 2016;**10**(7):e0004828

[270] Chen HR, Chao CH, Liu CC, Ho TS, Tsai HP, Perng GC, et al. Macrophage migration inhibitory factor is critical for dengue NS1-induced endothelial glycocalyx degradation and hyperpermeability. PLoS Pathogens. 2018;**14**(4):e1007033

[271] Singh S, Anupriya MG, Modak A, Sreekumar E. Dengue virus or NS1 protein induces trans-endothelial cell permeability associated with VE-Cadherin and RhoA phosphorylation in HMEC-1 cells preventable by Angiopoietin-1. The Journal of General Virology. 2018;99(12):1658-1670

[272] Barbachano-Guerrero A, Endy TP, King CA. Dengue virus non-structural protein 1 activates the p38 MAPK pathway to decrease barrier integrity in primary human endothelial cells. The Journal of General Virology. 2020;**101**(5):484-496

[273] Niranjan R, Sumitha MK, Sankari T, Muthukumaravel S, Jambulingam P. Nonstructural protein-1 (NS1) of dengue virus type-2 differentially stimulate expressions of matrix metalloproteinases in monocytes: Protective effect of paracetamol. International Immunopharmacology. 2019;**73**:270-279

[274] Adikari TN, Gomes L, Wickramasinghe N, Salimi M, Wijesiriwardana N, Kamaladasa A, et al. Dengue NS1 antigen contributes to disease severity by inducing interleukin (IL)-10 by monocytes. Clinical and Experimental Immunology. 2016;**184**(1):90-100

[275] Chao CH, Wu WC, Lai YC, Tsai PJ, Perng GC, Lin YS, et al. Dengue virus nonstructural protein 1 activates platelets via toll-like receptor 4, leading to thrombocytopenia and hemorrhage. PLoS Pathogens. 2019;**15**(4):e1007625

[276] Calisher CH, Gould EA. Taxonomy of the virus family Flaviviridae. Advances in Virus Research. 2003;**59**:1-19

[277] Gould EA, Solomon T. Pathogenic flaviviruses. Lancet. 2008;**371**(9611):500-509

[278] Counotte MJ, Meili KW, Taghavi K, Calvet G, Sejvar J, Low N. Zika virus infection as a cause of congenital brain abnormalities and Guillain-Barre syndrome: A living systematic review. F1000Res. 2019;**8**:1433

[279] Wang C, Puerta-Guardo H, Biering SB, Glasner DR, Tran EB, Patana M, et al. Endocytosis of flavivirus NS1 is required for NS1-mediated endothelial hyperpermeability and is abolished by a single N-glycosylation site mutation. PLoS Pathogens. 2019;**15**(7):e1007938

[280] Weinbaum S, Tarbell JM, Damiano ER. The structure and function of the endothelial glycocalyx layer. Annual Review of Biomedical Engineering. 2007;**9**:121-167

[281] Connolly-Andersen AM, Thunberg T, Ahlm C. Endothelial activation and repair during hantavirus infection: Association with disease outcome. Open Forum Infectious Diseases. 2014;**1**(1):ofu027

[282] Somnuke P, Hauhart RE, Atkinson JP, Diamond MS, Avirutnan P. N-linked glycosylation of dengue virus NS1 protein modulates secretion, cell-surface expression, hexamer stability, and interactions with human complement. Virology. 2011;**413**(2):253-264

[283] Pryor MJ, Wright PJ. Glycosylation mutants of dengue virus NS1 protein. The Journal of General Virology. 1994;**75**(Pt. 5):1183-1187

[284] Crabtree MB, Kinney RM, Miller BR. Deglycosylation of the NS1 protein of dengue 2 virus, strain 16681: Construction and characterization of mutant viruses. Archives of Virology. 2005;**150**(4):771-786

[285] Annamalai AS, Pattnaik A, Sahoo BR, Guinn ZP, Bullard BL, Weaver EA, et al. An attenuated Zika virus encoding non-glycosylated envelope (E) and non-structural protein 1 (NS1) confers complete protection against lethal challenge in a mouse model. Vaccines (Basel). 2019;7(3):112

[286] Whiteman MC, Wicker JA, Kinney RM, Huang CYH, Solomon T, Barrett ADT. Multiple amino acid changes at the first glycosylation motif in NS1 protein of West Nile virus are necessary for complete attenuation for mouse neuroinvasiveness. Vaccine. 2011;**29**(52):9702-9710

[287] Li F, Wang Y, Yu L, Cao S, Wang K, Yuan J, et al. Viral infection of the central nervous system and Neuroinflammation precede blood-brain barrier disruption during Japanese encephalitis virus infection. Journal of Virology. 2015;**89**(10):5602-5614

[288] Basu A, Chaturvedi UC. Vascular endothelium: The battlefield of dengue viruses. FEMS Immunology and Medical Microbiology. 2008;**53**(3):287-299

[289] Xu X, Vaughan K, Weiskopf D, Grifoni A, Diamond MS, Sette A, et al. Identifying candidate targets of immune responses in Zika virus based on homology to epitopes in other *Flavivirus* species. PLoS Currents. 2016;**8**:1-38

Section 3

Molecular Biology Diagnosis and Control Strategies

Chapter 6

Dengue Virus and the Relationship with MicroRNAs

Samir Casseb and Karla de Melo

Abstract

Dengue is an acute febrile disease caused by a virus of the genus *Flavivirus*, family Flaviviridae, endemic in tropical regions of the globe. The agent is a virus with single-stranded RNA, classified into four distinct dengue virus (DENV) serotypes: DENV-1, DENV-2, DENV-3, and DENV-4. The host's innate and adaptive immune responses play an essential role in determining the natural history of viral infections, especially in dengue. In this context, it has observed in recent years that the presence of RNA interference (RNAi) in viral infection processes is increasing, as well as immune defense. The context microRNAs (miRNAs) go for stood out, as their presence during viral infection, both in the replication of the virus and in the defense against these infections, becomes increasingly noticeable, therefore, making it increasingly necessary to better understand the role of these small RNAs within viral infection by DENV and what their consequences are in aggravating the consequences of patients affected by this disease.

Keywords: dengue, miRNA, genetics, immunology, *Flavivirus*

1. Introduction

RNA interference (RNAi) is understood as the mechanism of gene silencing through transcription or post-transcription. Post-transcription gene silencing (PTGS) operates through translational repression induced by microRNAs (miRNAs), from precursors transcribed in the nucleus [1].

The silencing machinery by microRNAs directs mRNA to the P bodies present in the cytoplasm. They are deprived of the translation machinery and conserve proteins involved in the degradation of the target mRNA [2].

The natural functions of RNAi and their related processes appear to be the protection of the genome against invasion by mobile genetic elements, such as viruses and transposons, as well as the functioning of eukaryotic organism development programs [3, 4].

These analyses led to the identification of proteins encoded by the host involved in gene silencing. Also, they revealed that several enzymes or essential factors are common to these processes. Some components have identified to serve as initiators. In contrast, others serve as effectors, amplifiers, and transmitters for the gene silencing process [5].

The RNAi is widely used to fight viruses, due to the exposure of their genetic material in the intracellular environment at various stages of their replication cycle [6, 7]. Due to the distinction between viral and cellular genomes, the chances of cross-silencing are low. In contrast, mutational changes in the viral genome allow mechanisms to escape interference pathways [8, 9].

2. miRNA

The microRNAs are defined as small single-stranded RNA molecules with approximately 19–25 nucleotides, not protein encoders, that act as mediators for the regulation of the posttranscriptional gene expression [10].

The first miRNA was described in 1993 and related to the regulation of larval development in *Caenorhabditis elegans*. However, understand that the miRNA class is the largest class of gene regulators, with around 1000 miRNAs. Promoting regulation is necessary to bind the 3'untranslated region of the target mRNA [11].

There are more than 2500 miRNAs identified in the human genome. Although transcriptional targets are predicted, most of these have not been validated, which makes this area for investigation rich [6, 12]. Studies revealed that viruses encode miRNA, for example, Epstein-Barr virus (EBV), human cytomegalovirus (HCMV), and human immunodeficiency virus type 1 (HIV-1) [13].

miRNAs play essential roles in the cell, such as proliferation, differentiation, apoptosis, stress response, and transcriptional regulation. Studies have shown that miRNAs change their expression in several pathologies, increasing their importance and the need for a better understanding of this process [14].

2.1 miRNA biogenesis and mechanism of action

The miRNA biogenesis process consists of transcription, export, processing, and maturation, at the cytoplasmic and cellular levels. As a fundamental element of this miRNA transcription, RNA polymerases II and III are found, with the function of transcribing gene encoding proteins [12].

Currently, most of the identified miRNAs are intragenic and processed from introns. Simultaneously, the rest are intergenic and transcribed independently of a host gene and regulated by their promoters [15]. Sometimes, miRNAs are transcribed as a long transcript called "clusters," which can have similar regions, and, in this case, are considered a family. miRNA biogenesis can be classified into two pathways: canonical and noncanonical (**Figure 1**) [5].

What defines the choice of these mechanisms is the complementarity between the bases of miRNA and mRNA. When there is perfect parity between the bases, degradation of the mRNAs will occur [16]. On the other hand, incomplete pairings generate inhibition of the translation of the target mRNA. Since miRNAs are small molecules, there is no need for complete pairing for binding. Thus, a miRNA can act in the regulation of several target mRNAs, or several miRNAs regulate a single mRNA [17].

2.1.1 Canonical pathway

The canonical pathway of biogenesis is the dominant pathway by which miRNAs are processed. In this way, pri-miRNAs are transcribed from their genes and processed into pre-miRNAs by the microprocessor complex, consisting of a protein that binds RNA to the critical region of DiGeorge syndrome 8 (DGCR8) and a ribonuclease III enzyme, Drosha [18]. DGCR8 recognizes an N6-methyladenylated GGAC and other motifs within the pri-miRNA [19]. At the same time, Drosha cleaves the duplex pri-miRNA based on the characteristic structure of the pri-miRNA, resulting in the formation of an excess of 2 nt 3′ in the pre-miRNA [20]. Once pre-miRNAs

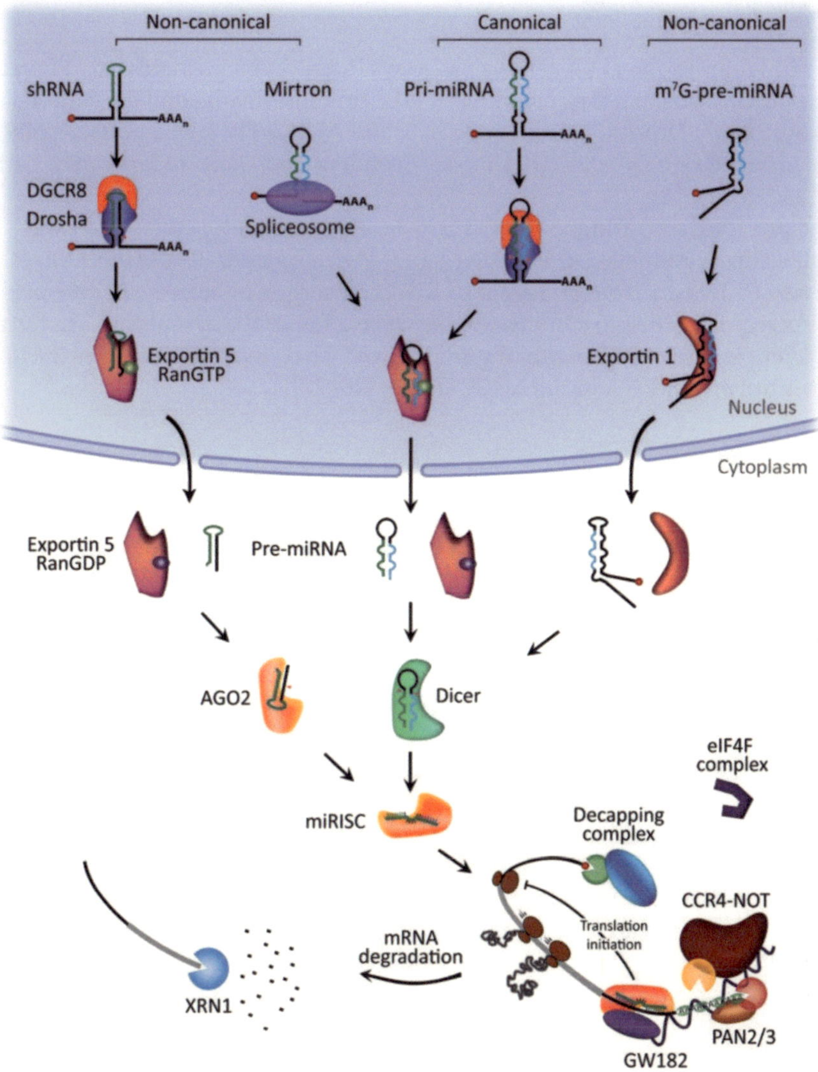

Figure 1.
MicroRNA biogenesis and mechanism of action. The canonical miRNA biogenesis begins with the generation of the pri-miRNA transcript passing through the microprocessor complex, composed of the critical region 8 of Drosha and DiGeorge syndrome (DGCR8), and cleaves the pri-miRNA to produce the precursor miRNA (pre-miRNA). The mature miRNA is associated with the Argonaute (AGO) protein family forming a miRNA-induced silencing complex (miRISC). In noncanonical pathways, small hairpin RNA (shRNA) is initially cleaved by the microprocessor complex and exported to the cytoplasm via exportin 5/RanGT, cleaved by AGO2, but this action is independent of Dicer (modified by Tanzer et al.) [21].

are generated, they are exported to the cytoplasm by an exportin 5 (XPO5)/RanGTP complex and processed by the RNase III Dicer endonuclease [5, 22].

This processing involves removing the loop from the terminal, resulting in a mature miRNA duplex. The directionality of the miRNA chain determines the name of the mature miRNA form. The 5p chain emerges from the 5′ end of the pre-miRNA hairpin, while the 3p chain originates from the 3′ end. Both chains derived from the mature miRNA duplex can carry in the Argonaute family of proteins. miRNA chains that do not contain incompatibilities are cleaved by AGO2 and degraded by cellular machinery that can produce a strong chain bias. Otherwise, miRNA duplexes with central mismatches or miRNA not loaded with AGO2 are passively unwound and degraded [23].

2.1.2 Noncanonical pathway

Several noncanonical biogenesis pathways in miRNA are elucidated (**Figure 1**). These pathways make use of combinations of proteins involved in the canonical pathway, mainly Drosha, Dicer, exportin 5, and AGO2. The noncanonical miRNA can be grouped into Drosha-/DGCR8-independent and Dicer-independent pathways [24, 25].

The pre-miRNAs produced by the Drosha-/DGCR8-independent pathway resemble Dicer products. On the other hand, Dicer-independent miRNAs are processed by Drosha from endogenous RNA transcripts of hairpins. These pre-miRNAs require AGO2 to complete their maturation in the cytoplasm. They are of insufficient length to be the substrates for Dicer. That, in turn, promotes the loading of the entire pre-miRNA in the AGO2 slicing [26, 27].

2.1.3 Argonaute and TNRC6 proteins

The proteins of the Argonaute family are related to the RISC complex, as a member of the machinery of the RNAi pathways [28]. The highly conserved between species and several organisms encode several members of the family. Usually found in the cytoplasm are concentrated close to the P bodies [29].

Such proteins, therefore, act with the transcriptional and posttranscriptional silencing pathways. The main stage of the interference mechanism is the cleavage of mRNAs; the Argonaute protein in the RISC complex catalyzes this process [28].

Argonautes are applied in transcriptional and posttranscriptional gene silencing, acting through the modulation of the degradation or inhibition of the translation of specific mRNAs, when associated with miRNAs [18].

The miRNAs associated with Argonaute proteins constitute a more massive complex called the miRNA-induced silencing complex, which will suppress the expression of mRNAs. In addition to interference at the translational level, it shows that miRNAs can induce poly(A) tail deadening [18, 19]. Studies suggest that proteins of the TNRC6 family are essential components when associated with miRISCs, for the location of cytoplasmic P bodies and the gene silencing of mRNAs [19, 20].

3. miRNA and dengue virus

The dengue virus is a virus composed of a single-stranded positive RNA belonging to the family Flaviviridae. DENV serotypes have been identified (DENV-1 to DENV-4). All serotypes are causing similar diseases and similar symptoms, without significant severity and serious diseases, such as dengue hemorrhagic fever and dengue shock syndrome. The DENV genome is approximately 11 kb in length that encodes a single polyprotein. This polyprotein is cleaved posttranslationally by the host and viral proteases into three structural proteins (capsid C; pre-membrane/membrane, prM/M; envelope, E) and seven nonstructural proteins (NS1, NS2A, NS2B, NS3, NS4A, NS4B, and NS5) [30, 31].

The DENVs enter their target cells via receptor-mediated endocytosis in a clathrin-dependent manner. An acidified endosomal vesicle, virion, undergoes conformational changes that allow fusion and endosomal membrane and release RNA from the genome into the cytosol. After initial translation and cleavage of polyprotein, DENV triggers the formation of a replication complex in the perinuclear endoplasmic reticulum, and RNA replication and protein translation occur. Protein C then packages the newly synthesized positive RNA assembled into a virion, which is covered with prM/E heterodimers. When the vesicles containing the immature virions move through the Golgi apparatus, the prM is cleaved by a furin protease. Finally, immature virions become mature or partially mature virions, which are secreted [32, 33].

3.1 Mosquitoes, miRNAs, and dengue

The functions that miRNA is involved in mosquitoes are related to posttranscriptional regulation of gene expression in physiological and immunological pathways and affect development, metabolism, host-pathogen interactions, and resistance to insecticides [34].

3.1.1 Development and metabolism

The specific expression of the miRNA stage in the four stages of development (eggs, larvae, pupae, and adults) was confirmed using sequencing. Understand the role of regulated miRNAs in the development of the mosquito and the action of knocking down the expressed miRNAs in a specific way carried out in *Ae. albopictus*. The knockdown of aal-miR-286b and aal-miR-2942 decreased the hatching of embryos and the hatching rate of larvae, respectively, compared to the knock-in groups. Reduced longevity and fertility (aal-miR-1891) were observed in the knockdown groups for miR-1891 compared to the knock-in and control groups in adults. Female mosquitoes require sugar for energy metabolism and a blood meal for egg development. Recent studies have indicated that blood supply leads to the differential expression of many genes, proteins, and miRNAs. The abundance of miRNA differs under sugar-fed and blood-fed conditions; ast-miR-2796-5p was observed exclusively in sugar-fed. The depletion of aae-miR-275 in *Ae. aegypti* females led to severe defects in blood digestion, fluid excretion, and egg development. aae-miR-1890 is induced after blood feeding and reaches a peak of 24 PMB. The systemic depletion of aae-miR-1890 resulted in less egg development and deposition, suggesting that miR-1890 may be the key to mosquito blood digestion. In contrast to the upregulated miRNAs after blood feeding, some miRNAs were downregulated. For example, reduced ast-miR-989 was observed 72 h after a blood meal. aga-let7 decreased in the midgut and other parts/leftovers, but most miRNAs increased after blood feeding [35–37].

3.1.2 Mosquitoes and dengue infection

The viruses of the *Flavivirus* genus are transmitted by mosquitoes and cause diseases, including dengue. It is observed that *Cx. quinquefasciatus* mosquitoes with West Nile virus (WNV) showed altered miR-92 and miR-989 expressions. In *Aedes albopictus*, the aae-miR-2940 miRNA is downregulated in response to WNV infection to restrict viral replication. In studies, the expressions of 35 miRNAs of mosquitoes modulating DENV infection in *Aedes aegypti* and more than 66 miRNAs were reported. *Ae. albopictus* is differentially expressed after DENV-2 infection. Therefore, aal-miR-34-5p and aal-miR-87 contribute to antipathogenic and immunological responses during DENV-2 infection. ae-miR-375 is the key to DENV replication, which can improve DENV-2 infection in an *Ae. aegypti* cell line. aae-miR-252 is three times more expressed after DENV-2 infection in *Ae. albopictus* cell line (C6/36); this inhibited DENV replication by suppressing the expression of the envelope protein of DENV. Regarding aal-miR-281, an abundant miRNA specific to the midgut, it was found that it facilitates the replication of DENV-2 in *Ae. albopictus* [36, 37].

4. miRNA impact on DENV infection

Studies have demonstrated the importance of miRNAs in viral infections. Mutations in the main catalytic components of the RNA interference pathway led to an increase in DENV replication in mammalian cells (**Figure 2**) [38]. Studies that analyzed the expression of miRNA in the blood of patients with dengue demonstrated a large number of miRNAs expressed differently in response to dengue infections [35]. About 348 miRNAs were described with different expressions in patients with dengue. Interestingly, studies have also identified 17 miRNAs that could use to distinguish between mild and severe dengue with complications [39].

The expressions of miR-24-1-5p, miR-512-5p, and miR-4640-3p were able to distinguish mild dengue from those with liver complications. At the same time, miR-383 was significantly more expressed in dengue with mild clinical status than those diagnosed with severe dengue and accumulation of body fluids [40, 41].

Studies have also shown 12 miRNAs with negative regulation and 41 with positive regulation in the serum of patients infected with DENV-1 when compared to the control group. Among these miRNAs we highlight hsa-miR-21-5p, hsa-miR-146a-5p, hsa-miR-590-5p, hsa-miR-188-5p, and hsa-miR-152-3p that were identified as promising invasive molecular markers for the detection of DENV infection [42, 43].

The microRNAs miR-21-5p and miR146a-5p are involved in inflammation and cell proliferation. They are expressed significantly concerning the control group, indicating their sensitivity and specificity as indicators of DENV infection. Besides, both miRNAs are correlated with the number of leukocytes and neutrophils. These findings suggested that some miRNAs could be used as diagnostic markers for DENV infections [44].

Effective disruption of host RNAi machinery is one of the pathogenic strategies of viruses to mitigate the host's response. Several viruses have reported producing protein suppressors through RNAi to cause silencing in infected cells, thereby

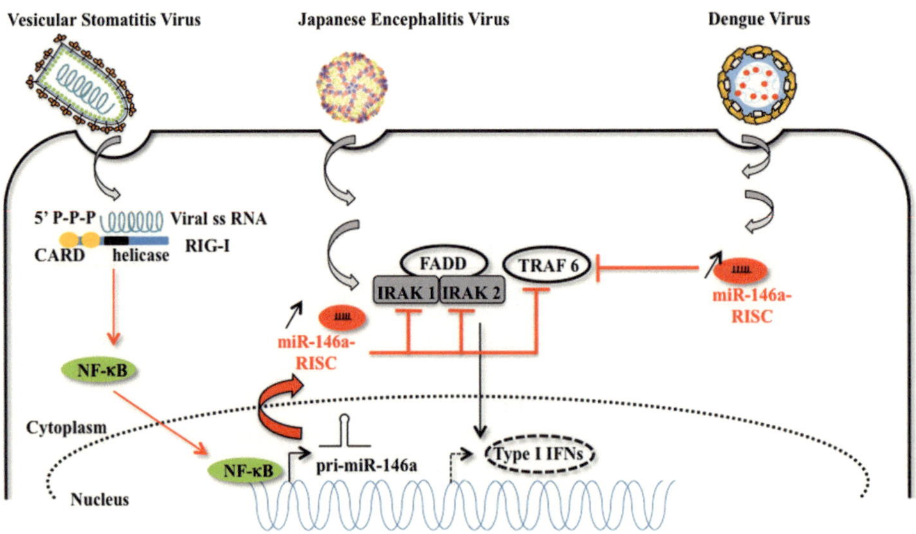

Figure 2.
An example of increased miRNA expression after the entry of vesicular stomatitis virus (VSV), Japanese encephalitis virus (JEV), and dengue virus in mammalian cells. miRNA expression increased in a RIG-I-dependent manner. The RIG-I protein interacts with viral RNA through its helicase domain, leading to nuclear transcription of the pri-miRNA by NF-kB. The reduction of target mRNAs explains the proviral function of this miRNA as the response of interferon type I (adapted from Bruscella et al.) [45].

interfering with RISC's loading or inhibiting the cutting activity of the AGO protein, a component of RISC and the biogenesis of miRNAs. DENV also has such suppressors that could neutralize the host's RNAi response. NS4B has reported suppressing host RNAi, interfering with the processing of Dicer, a key protein in miRNA biogenesis [38]. It has also reported that NS1 protein can interfere with apoptosis through miRNA-15 and miRNA-16 [5]. The NS3 protein has shown to interfere with the AGO1 protein [46].

5. miRNAs and the inhibition of viral replication

The miRNAs generally induce translational repression by binding to target mRNAs. Thus, it is not surprising that most of the miRNAs identified so far have DENV replication. The evidence points to the fact that miRNAs bind complementarily to the DENV 5'UTR or 3'UTR genome and thus inhibit DENV replication. The miR-548 g-3p represented the first evidence that a miRNA suppresses DENV multiplication by directly linking it to the viral genome. In the study, they showed that miR-548 g-3p was able to bind to the stem-loop A (SLA) promoter at 5'UTR, which is a crucial element for DENV RNA synthesis and replication, and uncontrolled replication of DENV-1. This inhibitory effect was proposed to arise from the binding of miR-548 g-3p to SLA, which could make it physically difficult, and thus attenuated the interaction between the SLA promoter and NS5. This DENV protein contains a C-dependent RNA-terminal RNA polymerase domain [45, 47].

Their hypothesis suggests that a functional miRNA has been preserved among all DENV serotypes and is present in the 3'UTR. The three dengue serotypes, miR-133a, miR-484, and miR-744, are involved in DENV replication, genome circularization, and viral viability. The overexpression of miR-133a, miR-484, and miR-744 in Vero cells had been experimentally validated to show the potencies of these three miRNAs in inhibiting DENV replication [48]. In another study, it found that miR-252 can inhibit DENV-2 replication in cell culture. The identification of protein E as a target for this miRNA is interesting since it has an indispensable role for viral entry [49, 50].

6. miRNAs that modulate host factors to inhibit or facilitate DENV replication

The DENV virus depends on its host's machinery for replication and infection, and it is not surprising that several miRNAs have shown to indirectly regulate DENV replication through modulation of host factors or the immune response. These indirect effects included modulation of the expression of a cell transcript that encodes a host factor necessary for one or a few stages of the viral cycle. The modulation of receptor expression can regulate virus entry, tropism, and essential cofactors for replication or translation that can impair or increase viral replication and the production of viral proteins. Also, miRNAs can increase or restrict cellular responses to viral infection, such as immune response or defense mechanisms [51].

The miRNA let-7c is highly expressed in Huh-7 cells and may be related to the protection of infected cells from oxidative stress and the response to inflammation after DENV infection. Let-7c has shown to bind directly to the basic transcription factor-1 of the leucine zipper (BACH1), a potent repressor of the anti-inflammatory and antioxidant protein heme oxygenase-1 (HO-1), and to dysregulate infection by DENV-2 and DENV-4. In this way, let-7c is probably able to protect the host from virus-induced infection [49].

In addition to modulating the host's immune response, miRNA may have antiviral actions. An example is miR-223, capable of inhibiting DENV-2 replication; its antiviral effect is probably associated with attenuated expression of the microtubule-destabilizing protein, stathmin 1 (STMN1), a key regulator of protein microtubules that controls microtubule dynamics [52]. The exact mechanism of how STMN1 affected DENV-2 replication is not yet known. However, studies have shown that an intact microtubule network involved in STMN1 sequestration was essential for HMCV to establish an infection. As such, it is highly likely that STMN1 is playing a similar role in establishing controlled microtubule dynamics in the context of DENV infection [53].

It is important to emphasize that despite all studies and the discovery of several miRNAs associated with cell regulation positively or negatively, better clarification of the processes involving miRNAs and DENV is still needed.

6.1 Perspective

6.1.1 Diagnostic using miRNA

As already reported in this chapter, several human diseases were induced due to differential miRNA expressions. Recently, several studies have confirmed the vibrant role of miRNAs in the successful regulation of various biological processes through the synergistic effects of the multiple miRNA networks, an integrated way to control an individual gene [17].

Also, several physiological functions (such as development, infection, immune response, inflammation, tumor genesis, and regulation of bone mass) have suggested being controlled by miRNAs. The miRNAs can regulate gene expression at the posttranscriptional level of more than 50% of the protein-coding genes in humans.

The miRNAs were found to play roles in helping and defending viruses. Mammalian miRNA genes generally exist in the noncoding region of the genes. However, they also occur both in the exonic regions of the gene encoding protein 16, and in alternative exon splicing, it can also regulate the expression of miRNA interionic genes. Study results show a role for unregulated autophagy in the pathogenesis of some RNA viruses. In this context, the positive regulation of hsa-miR-31 and the negative regulations of hsa-miR-493, hsa-miR-889, hsa-miR-655, hsa-miR-656, hsa-miR-26a-1, hsa-miR-154, hsa-miR-335, hsa-miR-1197, and hsa-miR-146a improve innate antiviral responses in cells infected by the virus [26].

Thus, this study aimed at the expression of these miRNAs during dengue infection; in this way, monitoring possible changes can be used as a complementary diagnostic method for faster interventions that can prevent more severe clinical conditions in patients infected with dengue.

6.1.2 Role of RNAi in dengue therapy

To date, miRNAs are used against some viruses that cause disease in humans, including influenza viruses, hepatitis C viruses, hepatitis B viruses, human immunodeficiency virus type 1, polio, and DENV. These viruses are characterized by the presence of ssRNA genomes, which are potential targets for RNAi in the cytoplasm. This functional interaction occurred during the removal and replication of viral RNA [15, 54].

Any changes in the miRNA pathway may shed light on why some mosquitoes are specific vectors for arthropod-borne virus infections (arboviruses), while others are not. The first evidence is the interference of Sindbis viruses that express the recombinant part of the non-inconsequential unrelated RNA (DENV-2), with the replication of DENV-2 in mosquitoes (Egyptian Aedes) through a system such as the silencing mechanism in plants [55].

Potential evidence may be involved with the interaction of dsRNA or siRNA derived from the arbovirus genome. Mammals have thousands of Piwi-interacting RNA genes from producer types of microRNA regulation expression to control the various stages of cell development and physiology. The critical role of RNAi is a defense against viruses in primary organisms, but in mammals, it is the antiviral defense mechanism hitherto controversial. Currently, it is a conserved mechanism of RNAi in mammals, where its introduction to siRNA affects the silent replication of viruses. Currently, the most significant therapeutic attempt using miRNA is to block the "shutdown" actions of genes that end up facilitating viral replication [41, 42].

7. Conclusions

It is possible to conclude that miRNA has an important relationship during DENV infection, and this regulation can be positive for the virus, that is, facilitating the entry of the virus and helping in the replication process, but it is important to emphasize that there are miRNAs that can also have antiviral action, thereby blocking viral replication.

The miRNA studies demonstrate how important this small RNAi is for viral infections, whether in arthropod vectors like mosquitoes or mammals like humans.

One of the significant difficulties in the study of miRNA is the difficulty of understanding all of its relationships within the cell. Thus, further studies are needed to elucidate more forcefully what the functions of each miRNA are with the cell cycle and the viral replication cycle. Nevertheless, these RNAs have been bringing great perspectives both in treatment and as markers for DENV.

Acknowledgements

I thank the colleagues who contributed to this work and the institutions that helped in the preparation of this text.

Conflict of interest

The authors declare no conflict of interest.

Notes/thanks/other declarations

The authors thank everyone who contributed to the elaboration of this text.

Author details

Samir Casseb* and Karla de Melo
Evandro Chagas Institute, Ananindeua, Brazil

*Address all correspondence to: samircasseb@iec.gov.br

References

[1] Wiesen JL, Tomasi TB. Dicer is regulated by cellular stresses and interferons. Molecular Immunology. 2010;**46**(6):1222-1228. DOI: 10.1016/j.molimm.2008.11.012

[2] Liu J, Rivas FV, Wohlschlegel J, Yates JR, Parker R, Hannon GJ. A role for the P-body component GW182 in microRNA function. Nature Cell Biology. 2005;**7**(12):1261-1266. DOI: 10.1038/ncb1333

[3] Almeida R, Allshire RC. RNA silencing and genome regulation. Trends in Cell Biology. 2005;**15**(5):251-258. DOI: 10.1016/j.tcb.2005.03.006

[4] Matskevich A, Jung JS, Schümann M, Cascallo M, Moelling K. Vero cells as a model to study the effects of adenoviral gene delivery vectors on the RNAi. Journal of Innate Immunity. 2009;**1**:389-394. DOI: 10.1159/000191408

[5] Casseb SMM, Simith DB, Melo KFL, Mendonça MH, Santos ACM, Carvalho VL, et al. Drosha, DGCR8, and Dicer mRNAs are down-regulated in human cells infected with dengue virus 4, and play a role in viral pathogenesis. Genetics and Molecular Research [Internet]. 2016;**15**(2). DOI: 10.4238/gmr.15027891

[6] Ricarte Filho JCM, Kimura ET. MicroRNAs: Nova classe de reguladores gênicos envolvidos na função endócrina e câncer. Arquivos Brasileiros de Endocrinologia e Metabologia. 2006;**50**(6):1102-1107. DOI: 10.1590/S0004-27302006000600018

[7] Lin H-R, Ganem D. Viral microRNA target allows insight into the role of translation in governing microRNA target accessibility. Proceedings of the National Academy of Sciences of the United States of America. 2011;**108**(13):5148-5153. DOI: 10.1073/pnas.1102033108

[8] Ooi YS, Stiles KM, Liu CY, Taylor GM, Kielian M. Genome-Wide RNAi screen identifies novel host proteins required for alphavirus entry. In: Dermody TS, editor. PLoS Pathogens [Internet]. Public Library of Science (PLoS). 19 December 2013;**9**(12):e1003835. DOI: 10.1371/journal.ppat.1003835

[9] Olson KE, Blair CD. Arbovirus-mosquito interactions: RNAi pathway. Current Opinion in Virology. 2015;**15**:119-126. DOI: 10.1016/j.coviro.2015.10.001

[10] Dalmay T, Itgb S. MicroRNAs and the hallmarks of cancer. Oncogene. 2006;**25**:6170-6175. DOI: 10.1038/sj.onc.1209911

[11] Brennecke J, Stark A, Russell RB, Cohen SM. Principles of microRNA-target recognition. PLoS Biology. 2005;**3**(3):85. DOI: 10.1371/journal.pbio.0030085

[12] Brandenstein MV, Richter C, Fries JWU. MicroRNAs: Small but amazing , and their association with endothelin. Life Sciences. 2012;**91**(13-14):475-489. DOI: 10.1016/j.lfs.2012.06.025

[13] Qi Y, Li Y, Zhang L, Huang J. microRNA expression profiling and bioinformatic analysis of dengue virus-infected peripheral blood mononuclear cells. Molecular Medicine Reports. 2013;**7**(3):791-798. DOI: 10.3892/mmr.2013.1288

[14] Zhang P, Zhang H. Autophagy modulates miRNA-mediated gene silencing and selectively degrades AIN-1/GW182 in *C. elegans*. EMBO Reports. 2013;**14**(6):568-576. DOI: 10.1038/embor.2013.53

[15] Yen P-S, Chen C-H, Sreenu V, Kohl A, Failloux A-B. Assessing the

Potential Interactions between Cellular miRNA and Arboviral Genomic RNA in the Yellow Fever Mosquito, Aedes aegypti. Viruses [Internet]. MDPI AG. 10 June 2019;**11**(6):540. DOI: 10.3390/v11060540

[16] Makarova JA, Ivanova SM, Tonevitsky AG, Grigoriev AI. New functions of small nucleolar RNAs. Biochemistry. 2013;**78**(6):638-650. DOI: 10.1134/S0006297913060096

[17] Taft RJ, Glazov EA, Lassmann T, Hayashizaki Y, Carninci P, Mattick JS. Small RNAs derived from snoRNAs. RNA. 2009;**15**(7):1233-1240. DOI: 10.1261/rna.1528909

[18] Höck J, Meister G. The Argonaute protein family. Genome Biology. 2008;**9**(2):210. DOI: 10.1186/gb-2008-9-2-210

[19] Baillat D, Shiekhattar R. Functional dissection of the human TNRC6 (GW182-related) family of proteins. Molecular and Cellular Biology. 2009;**29**(15):4144-4155. DOI: 10.1128/MCB.00380-09

[20] Castilla-llorente V, Spraggon L, Okamura M, Naseeruddin S, Adamow M, Qamar S. Mammalian GW220/TNGW1 is essential for the formation of GW/P bodies containing miRISC. The Journal of Cell Biology. 2012;**198**(4):529-544. DOI: 10.1083/jcb.201201153

[21] Tanzer A, Stadler PF. Molecular evolution of a microRNA cluster. Journal of Molecular Biology. 2004;**339**(2): 327-335. DOI: 10.1016/j.jmb.2004.03.065

[22] Xiao C, Rajewsky K. MicroRNA control in the immune system: Basic principles. Cell. 2009;**136**(1):26-36. DOI: 10.1016/j.cell.2008.12.027

[23] Zheng GXY, Do BT, Webster DE, Khavari PA, Chang HY. Dicer-microRNA-Myc circuit promotes transcription of hundreds of long noncoding RNAs. Nature Structural & Molecular Biology. 2014;**21**(7):585-590. DOI: 10.1038/nsmb.2842

[24] Harris E, Holden KL, Edgil D, Polacek C, Clyde K. Molecular biology of flaviviruses. Novartis Found Symposium. 2006;**277**:23-39. DOI: 10.1002/0470058005.ch3

[25] Bernier A, Sagan S. The Diverse Roles of microRNAs at the Host–Virus Interface. Viruses [Internet]. MDPI AG; 19 August 2018;**10**(8):440. DOI: 10.3390/v10080440

[26] Al-Janabi O, Wach S, Nolte E, Weigelt K, Rau TT, Stöhr C, et al. Piwi-like 1 and 4 gene transcript levels are associated with clinicopathological parameters in renal cell carcinomas. Biochimica et Biophysica Acta. 2014;**1842**(5):686-690. DOI: 10.1016/j.bbadis.2014.01.014

[27] Stroynowska A, Agnieszka C, Krzyzosiak WJ. The panorama of miRNA-mediated mechanisms in mammalian cells. Cellular and Molecular Life Sciences. 2014;**71**:2253-2270. DOI: 10.1007/s00018-013-1551-6

[28] Faehnle CR, Joshua-Tor L. Argonautes confront new small RNAs. Current Opinion in Chemical Biology. 2008;**148**(4):825-832. DOI: 10.1038/jid.2014.371

[29] Zipprich JT, Bhattacharyya S, Mathys H, Filipowicz W. Importance of the C-terminal domain of the human GW182 protein TNRC6C for translational repression. RNA. 2009;**15**(5):781-793. DOI: 10.1261/rna.1448009

[30] Diniz DG, Fôro CAR, Turiel MCP, Sosthenes MC, Demachki S, Gomes GF, et al. Environmental influences on antibody-enhanced dengue disease outcomes. Memórias do Instituto Oswaldo Cruz [Internet]. FapUNIFESP (SciELO). Dec 2012;**107**(8):1021-1029. DOI: 10.1590/s0074-02762012000800010

[31] Huang YJS, Higgs S, Horne KM, Vanlandingham DL. Flavivirus-mosquito interactions. Viruses. 2014;**6**(11):4703-4730. DOI: 10.3390/v6114703

[32] Davis-Dusenbery BN, Hata A, Qi Y, Li Y, Zhang L, Huang J. Mechanisms of control of microRNA biogenesis. Molecular Medicine Reports. 2013;**148**(3):791-798. DOI: 10.3892/mmr.2013.1288

[33] Gubler DJ. Dengue and dengue hemorrhagic fever. Clinical Microbiology Reviews. 1998;**11**(3):480-496. DOI: 10.1016/S0140-6736(97)12483-7

[34] Smith JL, Jeng S, McWeeney SK, Hirsch AJ. A MicroRNA screen identifies the Wnt signaling pathway as a regulator of the interferon response during flavivirus infection. In: Diamond MS, editor. Journal of Virology [Internet]. American Society for Microbiology; 1 February 2017;**91**(8). DOI: 10.1128/jvi.02388-16

[35] Feng X, Zhou S, Wang J, Hu W. microRNA profiles and functions in mosquitoes. PLOS Neglected Tropical Diseases. 2018;**12**(5):6463. DOI: 10.1371/journal.pntd.0006463

[36] Asgari S. Role of microRNAs in Arbovirus/vector interactions. Viruses. 2014;**6**(9):3514-3534. DOI: 10.3390/v6093514

[37] Lima-Camara TN. Arboviroses emergentes e novos desafios para a saúde pública no Brasil. Rev Saúde Pública. 2016;**50**(36):1-7. DOI: 10.1590/S1518-8787.2016050006791

[38] Kakumani PK, Ponia SS, Rajgokul KS, Sood V, Chinnappan M, Banerjea AC, et al. Role of RNA interference (RNAi) in dengue virus replication and identification of NS4B as an RNAi suppressor. Journal of Virology. 2013;**87**(16):8870-8883. DOI: 10.1128/JVI.02774-12

[39] Tambyah PA, Ching CS, Sepramaniam S, Ali JM, Armugam A, Jeyaseelan K. microRNA expression in blood of dengue patients. Annals of Clinical Biochemistry. 2016 Jul;**53**(4):466-476. DOI: 10.1177/0004563215604001

[40] Pong LY, Parkkinen S, Dhanoa A, Gan HM, Wickremesinghe IAC, Syed HS. MicroRNA profiling of mouse liver in response to DENV-1 infection by deep sequencing. PeerJ. 2019;**7**(4):6697. DOI: 10.7717/peerj.6697

[41] Mishra R, Lata S, Ali A, Banerjea AC. Dengue haemorrhagic fever: A job done via exosomes? Emerging Microbes & Infections. 2019;**8**(1):1626-1635. DOI: 10.1080/22221751.2019.1685913

[42] Castillo JA, Castrillón JC, Diosa-Toro M, Betancur JG, St Laurent G, Smit JM, et al. Complex interaction between dengue virus replication and expression of miRNA-133a. BMC Infectious Diseases. 2016;**16**(1):29. DOI: 10.1186/s12879-016-1364-y

[43] Mishra R, Sood V, Banerjea AC. Dengue NS5 modulates expression of miR-590 to regulate ubiquitin-specific peptidase 42 in human microglia. FASEB BioAdvances. 2019;**1**(4):265-278. DOI: 10.1096/fba.2018-00047

[44] Ouyang X, Jiang X, Gu D, Zhang Y, Kong SK, Jiang C, et al. Dysregulated serum MiRNA profile and promising biomarkers in dengue-infected patients. International Journal of Medical Sciences. 2016;**13**(3):195-205. DOI: 10.7150/ijms.13996

[45] Bruscella P, Bottini S, Baudesson C, Pawlotsky JM, Feray C, Trabucchi M. Viruses and miRNAs: More friends than foes. Frontiers in Microbiology. 2017;**8**:1-11. DOI: 10.3389/fmicb.2017.00824

[46] Kakumani PK, Rajgokul KS, Ponia SS, Kaur I, Mahanty S, Medigeshi GR, et al. Dengue NS3, an RNAi suppressor, modulates the human miRNA pathways through its interacting partner. The Biochemical Journal. 2015;**471**(1):89-99. DOI: 10.1042/BJ20150445

[47] Wen W, He Z, Jing Q, Hu Y, Lin C, Zhou R, et al. Cellular microRNA-miR-548g-3p modulates the replication of dengue virus. The Journal of Infection. 2015;**70**(6):631-640. DOI: 10.1016/j.jinf.2014.12.001

[48] Castillo JA, Castrillón JC, Diosa-Toro M, Betancur JG, St. Laurent G, Smit JM, et al. Complex interaction between dengue virus replication and expression of miRNA-133a. BMC Infectious Diseases. 2015;**16**(1):29. DOI: 10.1186/s12879-016-1364-y

[49] Yan H, Zhou Y, Liu Y, Deng Y, Puthiyakunnon S, Chen X. miR-252 of the Asian tiger mosquito *Aedes albopictus* regulates dengue virus replication by suppressing the expression of the dengue virus envelope protein. Journal of Medical Virology. 2014;**86**(8):1428-1436. DOI: 10.1002/jmv.23815

[50] Castrillón-Betancur JC, Urcuqui-Inchima S. Overexpression of miR-484 and miR-744 in Vero cells alters dengue virus replication. Memórias do Instituto Oswaldo Cruz. 2017;**112**(4):281-291. DOI: 10.1590/0074-02760160404

[51] Girardi E, López P, Pfeffer S. On the importance of host microRNAs during viral infection. Frontiers in Genetics. 2018;**9**:1-17. DOI: 10.1186/s12929-019-0614-x

[52] Wu N, Gao N, Fan D, Wei J, Zhang J, An J. miR-223 inhibits dengue virus replication by negatively regulating the microtubule-destabilizing protein STMN1 in EAhy926 cells. Microbes and Infection. 2014;**16**(11):911-922. DOI: 10.1016/j.micinf.2014.08.011

[53] McCartney EM, Helbig KJ, Narayana SK, Eyre NS, Aloia AL, Beard MR. Signal transducer and activator of transcription 3 is a proviral host factor for hepatitis C virus. Hepatology. 2013;**58**(5):1558-1568. DOI: 10.1002/hep.26496

[54] Omoto S, Ito M, Tsutsumi Y, Ichikawa Y, Okuyama H, Brisibe EA, et al. HIV-1 nef suppression by virally encoded microRNA. Retrovirology. 2004;**1**:44. DOI: 10.1186/1742-4690-1-44

[55] Scaria V, Hariharan M, Maiti S, Pillai B, Brahmachari SK. Host-virus interaction: A new role for microRNAs. Retrovirology. 2006;**3**:68. DOI: 10.1186/1742-4690-3-68

Chapter 7

Phage Display as a Strategy to Obtain Anti-flavivirus Monoclonal Antibodies

Isaura Beatriz Borges Silva,
Renato Kaylan Alves de Oliveira França,
Jacyelly Medeiros Silva, Andrea Queiroz Maranhão
and Carlos Roberto Prudencio

Abstract

Arbovirus of the *Flaviviridae* family represents an issue worldwide, particularly because it can lead to serious illness and death in some countries. There is still a great complexity in obtaining effective therapies and specific and sensitive diagnostic tests, due to the high antigenic similarity between them. This similarity may account for antibodies cross reactivity which has positive and negative consequences for the course of infectious diseases. Among dengue virus (DENV) serotype infections, the cross-reactivity can increase virus replication and the risk of a severe disease by a mechanism known as an antibody-dependent enhancement (ADE). The search for serological biomarkers through monoclonal antibodies (MAbs) that identify unique viral regions can assist in the differential detection, whereas the development of recombinant antibodies with a neutralizing potential can lead to the establishment of efficacious treatments. The Phage Display methodology emerged as one of the main alternatives for the selection of human MAbs with high affinity for a specific target. Therefore, this technology can be a faster alternative for the development of specific diagnostic platforms and efficient and safe treatments for flavivirus infections. In this context, we propose for this chapter a discussion about Phage Display as a strategy to obtain MAbs for DENV and other flaviviruses.

Keywords: antibody, Phage Display, dengue virus, flavivirus, therapy, diagnosis

1. Introduction

When thinking about the development of virus detection and neutralization technologies whose bases of action are immunoglobulins, it is necessary to understand the structure of the viral particle of interest. In addition to the sequence of amino acid residues that make up the target epitopes, their position in the particle and their function in the process of infection and viral replication influence the design experiments aiming the obtantion of antibodies with a diagnostic and therapeutic potential.

The structures of flavivirus have been determined and studied, mainly, by combining cryo-electron microscopy with data from X-ray diffraction experiments using crystallography of viral proteins in the presence or not of antibody molecules. Results of this combination showed that the flavivirus is composed of a dense icosahedral electron nucleus and a lipid bilayer surrounding it. The genome comprises a sequence of ~10,700 nucleotides of a positive-sense RNA that encodes a polyprotein that is cleaved in 3 structural proteins, capsid protein (C), membrane protein (M), and envelope protein (E), and in 7 nonstructural proteins, NS1, NS2A, NS2B, NS3, NS4A, NS4B, and NS5 [1]. The NS1 protein plays a role in viral replication and is often shown to be a soluble antigen secreted into the bloodstream, interacting with components of the immune system. NS5 is the largest and most conserved nonstructural protein and acts in the transcription process of viral RNA [2, 3].

The icosahedral capsid is small and poorly organized, but it provides enough space for the genome and is surrounded by the envelope, so there are few connections between these structures, unlike what is found in other viruses. The viral envelope consists of two internal and concentric layers of phospholipids and an outer protein shell formed by regions of protein M and ectodomains of glycoprotein E organized in dimers which present protein determinants for the binding of the virus to the host cell (hemagglutination). Protein E contains three domains: domain I (DI), which is related to cell tropism and envelope organization; domain II (DII), which comprises the dimerization region and the fusion peptide; and domain III (DIII) with the function of binding to cell receptors, in the initial stage of viral infection [4, 5].

The fusion loop is a highly conserved region between dengue virus (DENV) serotypes and all flaviviruses, responsible for the late stage of infection, in which the virus interacts with the endosomal membrane, resulting in the release of the nucleocapsid in the cytoplasm. When the particle is in the lysosomal vesicle during the infection process, a structural reorganization of the viral envelope occurs; the fusion loop is exposed and inserted in the lysosomal membrane. After the formation of the fusion loop contact, protein E starts to organize itself into trimmers, resulting in the expansion of the viral particle and the approximation of the viral and lysosomal membranes, forming the fusion lipid pore that allows the release of the viral genome to the cytoplasm [3, 6, 7].

DENV serotypes show great heterogeneity in the structure of viral proteins. However, there is also antigenic similarity between DENV serotypes and, for some peptide sequences, between flaviviruses. Phylogeny studies of virus sequences, by estimating the antigenic distance between them, concluded that serotypes 1 and 3 are the most similar, serotype 2 was the second to diverge evolutionarily, and serotype 4 is the one that presents greater genetic difference. There is a 32% difference in the structure of protein E of the four DENV serotypes. Specific mutations in the genome result in the antigenic variability found in each serotype [7–9].

Much of the genetic difference between flaviviruses is due to protein E, which can show up to 60% difference in its amino acid sequence. In the phylogenetic analysis of the viruses, the DENV serotypes are closer to the Zika virus (ZIKV), with approximately 45% difference, and have 50 and 60% dissimilarity with West Nile virus (WNV) and yellow fever virus (YFV), respectively. DENV and other flaviviruses vary dramatically in terms of the amino acid sequence of the glycosylation region and the content of glycans added to the surface of E and precursor membrane protein (prM). Many epitopes of protein E are unique to a DENV serotype [4, 9–11]. It can also be observed in ZIKV, which has the glycosylation site, in the DI of protein E, different in conformation and length of the loop that contains this glycosylation site. The carbohydrate associated with this residue can act as a virus binding site in host cells. Thus, differences in this region of glycosylation can influence cell tropism, infection, and pathogenesis of these viruses [12]. Another important characteristic of ZIKV is the insertion of an alanine residue in the carboxyl termination of DIII, which is associated with an increased stability of this virus [13].

The hydrophobic sequence of the fusion loop appears to be the only epitope that is conserved among all flaviviruses; however, the degree of exposure in this region varies substantially among viruses [6]. Nonstructural proteins, NS1 and NS5, also present some epitopes conserved among the DENV serotypes and other members of the flavivirus genus, but their position also varies between viral strains. The relationships of antigenic similarity between flaviviruses generate immune responses that are configured as cross-reactions with protective or pathological characteristics [5, 14, 15].

2. Immunoglobulins

Immunoglobulins, or antibodies, are glycoproteins, expressed on the surface of B cells or secreted, that act in the neutralization and elimination of pathogens [16]. Antibodies are relatively flexible "Y"-shaped molecules made up of two heavy chains and two light chains, joined by an extensive network of non-covalent interactions, stabilized by disulfide bonds. Both types of chains are composed of constant and variable domains. The constant regions determine the functional properties of the antibody, and the variable regions determine the antigen-binding site. The light chain consists of a variable portion (VL) and a constant portion (CL) that can have two types of domains, kappa (ƙ) or lambda (λ). The heavy chain consists of a variable portion (VH) and three or four constant portions, depending on the class of the antibody, which are CH1, CH2, CH3, and CH4. The type of heavy chain determines the class, or isotype, of antibody, such as IgA, IgG, IgD, IgE, and IgM [17].

The antibody molecule can be subdivided into portions of the crystallizable fragment (Fc) and antigen-binding fragment (Fab) region. The Fc portion has the constant domains (CH2, CH3, CH4), and the Fab portion consists of the VH-CH1 and VL-CL domains. The Fab portion retains the ability to bind to the antigen, and the Fc portion acts to mediate the effector functions of antibodies [17].

Three segments containing variability can be identified in both the VH and VL domains. These segments are the hypervariable regions that determine antigen specificity and are more commonly called complementarity-determining regions (CDRs)—CDR1, CDR2, and CDR3. The combination of CDRs from a VH with CDRs from a VL forms the region of interaction with the epitope, called the paratope [17]. The variability of the antigen-binding regions is responsible for the ability of different antibodies to bind to many structurally diverse antigens [18]. **Figure 1** represents the structure of an IgG immunoglobulin and its domains.

In cognate antigen recognition, some naïve B cells can initiate somatic hypermutation, generating new variable domains, that can be selected based on their ability of antigen binding, usually with high affinity compared to germinal domains. After antigen recognition, naïve B cells differentiate into antibody-secreting plasma cells. These plasma cells secrete antibodies with high affinity and, can differentiate into memory B cells. Memory B cells are highly specialized cells for quickly recognizing the antigen in subsequent exposure, can persist for years, and provide long-term humoral protection for decades. These functional features of memory B cells are the basis of effective vaccines [19].

The knowledge about the mechanisms of antibody production and clonal selection of B cells led to the development of innovative hybridoma technology in 1975 [20]. The technique is based on the fusion of B lymphocytes with myeloma cells giving rise to hybrid cells that produce monoclonal antibodies (MAbs) continuously in vitro [21]. Therefore, MAbs are monovalent antibodies, which bind to the same epitope and are produced from a single B lymphocyte clone.

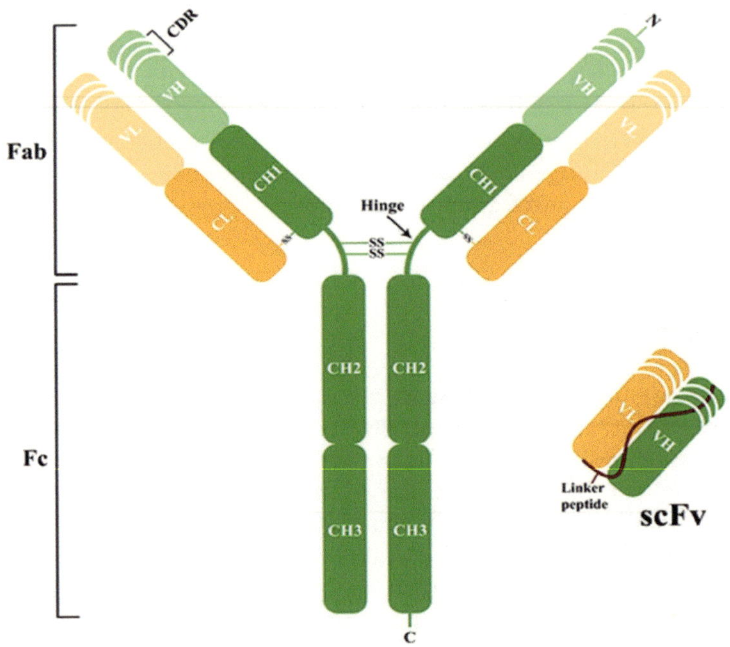

Figure 1.
Classical structure of an antibody. Structure of a class G immunoglobulin, representing the two portions of the molecule: two Fabs that correspond to the antigen-binding fragment and an Fc that corresponds to the crystallizable fragment. A type G antibody consists of two heavy polypeptide chains, each containing a VH and three constant domains (CH1, CH2, and CH3), and two light chains, each containing a VL and a CL. CDRs are three regions of hypervariability present in each of the variable domains. In addition to the natural format of the antibody, it is possible to generate recombinant antibodies such as the single-chain variable fragment (scFvs).

MAbs interact with a single epitope allowing a specific reactivity and affinity for target antigens. This feature is a great advantage over polyclonal antibodies, which have different epitope specificities and affinities [22, 23]. For this reason, MAbs have a broad clinical applicability in therapy for various illness, including cancer, transplant rejection, and autoimmune, infectious, hematologic, and cardiovascular diseases. Moreover, MAbs can play a significant role in the diagnosis and as antibody-drug conjugate for drug delivery. Thus, MAbs are considered a powerful tool for a wide range of medical applications.

2.1 Cross-reactivity of antibodies

Antibodies that bind to different flaviviruses are able to promote both the neutralization of the infection and the increase of the virus capture, such as by the interaction of immune complexes with Fc receptors expressed in certain cell types. The creation of alternative routes of entry of the viral particle into cells by low-neutralizing antibodies, during secondary infections of flavivirus, results in increased levels of viral replication and pathogenicity. This mechanism constitutes a phenomenon called antibody-dependent enhancement (ADE) [24, 25].

Different studies have been conducted to understand the effects of cross-reactive memory antibodies on subsequent flavivirus exposures. Many of them reported that the opsonization of the virus with weakly neutralizing antibodies led to the increase of the viral production and of pro-inflammatory mediators. This could lead to the suppression of the antiviral immune response, worsening the clinical condition of the disease [5, 7]. ADE has already been reported in in vitro experiments of infection of cells that express Fc receptors and in vivo experiments of vaccination with flavivirus [11, 26]. From the results of these experiments, ADE is pointed out as one of the main causes of severe forms of DENV infection and of the low protection induced by vaccines targeting DENV serotypes [27].

An opposite effect of cross-reacting antibodies has also been demonstrated, an increase in protection against secondary infections by flavivirus, which has resulted in potent neutralization and rapid induction of affinity maturing immune responses against heterologous flaviviruses. Studies in endemic areas of flavivirus showed protection against Zika virus infection in patients with a previous experience with DENV. A humoral response capable of potentially neutralizing both species of flavivirus was assembled from the expansion of cross-reaction memory B cell clones, even in the absence of DENV circulation. Thus, previous flavivirus infections can lead to both cross-neutralization and increased pathogenicity of the virus through the formation of interspecific antibody memory [28, 29].

The potential of cross-reaction immunity to trigger protection or pathology depends on the profile, quality, and magnitude of the immune responses induced by antibodies. The ADE reaction is a factor that should be considered in the development of therapeutic antibodies and vaccines for infections by flavivirus. Different approaches have been tested to shift the ADE profile to a cross-protection profile in heterogeneous infections of these viruses.

3. Phage Display

The principle of the Phage Display is the presentation of libraries of molecules on the surface of a bacteriophage (phage), allowing the identification of a wide range of biomolecules, including peptides, antibodies, and other proteins. The Phage Display methodology was first described in 1985, by George Smith and colleagues. Through the expression (display) of polypeptides on the phage surface (phage) M13, it was possible to perform the mapping of antibody epitopes by screening them using random peptide libraries [30]. In 1990, McCafferty and colleagues [31] demonstrated that it was also possible to fuse genes that encode an entire antibody domain, in the form of a scFv to the sequence of one of the bacteriophage's coat proteins. This approach allowed that this methodology could also be used for the selection of bacteriophages that recognize antigens.

Later, in 1994, Winter refined the Phage Display technology through a guided selection strategy of human antibody fragments from Phage Display repertoires for a single-antigen epitope, using rodent MAbs as a model [32]. The first all-human antibody produced, using Winter's Phage Display technique, to be marketed for use in humans was adalimumab (Humira), approved by the United States Food and Drug Administration (FDA) in 2002 for the treatment of rheumatoid arthritis [33]. It is noteworthy that George P. Smith and Gregory P. Winter received the Nobel Prize in chemistry in 2018 for the Phage Display of peptides and antibodies (Nobel Prize, 2018), a true tool for molecular evolution *in vitro* emphasizing the importance of this technique in obtaining biomolecules for various applications.

Phages are single-stranded viruses that infect Gram-negative bacteria and are used mainly for the purpose of gene cloning and expression of recombinant proteins, in addition to basic molecular biology studies. The particle coating is composed of five different proteins, pIII, pVI, pVII, pVIII, and pIX; proteins responsible for DNA replication include pII, pV, and pX; and the assembly proteins are pI, pIV, and pXI. All of the five proteins contribute to the stability of the phage particle; however, pIII is also necessary for the recognition and infection of the host cell [33]. Through genetic manipulation, sequences of billions of peptides, protein variants, and antibody fragments can be cloned into a vector associated with the phage coat protein gene, the pIII protein being the most commonly used [34]. Thus, the Phage Display methodology explores the possibility of direct binding of a certain protein (phenotype) with its cognate gene (genotype) by means of a phage [35].

3.1 Antibody Phage Display

Beyond the Phage Display and hybridoma technique, other strategies used for MAb production include immortalization of human B lymphocyte isolated from naturally infected or immunized individuals. One of the approaches for B lymphocyte immortalization is using Epstein-Barr virus (EBV). EBV is a human tumor virus that was shown to infect efficiently human B lymphocytes and induce continuous proliferation in vitro, opening a new perspective for the production of human MAbs [36]. Another relevant alternative for MAb production involves transgenic animals where mice are genetically manipulated to produce human immunoglobulin. In this strategy, genes of human immunoglobulins are inserted into mice genome replacing the endogenous sequences, making these animals capable to produce fully human antibodies when immunized with an antigen [37].

Among the existing methodologies of antibody production, the hybridoma technique remains the most widely used. However, the production steps are laborious and dependent on the animal immune system. In addition, the heterologous character of these proteins often makes them immunogenic to humans, provoking the response of human anti-mouse antibodies (HAMA), which restrict their therapeutic use [34]. Therefore, the Phage Display has emerged as one of the main alternatives for the generation of human recombinant MAbs. The major advantages of using the Phage Display, in contrast to the hybridoma technique, are clearly the absence of the use of animals in the process and the less time to obtain antibodies. The conventional method requires immunization which, depending on the type of antigen, can take weeks to produce sufficient immune response to produce specific antibodies [38].

There are important advantages and disadvantages between techniques for obtaining human MAbs. With the Phage Display technology, it is possible to isolate antibodies against all types of antigens, even those with high complexity; differently, the immortalization technique of human lymphocytes does not allow the isolation of antibodies against own antigens or non-immunogenic antigens [39]. In addition, only the Phage Display allows the optimization of MAbs, for example, by affinity maturation, and in general, the development of antibodies on the Phage Display tends to be faster than in other methods [40].

In addition to being robust due to the high stability of the phage, the Phage Display also allows control over biochemical parameters throughout the selection process. The particular advantage of having control over biochemical parameters during the time of selection can also be used to shape the specificity profile of an antibody from the start [41]. **Table 1** described the MAbs with FDA approval that was developed using the Phage Display technique.

Since 1990, different antibody formats have been employed in the construction of antibody Phage Display libraries (APDLs). Although antibody libraries are one of the most successful tools of Phage Display, the appropriate choice of antibody library is an important step for the success of antibody selection. Full-length antibodies in the immunoglobulin format are large (150 kDa), complex, and not suitable for Phage Display. Therefore, smaller antigen-binding fragments are used. For this reason, APDLs are in most cases constructed in either scFv (25 kDa), Fab (50 kDa), or single-domain antibody (sdAb) formats which are smaller and more effective, although each antibody format has its own advantages and limitations [42]. Particularly, sdAbs have received a growing interest as a promising antibody

Antibody	Target	Format	Indication	Company	Year
Humira adalimumab	TNF-α	Human	Rheumatoid arthritis and Crohn's disease	Abbott	2002
Lucentis Ranibizumab	VEGF-A	Humanized	Macular degeneration	Genentech	2006
Simponi Golimumab	TNF-α	Human	Rheumatoid arthritis	Johnson & Johnson	2009
Benlysta Belimumab	BLys	Human	Systemic lupus erythematosus	GSK	2011
Pending Raxibacumab	PA	Human	Anthrax infection (*Bacillus anthracis*)	GSK	2012
Cyramza Ramucirumab	VEGFR2	Human	Gastric cancer	Lilly	2014
Bavencio Avelumab	PD-L1	Human	Merkel cell carcinoma	Serono	2017
Tremfya Guselkumab	IL-23	Human	Plaque psoriasis	Janssen Biotech	2017
Gamifant Emapalumab	IFNγ	Human	Hemophagocytic lymphohistiocytosis	Swiss	2018

TNF-α, tumor necrosis factor alpha; VEGF-A, vascular endothelial growth factor A; BLys, B lymphocyte stimulator; PA, protective antigen; VEGFR2, vascular endothelial growth factor receptor 2; PD-L1, programmed death-ligand 1; IL-23, interleukin-23; IFNγ, interferon-γ

Table 1.
Monoclonal antibodies obtained by Phage Display with FDA approval.

class compared with those conventional. Their more hydrophilic structure, easy molecular manipulation, convex surface, and long CDRs enable them to recognize cryptic and inaccessible epitopes for typical antibody fragments [43].

There are many kinds of APDLs; they can be classified into two main types: natural APDL and synthetic APDL. This classification is based on the source of VH and VL genes. Natural APDL comprises immune libraries and naïve libraries, while synthetic APDLs comprise semisynthetic libraries and fully synthetic libraries [44]. The immune libraries use V-genes that already passed to the clonal selection and encode antibodies with high affinity and specificity against the target antigen. The immune APDLs have some advantages compared to other libraries, once they have the possibility to be explored for understanding the humoral responses in the specific disease. However, some limitations regarding this library are associated with the toxicity of some antigens and some ethical issues, which consequently impair the feasibility to active immunization of humans or other animals for obtention of antibody repertoires [41, 44].

The naïve APLD involves the generation of libraries that allows the discovery of MAbs against all types of antigen. These libraries are produced through the repertoires of healthy donors, and antibody genes contained have much more diversity than immune libraries. The main advantage of using naïve libraries is the possibility to isolate MAbs against non-immunogenic and toxic antigens. However, the major drawback is that the selected MAbs often have low affinities compared with antibodies from immune libraries [33]. The semisynthetic APLD is based on the display of artificially made diversity in V-gene segments, usually by in vitro randomization of CDRs from a limited number of naïve variable regions, reconstructing the V-gene repertoires [41]. One of the characteristics of these libraries is the absence of natural biases and redundancies usually found in a naïve library. Unlike semisynthetic APDLs, the fully synthetic library is constructed through the incorporation of nucleotide randomization based on in silico design and de novo synthesis. This refined synthesis appears to increase the functional size of library and consequently the isolation of MAbs with a great range of affinity. However, they still need to be optimized regarding their binding sites, affinity, valency, and other characteristics [41, 44].

Except in the case of fully synthetic libraries, generally, the construction of an antibody library is based on the amplification of the repertoire of the variable chain genes of one or more individuals using primers that cover all families of this gene. Subsequently, a random combination of the VL and VH chain is generated. In the case of the production of Fab libraries, a step is taken to join each variable chain fragment with its respective constant region. The PCR products of these amplifications, representing the antibody repertoire, are ligated into a phagemid vector and transformed into *E. coli*. However, phage vectors generally have only the origin of replication of the phage; they do not contain all the genes necessary for replication and assembly of these phages. Thus, screening libraries using this phagemid requires a helper phage to provide replication and assembly proteins. The addition of the phage to the bacterial cells transformed with the phagemid will result in the production of a mixture of phages that will present predominantly the phagemid vector [45].

Once assembled, each phage exposes a fragment of functional antibody fused to one of the phage surface proteins [46, 47]. A determining factor for the quality of a library and consequently the success of a biopanning by Phage Display is its initial diversity, given by the number of different antibodies in the library. The greater the initial diversity of clones within the library, the greater the likelihood of containing sequences that will bind to a given target with greater affinity [45]. The capacity to produce very large libraries (1012 different clones) has turned the Phage Display into a fast and reliable high-throughput screening methodology [43].

Most biopanning methods are based on four main steps, preparing a library; incubation of that library with a given antigen; removal of nonspecific or low-affinity phages; and recovery of binding targets, which will be amplified after infection in *E. coli* and used in the next biopanning cycle (**Figure 2**). The Phage Display biopanning process is characterized by an increase in the number of clones with affinity for the target molecule through successive selection cycles, with a consequent reduction in the diversity of clones and in the presence of clones with low affinity [48]. Thus, the biopanning results in the sequential enrichment of phages that have a specific binding to the antigen.

These biopanning steps are usually repeated three to five times, until a high specificity/affinity ligand is identified [34, 45, 46]. During biopanning, phage binding to the antigen is retained on the plate, and, after a series of washes, these phages are eluted and amplified. Subsequently, the phages are again incubated with the antigen in the next cycle. Phages with low affinity for antigens may stick to the plate, not interacting with the particle, or remain suspended in the solution. After the wash step, many of these nonspecific phages are removed. Generally, this step involves the application of a greater wash stringency in each subsequent round, which can be performed by increasing the number of washes or increasing the concentration of the nonionic detergent buffer used.

3.2 Post-selection step

During the biopanning stage, it is possible to monitor the enrichment of antibodies by measuring the phage titers that enter the selection and the phage titers that are eluted, assessing the enrichment ratio at each selection cycle. The enrichment follow-up provides the assurance that the selection was carried out

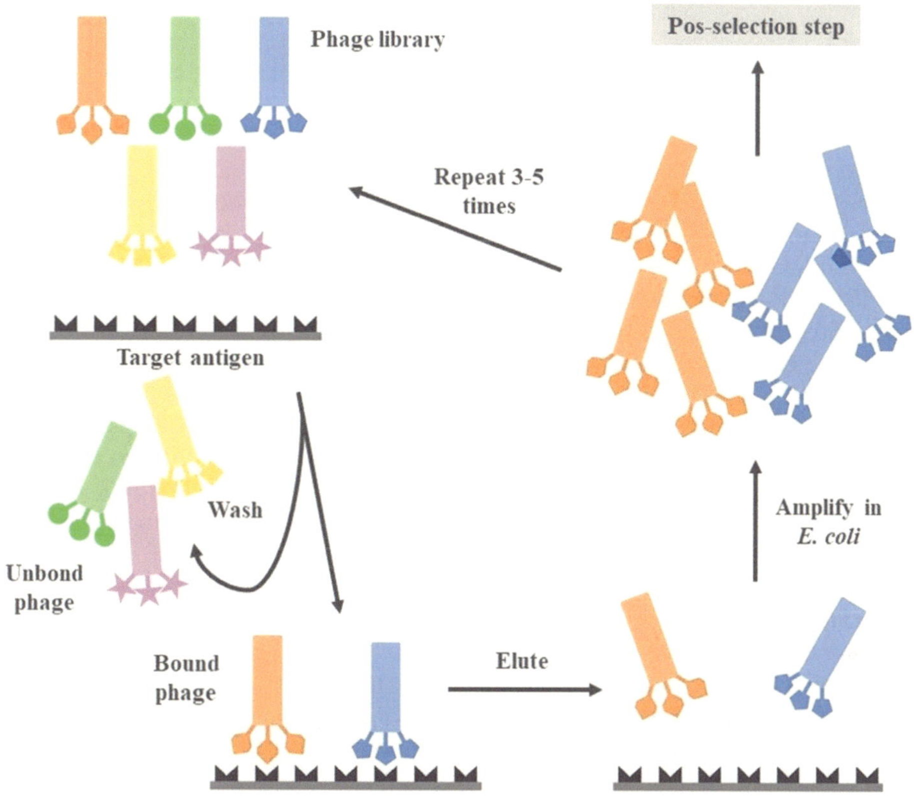

Figure 2.
Biopanning steps. Representation of a biopanning process characterized by a step of Phage Display library incubation with the target antigen, removal of unbound phages, elution of bound phages, and phage amplification in E. coli*, followed by another cycle. After 3–5 cycles post-selection step is carried out.*

efficiently and is followed by the analysis of the selection progress and the identification of the antibodies that have greater affinity to the target antigen [49]. Over the decades, different ways of analyzing selection have been reported, depending on the selection system employed, the antibody library used, and the antigen of interest. However, two methods stand out for the quality of the results they offer, a monoclonal analysis of a sample of the selected antibodies and a polyclonal analysis of the sequences of the entire antibody population.

From the population of selected phages or using cultures of the selected soluble antibodies, the specific binding of individual clones to the immobilized antigen is assessed in an ELISA assay. In this monoclonal ELISA, the binding of 30–100, or more, randomly chosen clones is compared with each other and with the negative control. Phages with the highest absorbance values are considered the ones that have displayed functionally antibodies of greater affinity. Positive clones for the binding analysis are subjected to a Sanger sequencing reaction to determine the sequences of the antibodies [50–52]. In this type of Phage Display analysis, the phenotypes (activity) of the antibodies are investigated first and then their genotype is determined. The disadvantage of this type of analysis is that it does not allow exploring the antibody population in depth and may not include all antibodies of greater affinity. In addition, it does not allow the study of the magnitude of selection and enrichment [53].

A high-throughput sequencing provides a tool for rapid analysis of the selection and direct identification of the most enriched antibodies, with greater affinity, without requiring a step of their expression. In addition to the speed of analysis, it is possible to investigate the original diversity of the library; identify all antibodies that enriched, the most enriched, and the rare in the population; and determine the frequency of increase throughout the selection. This is possible because sequencing technologies, called next-generation sequencing (NGS), are used, and they allow sequencing a large number of sequences, in the order of millions, in the same sequencing reaction [54]. The interpretation of NGS results from antibody libraries requires the use of a bioinformatics tool specialized in calculating the enrichment of variable domains in a selection of Phage Display. Different tools for this purpose are described in the literature, such as the recent ATTILA pipeline [55].

Despite providing a profound assessment of all antibodies in all cycles, two major problems arise in the analysis of biopanning by sequencing. The first corresponds to the noise in the identified final sequences that results from the sequencing process or the gene amplification reaction. However, more accurate pipelines for isolating DNA libraries for sequencing and more powerful bioinformatics analysis programs have been produced to overcome the artifacts introduced by PCR and sequencing errors. The second is the limitation of the high-performance sequencing methodology that, although it allows the sequencing of millions of sequences, can only properly read up to 400 base pairs. Therefore, this analysis requires that the variable domains of the heavy and light chain of antibodies, whose size ranges from 300 to 400 base pairs, be amplified and sequenced separately, resulting in the loss of the VH and VL pairs of the most enriched antibodies. Recently, studies have been carried out to provide a method of sequencing without losing the VH and VL pairs of antibodies. In the analysis of the selection process by a high-throughput sequencing, the antibody's genotype is first determined and then their phenotype is characterized [53, 56, 57].

4. Application of Phage Display in the context of DENV and other flavivirus infections

The use of MAbs against an infection pathogen is an area of great interest for research. In **Table 2** it is demonstrated MAbs developed for infection disease who have been approved by the FDA. As can be seen, few MAbs are approved for use in infectious diseases, although there is still a strong demand for development in this field. Some challenges involving MAb production against pathogens are their economic viability due to their high cost and if target an episodic disease, there is no supporting for continued production. Moreover, there is a concern about the selection of neutralization-escape mutants [58]. However, they may be notably effective for certain emerging infectious diseases, in which the process of vaccine development could be lengthened and difficult. Thus, MAbs should have more effectiveness for the first response against these diseases [57].

Small molecules are most antibiotic antivirals. However, Phage Display-derived MAbs have an overall success rate of 35% of passage from clinical phase I to launch, compared to an average of 12% for a small-molecule drug candidate [59]. In this regard, Phage Display-derived MAb is considered an important alternative approach to infectious disease treatment compared to classical small-molecule discovery. Raxibacumab is an example of a fast-track designation from the FDA, providing the expedition of the drug to use against *B. anthracis* infection. This bacterium secretes proteins, the lethal factor and the edema factor, that inhibit normal immune system functioning that ultimately cause cell death. The entry of these factors is mediated by the protective antigen (PA), also secreted by the bacteria. Raxibacumab is directed to *B. anthracis* PA and thus prevents the cellular

Antibody	Target	Format	Indication	Company	Year	Method
Pending Raxibacumab	PA	Human	Anthrax infection (*Bacillus anthracis*)	GSK	2012	Phage Display
Zinplava Bezlotoxumab	Toxin B	Human	*Clostridium difficile* infection	Merck/ Dohme	2016	Transgenic mice
Trogarzo Ibalizumab	CD4	Humanized	HIV infection	TaiMed	2018	Hybridoma
Synagis Palivizumab	RSV F	Humanized	Respiratory syncytial virus (RSV) prophylaxis	MedImmune	1998	Hybridoma

PA, protective antigen; CD4, cluster of differentiation 4; RSV F, respiratory syncytial virus fusion

Table 2.
Monoclonal antibodies for infectious diseases approved by the FDA.

uptake of the lethal factor and edema factor. The MAb was developed by the Phage Display, using a library licensed by Human Genome Sciences (HGS), which now is GlaxoSmithKline (GSK), from Cambridge Antibody Technology. Recombinant PA was used in the biopanning process to select candidates, which were then screened in assays for PA neutralization [60, 61].

The Phage Display technology provides a rapid methodology for building a high-affinity antibody library from immune repertoires. These antibodies can be used to generate diagnostic bases or be tested for therapeutic capability. For example, from the repertoire of B cells of patients who recovered from *influenza* virus infections or who received vaccination, it was possible to isolate, by Phage Display, several antibodies with the neutralization property of different *influenza* virus subtypes. Another example of antibody-based immunotherapy developed by Phage Display involves the identification of antibodies specific to different types of coronavirus. These studies are an example of how Phage Display enables the selection of antibodies by an in vitro process, especially for new or mutated pathogens in an outbreak of emergent infectious diseases, as it uses only pathogen-specific antigens [39, 62, 63].

Particularly, MAbs play an important role in antiviral immunity preventing viral replication and disease progress. Antibodies can interfere with virus infection by various mechanisms. The primary mechanism is by targeting the virus surface proteins; antibodies can inhibit virus attachment to cell surface receptors. Another main mechanism is targeting non-receptor-binding regions, such as in endosomal membrane fusion step where neutralization can occur by interfering virus conformational changes. In general, flavivirus particles tend to display on their surface continuum epitopes that induce potently neutralizing antibodies, blocking viral entry into cells [58].

From the understanding of the structure of each flavivirus, it was possible to determine the antibody targets most conducive to the diagnosis and protection of the disease [64]. It is important to note that flaviviruses are not static particles and viral proteins are in a constant dynamic movement, a process known as breathing, in order to transiently reveal new epitopes, and this characteristic influences the detection and neutralization capabilities of antibodies [10].

So far, no MAbs against flavivirus have reached the clinical stages, except for WNV. However, several studies have demonstrated potentially neutralizing MAbs that could be therapeutically used against these infections [65, 66]. Different antibodies have been generated exploring the characteristics of viral epitopes. The E glycoprotein is the main target of neutralizing antibodies, especially the E DIII has been described to be the most efficient to block adsorption of DENV in vitro [58]. In the field of DENV diagnosis, MAbs have been especially applied to distinguish DENV serotypes [67, 68]. For this purpose E and soluble NS1 proteins are the main targets of these MAbs using different assay formats, such as ELISA and rapid test based on immunochromatography [69].

The pre-existing cross-reactive antibodies can be boosted in a secondary infection with antigenically related molecules; consequently antibody to fusion loop tends to have dominance upon sequential infections with DENV or other flaviviruses. Antibodies to E-dimer epitope (EDE) are divided into two subclasses, EDE1 and EDE2, based on the recognition of the conserved glycan Asn-153 of DENV [58]. EDE1 has already been shown to potently neutralize ZIKV infection; this class of antibody does not require glycosylation for binding [70]. However, EDE2 have a reduced neutralization potential against ZIKV, once these antibodies have a strongly binding dependence on the glycan, which have different positioning between ZIKV and DENV [66].

The generation of monoclonal antibodies by Phage Display can help improve the speed at which new antibodies are produced. The freedom associated with recombinant antibodies also allows them to be customized for various applications, allowing the development of MAbs with binding, functional, and pharmacological characteristics suitable for a therapeutic and diagnostic use [37]. Thus, the use of Phage Display to identify antibodies against DENV, as well as for other flavivirus, can contribute to the knowledge of the specific antigenic properties of the virus, allowing to generate new perspectives for the development of efficient therapies, vaccines, and diagnostic platforms of this virus.

To obtain specific antibodies to the DENV, it is possible to employ different libraries of Phage Display and distinct selection approaches depending on the purpose. Using a llama immune library, a diagnostic methodology was developed based on antibodies capable of binding to the NS1 of the four DENV serotypes, without cross-reacting with NS1 of other flaviviruses. The panning was performed with immobilized antigen, so that in each round, the phage population was incubated with NS1 from one of the serotypes, resulting in phage specific to all forms of NS1. To characterize the diagnostic potential of the antibodies, MAbs were addressed [71]. Lebani et al. [72] isolate four serotype-specific human antibodies through a negative selection strategy. Each MAb was specific for NS1 from a DENV serotype, without cross-linking.

In another approach, Cabezas et al. [73] worked with human naïve library to obtain a panel of antibody fragments with different specificity toward DENV serotypes. The biopanning was made against inactivated DENV-containing supernatants harvested from infected Vero cells for 4 days with each serotype. These supernatants were directly used for Phage Display biopanning. A panel of nine scFvs, where seven were specific for DENV2, DENV3, and DENV4 while the other two were cross-reactive, was obtained. Silva [74] employed a subtractive biopanning, in which a human Fab Phage Display library was first incubated against ZIKV particles, to eliminate the majority of antibodies that binds to this viral particle, and nonbinding phages were then incubated against DENV2 particles, followed by elution of ligand phages. Analysis by NGS of the pool of phages retrieved after four rounds of this biopanning showed that the VH and VL sequences obtained may not have cross-reactivity between DENV2 and ZIKV.

Antibody-based DENV infection therapies developed by Phage Display have also been reported. Saokaew et al. [75] show that a human scFv specific for DIII was able to neutralize DENV2 infection at in vitro assays. The human MAb 5A, originated from a selection of Phage Display, has been shown to be specific to the fusion loop, both in its pre-fusion conformation to the endocytic membrane, before infection, and in its acid-dependent post-fusion conformation, during the final viral infection process, and proved to be a potent neutralizing antibody of different strains of yellow fever virus in vitro and in vivo. Thus, MAb 5A prevents both virus attachment and fusion. As the fusion loop is a highly conserved antigen, there is a high possibility that 5A neutralizes other flaviviruses [76]. In the same way, Wu et al. [77] identified a panel of human MAbs that target DIII of the ZIKV envelope protein from a large Phage Display naïve antibody library. These germline-like antibodies bound ZIKV DIII specifically with high affinities. These MAbs neutralized the currently circulating ZIKV strains and showed a synergistic effect in neutralizing ZIKV in vitro and in a mouse model of ZIKV infection.

As an example of Phage Display using immune libraries to select high-affinity MAbs, Mwale et al. [78] analyzed the immune response in chicken through the determination of the polyclonal immunoglobulin yolk (IgY) against a truncated Zika virus envelope protein. They induced an immune response in white leghorn laying hens against the ZIKV envelope protein. A high-level titer of anti-ZIKV envelope protein antibodies was detected and after constructed two antibody libraries; they found some scFvs that showed specific binding activities toward the ZIKV envelope protein.

Moreover, Phage Display has been used to find therapeutic antibody fragments against nonstructural proteins. A MAb fragment Fab NS3-specific obtained from a naïve human Fab Phage Display library was shown to inhibit the ATPase and helicase activities of NS3 protein and reduces DENV replication in vitro. The ability to inhibit in vitro DENV replication may be exploited in a therapeutic approach [79]. Using a human scFv Phage Display library, Poungpair et al. [80] obtained two scFv clones that bound specifically to the NS1 of DENV 2, used as antigen in phage biopanning. They observed that cells infected with DENV2 and treated with selected scFvs had significant reduction of the infectious viral particles in supernatant. Besides that, the analysis of mimotope/epitope mapping indicated that the NS1 sites bound by antibody fragments can lead to interference of the virus replication by affecting the virus release.

5. Final considerations

Over the years many discoveries have been made aiming for the control and treatment of emerging infectious diseases, some of those include the development of efficient drugs that could act specifically in the pathogen to eliminate efficiently. In this way, MAbs emerged as the main biological drugs for this purpose. Moreover, MAbs play an important role in the development of serological diagnostic test that could be used for tracking the spread of disease and determining public health prevention measures and clinical care. There are still great questions around the infection mechanisms by flavivirus, especially related to the cross-reactivity between them and the risk of complications. In this way, the use of effective, fast, and robust approaches to facilitate the development of flavivirus MAbs is a determinant factor.

The Phage Display technology presents a great potential to provide optimized strategies, allowing the obtention of high-affinity human antibodies for a specific target. Some of the main advantages that make this technology so promising are the possibility to obtain human MAbs without in vivo immunization; the enormous diversity of variant antibodies displayed within a single library; the ability to tailor MAbs with the desired properties by using different strategies such as depletion, guided selection, and biochemical control; and the possibility to be applied against practically any kind of target antigen [33]. However, some concerns about Phage Display are the dependence of the initial library quality, the difficulties in the post-selection step involving analysis and recombinant antibody production, and the possibility of obtention of low-affinity antibodies, especially in naïve libraries [35]. Considering the impact of infectious diseases on the health system and economy, mainly DENV and ZIKV, that co-circulate in tropical countries, MAbs obtained by Phage Display may overcome issues related to versatility and high throughputness compared to other approaches, playing a larger role in the actual and future public health response.

Acknowledgements

The authors would like to thank the Immunology Department of Adolfo Lutz Institute, the Coordination of Improvement of Postgraduate Level Personnel (CAPES), and the National Council for Scientific and Technological Development (CNPq). The authors also thank the Cellular Biology Department from the University of Brazilia, Post-Graduate Program in Molecular Biology (UNB), and Foundation for Scientific and Technological Enterprises (FINATEC) for the financial and technical support. This study was financed under grant CNPq/CAPES/MS-DECIT No. 440812/2016-0 and FINEP under sgrant No. 01.16.0075, under the coordination of Dr. Carlos R. Prudencio.

Conflict of interest

The authors declare no conflict of interest.

Author details

Isaura Beatriz Borges Silva[1,2], Renato Kaylan Alves de Oliveira França[3], Jacyelly Medeiros Silva[3], Andrea Queiroz Maranhão[3] and Carlos Roberto Prudencio[1*]

1 Center of Immunology, Adolfo Lutz Institute, São Paulo/SP, Brazil

2 Interunits Post-Graduate Program in Biotechnology, University of São Paulo, São Paulo/SP, Brazil

3 Molecular Biology Laboratory, CEL/IB, University of Brasília, Brasília/DF, Brazil

*Address all correspondence to: carlos.prudencio@ial.sp.gov.br

References

[1] Kuhn RJ, Zhang W, Rossmann MG, et al. Structure of dengue virus: Implications for flavivirus organization, maturation, and fusion. Cell. 2002;**108**(5):717-725. DOI: 10.1016/s0092-8674(02)00660-8

[2] Zeidler JD, Fernandes-Siqueira LO, Barbosa GM, Da Poian AT. Non-canonical roles of dengue virus non-structural proteins. Viruses. 2017;**9**(3):42. DOI: 10.3390/v9030042. [Published: 13 March 2017]

[3] Zonetti LFC, Coutinho MC, de Araujo AS. Molecular aspects of the dengue virus infection process: A review. Protein and Peptide Letters. 2018;**25**(8):712-719. DOI: 10.2174/0929866525666180709115506

[4] Heinz FX, Stiasny K. The antigenic structure of Zika virus and its relation to other Flaviviruses: Implications for infection and Immunoprophylaxis. Microbiology and Molecular Biology Reviews. 2017;**81**(1):e00055-e00016. DOI: 10.1128/MMBR.00055-16. [Published: 08 February 2017]

[5] Rathore APS, St. John AL. Cross-reactive immunity among Flaviviruses. Frontiers in Immunology. 2020;**11**:334. DOI: 10.3389/fimmu.2020.00334. [Published: 26 February 2020]

[6] Modis Y, Ogata S, Clements D, Harrison SC. Structure of the dengue virus envelope protein after membrane fusion. Nature. 2004;**427**(6972):313-319. DOI: 10.1038/nature02165

[7] Wen J, Shresta S. Antigenic cross-reactivity between Zika and dengue viruses: Is it time to develop a universal vaccine? Current Opinion in Immunology. 2019;**59**:1-8. DOI: 10.1016/j.coi.2019.02.001 10

[8] Bell SM, Katzelnick L, Bedford T. Dengue genetic divergence generates within-serotype antigenic variation, but serotypes dominate evolutionary dynamics. eLife. 2019;**8**:e42496. DOI: 10.7554/eLife.42496 11. [Published: 06 August 2019]

[9] Dai L, Song J, Lu X, et al. Structures of the Zika virus envelope protein and its complex with a Flavivirus broadly protective antibody. Cell Host & Microbe. 2016;**19**(5):696-704. DOI: 10.1016/j.chom.2016.04.013 12

[10] Sirohi D, Kuhn RJ. Zika virus structure, maturation, and receptors. The Journal of Infectious Diseases. 2017;**216**(suppl_10):S935-S944. DOI: 10.1093/infdis/jix515 13

[11] Malafa S, Medits I, Aberle JH, et al. Impact of flavivirus vaccine-induced immunity on primary Zika virus antibody response in humans. PLoS Neglected Tropical Diseases. 2020;**14**(2):e0008034. DOI: 10.1371/journal.pntd.0008034 14. [Published: 04 February 2020]

[12] Sirohi D, Chen Z, Sun L, et al. The 3.8 Å resolution cryo-EM structure of Zika virus. Science. 2016;**352**(6284):467-470. DOI: 10.1126/science.aaf5316 15

[13] Kostyuchenko VA, Lim EX, Zhang S, et al. Structure of the thermally stable Zika virus. Nature. 2016;**533**(7603):425-428. DOI: 10.1038/nature1799416

[14] Poonsiri T, Wright GSA, Diamond MS, Turtle L, Solomon T, Antonyuk SV. Structural study of the C-terminal domain of nonstructural protein 1 from Japanese encephalitis virus. Journal of Virology. 2018;**92**(7):e01868-e01817. DOI: 10.1128/JVI.01868-17.17. [Published: 14 March 2018]

[15] Batista ICA, Quinan BR, Rocha Alves ÉA, et al. Design and production of dengue virus chimeric proteins useful

for developing tetravalent vaccines. Vaccine. 2020;**38**(8):2005-2015. DOI: 10.1016/j.vaccine.2020.01.003 18

[16] Moser M, Leo O. Key concepts in immunology. Vaccine. 2010;**285**:2-13. DOI: 10.1016/j.vaccine.2010.07.022

[17] Abbas AK, Lichtman AH, Pillai S. Cellular and Molecular Immunology. 8ª ed. Philadelphia: Elsevier; 2015

[18] Janeway CA Jr, Travers P, Walport M, Shlomchik MJ. The generation of diversity in immunoglobulins. In: Immunobiology: The Immune System in Health and Disease. 5th ed. Nova Iorque: Garland Science; 2001

[19] Akaya M, Kwak K, Pierce SK. B cell memory: Building two walls of protection against pathogens. Nature Reviews Immunology. 2020;**20**:229-238. DOI: 10.1038/s41577-019-0244-2

[20] Köhler G, Milstein C. Continuous cultures of fused cells secreting antibody of predefined specificity. Nature. 1975;**256**(5517):495. DOI: 10.4049/jimmunol.174.5.2451

[21] Pandey S. Hybridoma technology for production of monoclonal antibodies. Hybridoma. 2010;**1**(2):88-94

[22] Zola H. Monoclonal antibodies. Encyclopedia of Life Sciences. 2001:1-9. DOI: 10.1002/9780470015902.a0001205.pub3

[23] Siddiqui MZ. Monoclonal antibodies as diagnostics; an appraisal. Indian Journal of Pharmaceutical Sciences. 2010;**72**(1):12-17. DOI: 10.4103/0250-474X.62229

[24] Stettler K, Beltramello M, Espinosa DA, et al. Specificity, cross-reactivity, and function of antibodies elicited by Zika virus infection. Science. 2016;**353**(6301):823-826. DOI: 10.1126/science.aaf8505

[25] Haslwanter D, Blaas D, Heinz FX, Stiasny K. A novel mechanism of antibody-mediated enhancement of flavivirus infection. PLoS Pathogens. 2017;**13**(9):e1006643. DOI: 10.1371/journal.ppat.1006643. [Published: 15 September 2017]

[26] Chan KR, Wang X, Saron WAA, et al. Cross-reactive antibodies enhance live attenuated virus infection for increased immunogenicity. Nature Microbiology. 2016;**1**(12):16164. DOI: 10.1038/nmicrobiol.2016.164. [Published: 19 September 2016]

[27] Dejnirattisai W, Supasa P, Wongwiwat W, et al. Dengue virus sero-cross-reactivity drives antibody-dependent enhancement of infection with zika virus. Nature Immunology. 2016;**17**(9):1102-1108. DOI: 10.1038/ni.3515

[28] Robbiani DF, Bozzacco L, Keeffe JR, et al. Recurrent potent human neutralizing antibodies to Zika virus in Brazil and Mexico. Cell. 2017;**169**(4):597-609.e11. DOI: 10.1016/j.cell.2017.04.024

[29] Dussupt V, Sankhala RS, Gromowski GD, et al. Potent Zika and dengue cross-neutralizing antibodies induced by Zika vaccination in a dengue-experienced donor. Nature Medicine. 2020;**26**(2):228-235. DOI: 10.1038/s41591-019-0746-2

[30] Smith GP. Filamentous fusion phage: Novel expression vectors that display cloned antigens on the virion surface. Science. 1985;**228**:1315-1317. DOI: 10.1126/science.4001944

[31] McCafferty J, Griffiths AD, Winter G, Chiswell DJ. Phage antibodies: Filamentous Phage Displaying antibody variable domains. Nature. 1990;**348**(6301):552-554. DOI: 10.1038/348552a0

[32] Jespers LS, Roberts A, Mahler SM, Winter G, et al. Guiding the selection of

human antibodies from Phage Display repertoires to a single epitope of an antigen. Bio/Technology. 1994;**2**(9):899. DOI: 10.1038/nbt0994-899

[33] Nixon AE, Sexton DJ, Ladner RC. Drugs derived from Phage Display: From candidate identification to clinical practice. MAbs. 2014;**6**(1):73-85. DOI: 10.4161/mabs.27240

[34] Barbosa CD, Brigido MM, Maranhao AQ. Antibody Phage Display libraries: Contributions to oncology. International Journal of Molecular Sciences. 2012;**13**(5):5420-5440. DOI: 10.3390/ijms13055420

[35] Ledsgaard L, Kilstrup M, Vellatt AK, McCafferty J, et al. Basics of antibody Phage Display technology. Toxins. 2018;**10**(6):1-15. DOI: 10.3390/toxins10060236

[36] Mrozek-Gorska P, Buschle A, Pich D, et al. Epstein-Barr virus reprograms human B lymphocytes immediately in the prelatent phase of infection. Proceedings of the National Academy of Sciences of the United States of America. 2019;**116**(32):16046-16055. DOI: 10.1073/pnas.1901314116

[37] MLD S, Quintilio W, Manieri TM, Tsuruta LR, et al. Advances and challenges in therapeutic monoclonal antibodies drug development. Brazilian Journal of Pharmaceutical Sciences. 2018;**54**:1-15. DOI: 10.1590/s2175-97902018000001007

[38] Ch'ng ACW, Choong YS, Lim TS. Phage Display-Derived Antibodies: Application of Recombinant Antibodies for Diagnostics. Proof and Concepts in Rapid Diagnostic Tests and Technologies. London: IntechOpen; 2016. pp. 107-135. DOI: 10.5772/63927

[39] Lu RM, Hwang YC, Liu IJ, et al. Development of therapeutic antibodies for the treatment of diseases. Journal of Biomedical Science. 2020;**27**(1):1. DOI: 10.1186/s12929-019-0592-z. [Published: 02 January 2020]

[40] Lonberg N. Fully human antibodies from transgenic mouse and Phage Display platforms. Current Opinion in Immunology. 2008;**20**(4):450-459. DOI: 10.1016/j.coi. 2008.06.004

[41] Frenzel A, Kügler J, Helmsing S, Meier D, et al. Designing human antibodies by Phage Display. Transfusion Medicine and Hemotherapy. 2017;**44**(5):312-318. DOI: 10.1159/000479633

[42] Reader RH, Workman RG, Maddison BC, Gough KC. Advances in the production and batch reformatting of phage antibody libraries. Molecular Biotechnology. 2019;**61**:801-815. DOI: 10.1007/s12033-019-00207-0

[43] Aghebati-Maleki L, Bakhshinejad B, Baradaran B, et al. Phage Display as a promising approach for vaccine development. Journal of Biomedical Science. 2016;**23**(1):66. DOI: 10.1186/s12929-016-0285-9

[44] Zhao A, Tohidkia MR, Siegel DL, et al. Phage antibody display libraries: A powerful antibody discovery platform for immunotherapy. Critical Reviews in Biotechnology. 2016;**36**(2):276-289. DOI: 10.3109/07388551.2014.958978

[45] Barbas CF, Burton DR, Scott JK, Silverman GJ. Phage Display: A Laboratory Manual. New York: Cold Spring Harbor Laboratory Press: Cold Spring Harbor; 2001

[46] Hammers CM, Stanley JR. Antibody Phage Display: Technique and applications. Journal of Investigative Dermatology. 2014;**134**(2):1-5. DOI: 10.1038/jid.2013.521

[47] Dal Ferro M, Rizzo S, Rizzo E, Marano F, et al. Phage Display Technology for Human Monoclonal Antibodies Methods. Molecular Biology. 1904;**2019**:319-338

[48] Konthur Z, Crameri R. High-throughput applications of Phage Display in proteomic analysis. Targets. Vol.2 n°. 6: 261-270, 2003. DOI: org/10.1016/S1477-3627(03)02383-3

[49] Frei JC, Lai JR. Protein and antibody engineering by Phage Display. Methods in Enzymology. 2016;**580**:45-87. DOI: 10.1016/bs.mie.2016.05.005

[50] Bagheri S, Yousefi M, Safaie Qamsari E, et al. Selection of single chain antibody fragments binding to the extracellular domain of 4-1BB receptor by Phage Display technology. Tumour Biology. 2017;**39**(3):1010428317695924. DOI: 10.1177/101042831 7695924

[51] Fahimi F, Sarhaddi S, Fouladi M, et al. Phage Display-derived antibody fragments against conserved regions of VacA toxin of helicobacter pylori. Applied Microbiology and Biotechnology. 2018;**102**(16):6899-6913. DOI: 10.1007/s00253-018-9068-4

[52] Chen J, Zhao Y, Feng W. Selection, preparation and characterization of scFv against human lipocalin 6 by Phage Display technology. Protein Expression and Purification. 2020;**171**:105627. DOI: 10.1016/j.pep.2020.105627

[53] Noh J, Kim O, Jung Y, et al. High-throughput retrieval of physical DNA for NGS-identifiable clones in Phage Display library. MAbs. 2019;**11**(3):532-545. DOI: 10.1080/19420862.2019.1571878

[54] Christiansen A, Kringelum JV, Hansen CS, et al. High-throughput sequencing enhanced Phage Display enables the identification of patient-specific epitope motifs in serum. Scientific Reports. 2015;**5**:12913. DOI: 10.1038/srep12913. [Published: 06 August 2015]

[55] Maranhão AQ, Silva HM, Da Silva WM, França KA, De Leo TC, Dias-Baruffi M, et al. Discovering selected antibodies from deep-sequenced phage-display antibody library using ATTILA. Bioinformatics and Biology Insights. 2020;**14**:1-8. DOI: 10.1177/1177932220915240

[56] Turner KB, Naciri J, Liu JL, Anderson GP, Goldman ER, Zabetakis D. Next-generation sequencing of a single domain antibody repertoire reveals quality of Phage Display selected candidates. PLoS One. 2016;**11**(2):e0149393. DOI: 10.1371/journal.pone.0149393. [Published: 19 February 2016]

[57] Hemadou A, Giudicelli V, Smith ML, et al. Pacific biosciences sequencing and IMGT/HighV-QUEST analysis of full-length single chain fragment variable from an In vivo selected phage-display combinatorial library. Frontiers in Immunology. 2017;**8**:1796. DOI: 10.3389/fimmu.2017.01796. [Published: 20 December 2017]

[58] Rey FA, Stiasny K, Vaney MC, Dellarole M, et al. The bright and the dark side of human antibody responses to flaviviruses: Lessons for vaccine design. EMBO Reports. 2017;**19**:1-19. DOI: 10.15252/embr.201745302

[59] Huang JX, Bishop-Hurley SL, Cooper MA. Development of anti-infectives using Phage Display: Biological agents against bacteria, viruses, and parasites. Antimicrobial Agents and Chemotherapy. 2012;**56**(9):4569-4582. DOI: 10.1128/AAC.00567-12

[60] Mazumdar S. Raxibacumab. MAbs. 2009;**1**(6):531-538. DOI: 10.4161/mabs.1.6.10195

[61] Chan CE, Lim AP, MacAry PA, Hanson BJ. The role of Phage Display in therapeutic antibody discovery. International Immunology. 2014;**26**(12):649-657. DOI: 10.1093/intimm/dxu082

[62] Sui J, Li W, Murakami A, et al. Potent neutralization of severe acute respiratory syndrome (SARS) coronavirus by a human mAb to S1 protein that blocks receptor association. Proceedings of the National Academy of Sciences of the United States of America. 2004;**101**(8):2536-2541. DOI: 10.1073/pnas.0307140101

[63] Wu Y, Li C, Xia S, et al. Identification of human single-domain antibodies against SARS-CoV-2. Cell Host & Microbe. 2020;**S1931-3128**(20):30250-X. DOI: 10.1016/j.chom.2020.04.023

[64] Messer WB, de Alwis R, Yount BL, et al. Dengue virus envelope protein domain I/II hinge determines long-lived serotype-specific dengue immunity. Proceedings of the National Academy of Sciences of the United States of America. 2015;**112**(20):E2738. DOI: 10.1073/pnas.1317350111

[65] Salazar G, Zhang N, Fu TM, et al. Antibody therapies for the prevention and treatment of viral infections. NPJ Vaccines. 2017;**2**(1):1-12. DOI: 10.1038/s41541-017-0019-3

[66] Barba-Spaeth G, Dejnirattisai W, Rouvinski A, et al. Structural basis of potent Zika–dengue virus antibody cross-neutralization. Nature. 2016;**536**(7614):48-53. DOI: 10.1038/nature18938

[67] Gelanew T, Hunsperger E. Development and characterization of serotype-specific monoclonal antibodies against the dengue virus-4 (DENV-4) non-structural protein (NS1). Virology Journal. 2018;**15**(1):30. DOI: 10.1186/s12985-018-0925-7

[68] Xu H, Di B, Pan YX, et al. Serotype 1-specific monoclonal antibody-based antigen capture immunoassay for detection of circulating nonstructural protein NS1: Implications for early diagnosis and serotyping of dengue virus infections. Journal of Clinical Microbiology. 2006;**44**(8):2872-2878. DOI: 10.1128/JCM.00777-06

[69] Bosch I, De Puig H, Hiley M. Rapid antigen tests for dengue virus serotypes and Zika virus in patient serum. Science Translational Medicine. 2017;**9**(409):eaan1589

[70] Fernandez E, Dejnirattisai W, Cao B, et al. Human antibodies to the dengue virus E-dimer epitope have therapeutic activity against Zika virus infection. Nature Immunology. 2017;**18**(11):1261

[71] Shriver-Lake LC, Liu JL, Zabetakis D, et al. Selection and characterization of anti-dengue NS1 single domain antibodies. Scientific Reports. 2018;**8**(1):18086. DOI: 10.1038/s41598-018-35923-1. [Published: 27 December 2018]

[72] Lebani K, Jones ML, Watterson D, et al. Isolation of serotype-specific antibodies against dengue virus non-structural protein 1 using Phage Display and application in a multiplexed serotyping assay. PLoS One. 2017;**12**(7):e0180669. DOI: 10.1371/journal.pone.0180669. [Published: 06 July 2017]

[73] Cabezas S, Rojas G, Pavon A, et al. Selection of phage-displayed human antibody fragments on dengue virus particles captured by a monoclonal antibody: Application to the four serotypes. Journal of Virological Methods. 2008;**147**(2):235-243

[74] Silva IBB. Prospecção de anticorpos monoclonais humanos anti-Zika por Phage Display. São Paulo: Dissertação [Mestrado em Biotecnologia] – Universidade de São Paulo; 2019

[75] Saokaew N, Poungpair O, Panya A, et al. Human monoclonal single-chain antibodies specific to dengue virus envelope protein. Letters in Applied Microbiology. 2014;**58**(3):270-277. DOI: 10.1111/lam.12186

[76] Lu X, Xiao H, Li S, et al. Double lock of a human neutralizing and protective monoclonal antibody targeting the yellow fever virus envelope. Cell Reports. 2019;**26**(2):438-446.e5. DOI: 10.1016/j.celrep.2018.12.065

[77] Wu Y, Li S, Du L, et al. Neutralization of Zika virus by germline-like human monoclonal antibodies targeting cryptic epitopes on envelope domain III. Emerging Microbes & Infections. 2017;**6**:e89. DOI: 10.1038/emi.2017.79

[78] Mwale PF, Lee CH, Lin LT et al. Expression, purification, and characterization of anti-Zika virus envelope protein: Polyclonal and chicken-derived single chain variable fragment antibodies. International Journal of Molecular Sciences. 2020;**21**(2). pii: E492. DOI: 10.3390/ijms21020492

[79] Moreland NJ, Tay MY, Lim E, et al. High affinity human antibody fragments to dengue virus non-structural protein 3. PLoS Neglected Tropical Diseases. 2010;**4**:e881. DOI: 10.1371/journal.pntd.0000881

[80] Poungpair O, Bangphoomi K, Chaowalit P, et al. Generation of human single-chain variable fragment antibodies specific to dengue virus non-structural protein 1 that interfere with the virus infectious cycle. MAbs. 2014;**6**:474-482. DOI: 10.4161/mabs.27874

Chapter 8

Novel Single Hematophagous Insect RNA Detection Method Supports Its Use as Sentinels to Survey Flaviviruses Circulation

Juliana Sá Teles de Oliveira Molina,
Andreia Moreira dos Santos Carmo, Gabriel Lopes Pereira,
Leticia Abrantes de Andrade, Felipe Trovalim Jordão,
Rodrigo Buzinaro Suzuki, Luana Prado Rolim de Oliveira,
Aline Diniz Cabral and Márcia Aparecida Sperança

Abstract

Anthropogenic actions, including deforestation, disorganized urbanization, and globalization, contribute to emergence and reemergence of arboviruses worldwide, where Flavivirus is the most prevalent, and its continuous monitoring can help in preventive control strategies. Thus, the aim of this study was to detect flavivirus RNA in single hematophagous insects, which are used as sentinels. Total RNA was extracted from six *Aedes aegypti* stored since 2003 and from 100 Culicidae and collected through CDC trap in a public park of a Brazilian Northwest city of São Paulo State. *Flavivirus* was detected through RT/PCR targeting 230–250 bp of the RNA polymerase coding sequence (NS5). PCR amplicons were sequenced by Sanger method, used in comparative analysis over Basic Local Alignment Search Tool (BLAST) in GenBank, and subjected to Neighbor-Joining phylogenetic analyses. Efficiency of *Flavivirus* diagnosis was confirmed by detection of Dengue virus serotype 2 in *Ae. aegypti*. From the 100 collected insects, 19 were positive for *Culex flavivirus* (CxFV). NS5 partial sequence phylogenetic analysis clustered all CxFV in one branch separated from vertebrate flaviviruses, being applicable to the identification of *Flavivirus* species. The dipteran RNA extraction methodology described in this work supports detection of flaviviruses in single insects maintained in 80% ethanol, which can be used to constant arbovirus surveillance.

Keywords: dipteran, *Flaviviruses*, hematophagous insect, molecular diagnosis, RNA extraction, single-insect virus diagnosis

1. Introduction

In recent years, due to anthropogenic actions, including deforestation, disorganized urbanization, and globalization, arboviruses have emerged as a major challenge to global health [1, 2]. The arboviruses (arthropod borne viruses) are transmitted to humans through the bite of infected hematophagous insects, causing febrile diseases [3], with a broad variety of clinical manifestations, ranging from the absence of symptoms to the severe hemorrhagic and encephalitic disorders [4, 5]. The arbovirus vectors include different species of mosquitoes, flies, and ticks. The most worldwide prevalent arboviruses encompass Dengue Virus (DENV), Yellow Fever Virus (YFV), West Nile Virus (WNV), and Zika Virus (ZIKV) from Flaviviridae family and *Flavivirus* genus, and Chikungunya Virus (CHIKV) from family Togaviridae and genus *Alphavirus* [6], which are transmitted through mosquitoes belonging to the Culicidae family, mainly from *Culex* and *Aedes* genera [2].

Arbovirus transmissions occur principally in tropical and subtropical areas, since the presence of vector mosquitoes is associated, mainly, with hot and humid environments, fundamental requirements for their reproduction [7]. Recently, with the global warming and increase in international traveling, the dispersion of arthropod vectors is rising, especially mosquitoes of the genus *Aedes*, and the dissemination of arboviruses is reaching regions considered nonendemic [8–10]. Besides, mosquitoes' high genetic plasticity enables its adaptation to colder environments and international tourism to tropical and subtropical endemic areas, which contributes to arbovirus vectors' global dissemination [11, 12].

Dengue is the most prevalent arbovirus and is responsible for an estimate of 390 million annual cases worldwide [13], and 3.9 billion people, living in 128 countries, are on risk of infection [14]. Since 2010, dengue cases have been reported in non-endemic countries in Europe, including France, Croatia, and Portugal, where in 2012, an outbreak occurred with more than 2000 reported cases. In this period, 10 other European countries were affected by dengue fever. Further, among European travelers returning from low incoming endemic countries, dengue fever is the most diagnosed disease, after malaria [10, 15]. In 2016, more than 3.34 million cases of dengue were reported in American countries, Southeast Asia, and the Western Pacific. Only in the Americas, approximately 2.38 million people were affected, with 1032 deaths, including Brazil, responsible for almost 1.5 million of the reported cases [15]. In addition to Dengue, in Brazil, a South American country with high international touristic activity, according to the Ministry of Health, occurred 216,207 cases of Zika fever, another important emerging *Flavivirus* [16], and 691 cases of yellow fever with 220 confirmed deaths, only in 2016 [17]. This panel entails the flaviviruses negative impact on public health and also causes the economic burden, having direct and indirect consequences [18]. Direct costs include hospitalization, medications, diagnostic tests, vector control, training of professionals, and health surveillance. Among indirect costs are loss of worker productivity and profits, and interference in trade and tourism in affected areas.

There are no effective vaccines available for Dengue, Zika, and Chikungunya fevers [19], and the control of these arboviruses is exclusively implemented by chemical arthropod vector elimination [1]. Therefore, active searching for vectors is necessary to prevent the circulation of known arboviruses. Detection of arboviruses occurs only after detection of human cases, which causes delay in the disease and vector dissemination controls. Thus, to prevent emergency and reemergence of arboviruses, very early detection of vectors and arbovirus and the understanding of their diversity and infection cycle are of great importance. These strategies include also the identification of factors related to the dispersion and entrance of arboviruses in previous indene areas and the identification of wild animal natural reservoirs [20]. Considering the current difficulties in detecting silent circulation of arboviruses and also in obtaining samples from arthropod vectors, human and animal febrile cases, principally in the forests areas, the use of sentinels could be an alternative surveillance approach. Hematophagous insects are present in different wild natural and urban environments, being an excellent group of animal to be used as sentinel. Thus, in this work, the single-insect nucleic acid extraction method [21] was evaluated in hematophagous dipterans collected in a Brazilian municipal public park using CDC traps, in order to detect RNA from flaviviruses.

2. Materials and methods

2.1 Specimens and ethical aspects

A total of 106 insects of the order Diptera were analyzed, of which 100 were collected in the Municipal Park of the city of Marília—São Paulo, and six were specimens of *Aedes aegypti*, RED strain, of which five were experimentally infected with DENV2. More detailed information on the specimens used in this study is shown in **Table 1**. The protocol of collection and transport of arthropods in the Municipal Park of the city of Marília-São Paulo was authorized by the Biodiversity Authorization and Information System (SISBIO), of the Chico Mendes Institute for Biodiversity Conservation (ICMBio), Brazilian Ministry of Environment (MMA), under number 64603-1 (10/18/2018). *Ae. aegypti* strain RED specimens infected with DENV2, maintained in a biosafety level 2 (BSL-2) insectary facility in Institute of Biomedical Sciences from University of São Paulo, were gently donated by Margareth de Lara Capurro Guimarães at the Department of Parasitology of the Institute of Biomedical Sciences of the University of São Paulo (USP), of which five were submitted to infection by DENV-2, while one sample was not submitted to infection and was used as a negative control for DENV. These insects were previously used for purposes that are not related to this study and had approval and permissions needed in their own respective study.

This work did not involve collection of human samples, total or partial, and specimens or tissue samples from vertebrate animals and/or embryos. In addition, no threatened or protected species were collected.

2.2 Single-insect nondestructive RNA extraction

For RNA extraction, each dipteran was digested for 16 h at 56°C, inserted in 200 μL of a lysis buffer composed of 200 mM Tris-HCl (pH 7.5), 250 mM NaCl, 25 mM EDTA (pH 8.0), 0.5% of SDS, and 400 μg/mL of proteinase K as described for DNA extraction [21]. Before digestion, ethanol from insects stored in 80% ethanol was removed after washing twice with 1 mL of 1× PBS (137 mM NaCl, 2.7 mM KCl, 10 mM Na_2HPO_4, and 1.8 mM KH_2PO_4). Following the incubation period,

Taxon	Storage method	Collection local, data	Number of specimens
Anopheles (Culicidae)	Ethanol 80%	Marília-SP, December 2017	3
Phlebotomus (Psychodidae)	Ethanol 80%	Marília-SP, December 2017	2
Ceratopogonidae	Ethanol 80%	Marília-SP, November 2017	3
Cecidomyiidae	Ethanol 80%	Marília-SP, December 2017	1
Culicinae (Culicidae)	Ethanol 80%	Marília-SP, June 2017	91
Aedes aegypti (Culicidae)	Frozen at −20 °C	USP-SP, March 2003	6

Table 1.
Specimens of dipteran included in the study.

the digestion buffer was transferred to 1.5 mL RNase free tube and submitted to RNA purification. One milliliter of 80% ethanol was added to the insect specimen, which was stored in freezer at −20°C. Total RNA purification for each insect from the obtained digestion solution was performed through Qiagen® RNA Mini Kit and PureLink® RNA Mini Kit according to the manufacturer's instructions.

2.3 RNA quality and *Flavivirus* nucleic acid detection

The quality and quantity of extracted RNA from each insect were done through agarose gel electrophoresis and by reverse transcription and polymerase chain reaction (RT/PCR), with oligonucleotides that amplify a 464 bp fragment encoding the 28S ribosomal RNA fraction (28S rRNA) of dipteran (**Table 2**). RNA from each insect was diluted into a final volume of 60 μL of RNase free water, and 4 μL was subjected to 1.5% agarose gel electrophoresis in 0.5× TBE buffer and stained with SafeBlue® according to manufacturer's instructions. Ten insect samples were used to verify quality by RT/PCR, and before RT reaction, 40 μL of the total RNA was treated with DNase I by means of the Biometra Kit from Analytik Jena, following manufacturer's instructions, being diluted in 40 μL of RNase free water. Subsequently, three complementary DNA (cDNA) syntheses were performed, each with a different oligonucleotide, detailed in **Table 2**, being 0.5 μM of oligonucleotide 28SD7r, six bases random primers from Promega, or Oligo dT_{18}. For each cDNA synthesis, 5.5 μL of one insect total extracted RNA, treated with DNase I, was submitted to RT reaction with 200 units of MMLV Reverse Transcriptase (Invitrogen) following fabricator's instructions, in a total volume of 20 μL. Two microliter of the obtained cDNAs was used in PCR to amplify a 464 bp fragment corresponding to 28S rRNA of Dipteran (**Table 2**) through Brazil Platinum Taq DNA polymerase (Invitrogen) according to producer's instructions. PCR condition was one cycle of 94°C for 3 min; 40 cycles of 94°C for 30 s, 50°C for 30 s, and 72°C for 30 s; and 72°C for 7 min. To control DNase I treatment, 5.5 μL of untreated RNA was used directly on PCR. Reaction products were subjected to 1.5% agarose gel electrophoresis in 0.5× TBE buffer, after staining with SafeBlue®.

For *Flavivirus* and DENV-specific detection, 5.5 μL of total RNA was used in RT/PCR with MMLV reverse transcriptase from Invitrogen, to amplify a 250 bp nonstructural protein 5 (NS5) fragment, with the oligonucleotides cFD2 and MAMD (**Table 2**), and a 511 bp fragment, corresponding the junction of the capsid protein (C) and the premembrane protein (prM) of DENV encoding region, through primers D1 and D2 (**Table 2**). The reaction conditions for RT reactions were incubation at 42°C for 1 h, followed by reverse transcriptase inactivation at 80°C for 5 min. PCR conditions for cFD2 and MAMD were 94°C for 3 min; 40 cycles at 94°C for 1 min, 53°C for 1 min, and 72°C for 1 min; and 72°C for 7 min. The same conditions were used with oligonucleotides D1 and D2, except for the association temperature with 50°C. As a positive control of *Flavivirus* amplification, RNA from the Zika Virus and from the vaccine strain of Yellow Fever Virus was used in RT/PCR. PCR products were subjected to 1.5% agarose gel electrophoresis in 0.5× TBE buffer, after staining with SafeBlue®.

2.4 Sequencing and phylogenetic analysis

PCR positive fragments were purified by using the Thermo Scientific GeneJET PCR Purification Kit and sequenced with BigDye 3.1 (Applied Biosystems®) and PCR fragment-specific oligonucleotides, according to manufacturer's instructions. Sequence cycle conditions were 96°C for 1 min; 39 cycles at 96°C for 15 s, 50°C for 15 s, and 60°C for 4 min. After DNA precipitation

Primers	Sequence 5′-3′	Amplicon size	Genomic region	Reference
28SD7forw	AGAGAGAGTTCAAGAGTACGTG	464 bp	28S rRNA (Diptera)	[22]
28SD7rev	TTGGTCCGTGTTTCAAGACGGG			
D1 forw	TCAATATGCTGAAACGCGCGAGAAACC	511 bp	C/prM (DENV)	[23]
D2 rev	TTGCACCAACAGTCAATGTCTTCAGGTTC			
cFD2 rev	GTGTCCCAGCCGGCGGTGTCATCAGC	220–250 bp	NS5 (Flavivirus)	[24]
MAMD forw	AACATGATGGGRAARAGRGARAA			
Oligo dT18	TTTTTTTTTTTTTTTTTT		Poly A tail	

Table 2.
Description of the oligonucleotides used in this study.

with 10% of NaOAc (3 M, pH 5.2), 10% of 1.5 μL of glycogen (1 mg/mL), and two volumes of ethanol, the reactions were pelleted by centrifugation and were washed with 70% of ethanol. The reactions were loaded in an ABI PRISM® 3130XL Genetic Analyzer /HITACHI (16 capillaries). The source and specificity of the obtained sequences were evaluated by BLAST in GenBank [25].

The nucleotide and amino acid partial 226 bp sequence corresponding to the NS5 protein of *Flavivirus* were used to infer the evolutionary history by the Neighbor-Joining method [26]. Phylogenetic trees of confidence value of phylogenetic trees was determined by bootstrap analysis with 1000 replicates, for individual branches [27]. The length of branches was calculated by using the Tamura-Nei method [28] for nucleotides and the Poisson corrected method for amino acid sequences [29]. The coding (first, second, and third codon) and non-coding regions were included in the analysis, and all positions containing gaps and lack of data were discarded only after pairwise comparisons. Phylogenetic analyses were conducted using MEGA4 software [30].

In analysis, partial 16 NS5 sequences of CxFV generated in this study from *Culicidae* mosquitoes from Marilia, São Paulo, were aligned with the corresponding sequences from YFV vaccine strain, Zika Virus, and DENV from serotype 2 and with the sequences deposited in GenBank from CxFV isolated from China in Shanghai (MG602497), Argentina (GenBank KU726615), Africa in Uganda (GenBank GQ165808), and the Brazilian States of Mato Grosso (GenBank KY349933) and São Paulo, and the city of São José do Rio Preto (GenBank KT726939), using the CLUSTAL X [31]. Two alignments were generated to Neighbor-Joining analysis: alignment 1, consisting of nucleotide sequences (226 characters) (S1), and alignment 2, containing amino acid sequences (75 residues) (S2).

3. Results

Agarose gel electrophoresis analysis of the total RNA extracted from 10 specimens of dipteran maintained in 80% ethanol by the nondestructive nucleic acid extraction method described before [21] showed integrity, and an approximately amount of 1 μg/mL, per specimen (**Figure 1**). The presence of RNA was also confirmed by RT/PCR to amplify a 464 bp corresponding to the 28S rRNA from dipteran, after treatment of RNA with DNase I (**Figure 2**). The presence of DNA was observed in all samples (**Figure 2**; DNA). After DNase I treatment, DNA was present in samples 1, 2, 6, and 8, corresponding to PCR products obtained from

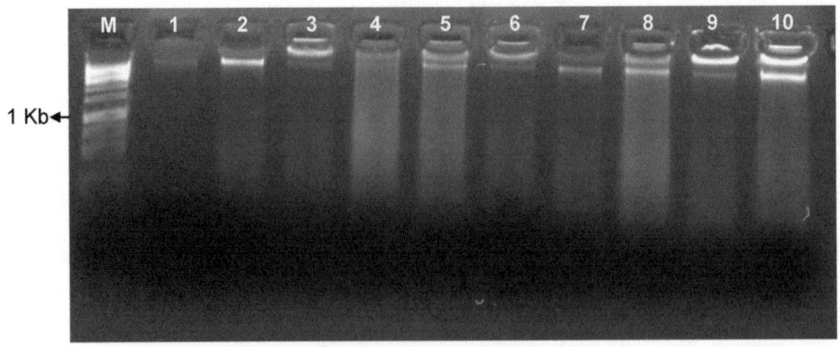

Figure 1.
1.5% Agarose gel electrophoresis containing 4 μL of extracted total RNA from a single dipteran. M, molecular size marker (O'GeneRuler DNA Ladder—1 kb). Lanes 1–10 correspond to different hematophagous dipterans collected in the Municipal Park of the city of Marília—São Paulo.

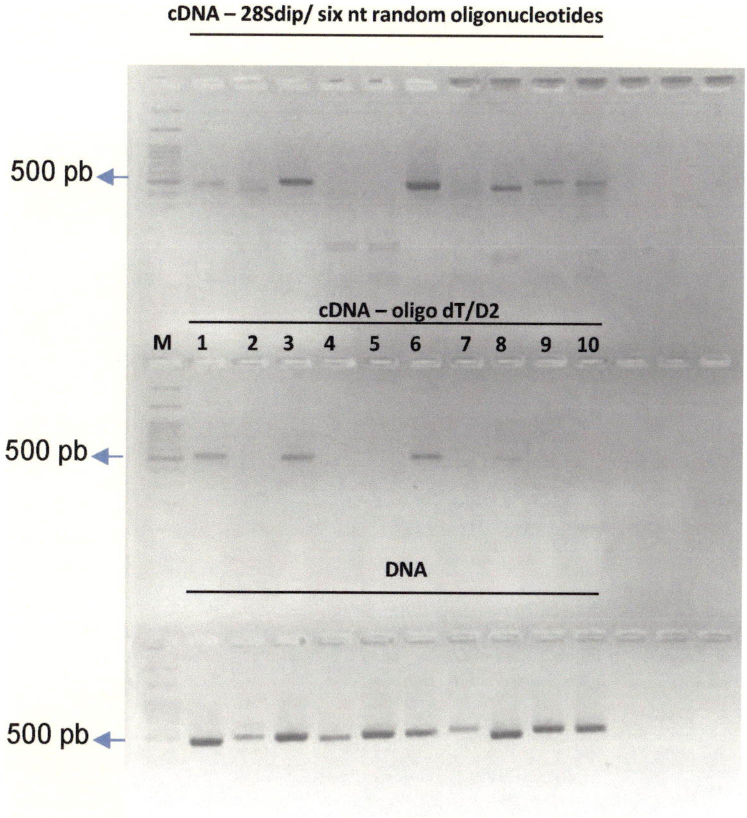

Figure 2.
1.5% Agarose gel electrophoresis containing 10 µL of PCR performed on cDNA and DNA of the dipteran samples. 28Sdip, 6 nt random oligonucleotides, Oligo (dT), and D2 correspond, respectively, to the gene coding for the 28S fraction of the dipteran rRNA, to six nucleotide random oligonucleotides, to a string of 18 deoxythymidylic acid residues that hybridize, and to the gene encoding the dengue virus prM protein, used in cDNA synthesis by reverse transcription reaction. ***DNA****, DNA samples from insects; M, molecular size marker (Sinapse Biotecnologia DNA 100 pb Ladder).*

cDNA synthesized with oligo (dT), which should amplify mRNA and not the 28S rRNA. Specific RNA amplification was observed in samples, 3, 4, 5, 7, 9, and 10, after 28S rRNA PCR performed on cDNA synthesized with random six nucleotides and 28S rRNA-specific oligonucleotides (**Figure 2**).

To verify the feasibility to use the dipteran extracted RNA for *Flavivirus* molecular diagnosis, initially, specimens of *Ae. aegypti* infected with DENV2 and frozen at −20°C, since 2003, were submitted to *Flavivirus* and to DENV-specific diagnostic methods by RT/PCR. **Figure 3** shows that from five *Ae. aegypti* infected with DENV2, four specimens were positive for NS5-based *Flavivirus* detection method. The specificity of the obtained PCR fragments, obtained from each *Ae. aegypti* specimen, was confirmed through Sanger sequencing. The DENV-specific diagnostic based on C/prM encoding gene was negative for all *Ae. aegypti* specimens tested (data not shown).

After *Flavivirus* molecular diagnosis standardization, the NS5-based detection method was applied to the total RNA extracted of the remaining Culicidae specimens included in the study (**Figure 4**), and 19 were positive for a 250 bp PCR fragment, which were sequenced by Sanger method. BLAST evaluation of the 19 amplicons showed 94–96% similarity to CxFV described in Africa, Argentina, China, and Brazil (Cuiabá in the State of Mato Grosso; São José do Rio Preto in the State of Sao Paulo).

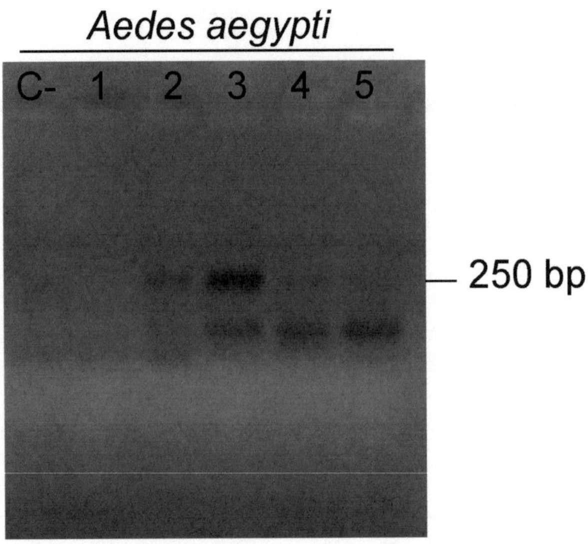

Figure 3.
1.5% Agarose gel electrophoresis stained with SafeBlue® for analysis of the RT/PCR products obtained from Ae. aegypti *infected with DENV-2. C−, PCR negative control performed with water; 1,* Ae. aegypti *uninfected; 2–5, samples of* Ae. aegypti *infected with DENV-2. The PCR reaction was done with primers cFD2 and MAMD, which amplify a 250 bp fragment corresponding to* Flavivirus *NS5 encoding gene.*

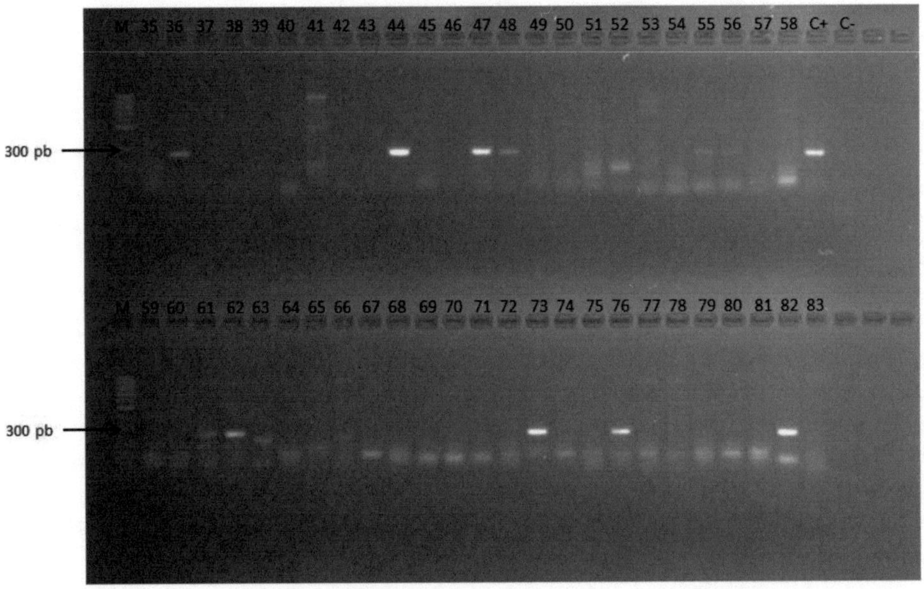

Figure 4.
2% Agarose gel electrophoresis for analysis of Flavivirus *molecular diagnosis based on the 250 bp PCR fragment corresponding to NS5 encoding gene. M, molecular size marker (Sinapse Biotecnologia 100 pb DNA Ladder); C−, negative control (water); C+, positive control (YFV); 35–83, samples of Culicidae mosquitoes collected in the Municipal Park of the city of Marília—São Paulo. Positive samples: 36, 44, 47, 48, 55, 56, 61, 62, 73, 76, and 82.*

Sixteen CxFV nucleotide (226 bp in length) and translated partial NS5 amino acid (75 residues) sequences, with good quality, were used for phylogenetic reconstruction by the Neighbor-Joining method (**Figures 5** and **6**). NS5 nucleotide and amino acidic partial sequence of CxFV obtained from culicids of Marilia

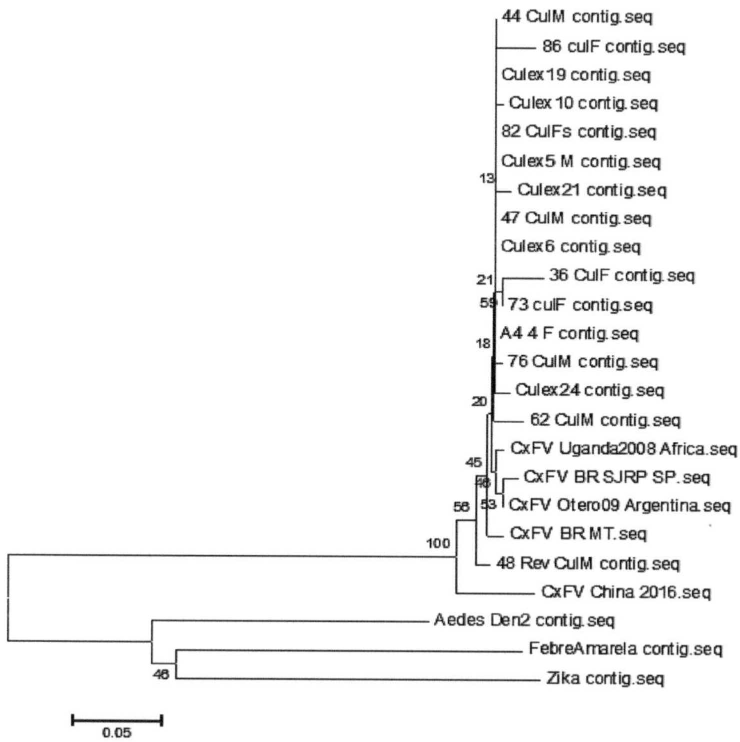

Figure 5.
Phylogenetic analysis based on partial nucleotide sequence of NS5 encoding gene from C. flavivirus. *The figure shows the best tree obtained after Neighbor-Joining phylogenetic analysis with the sum of branch lengths of 1.11310318. The tree was constructed after alignment of 226 nucleotides of 16 translated NS5 partial sequences of* C. flavivirus *obtained from Culicidae mosquitoes from Marilia—São Paulo, YFV vaccine strain, Zika Virus, and DENV2 and sequences recovered from GenBank of* C. flavivirus *isolated from China in Shanghai (MG602497), Argentina (KU726615), Africa in Uganda (GQ165808), and the Brazilian states of Mato Grosso (KY349933) and São Paulo, and the city of São José do Rio Preto (KT726939).*

city varied from 0 to 3% among the same virus species of other Brazilian regions, Africa, Argentina, and China.

The morphological characteristics of 19 CxFV infected dipterans were observed by optical microscopy in order to confirm the taxonomic position and to identify their gender. Nineteen specimens confirmed to belong to the genus *Culex* (Diptera: Culicidae); 9 specimens were females (47.37%), and 10 (52.63%) were males (**Figure 7**). The images were made after RNA extraction, showing the efficiency of the technique in preserving the specimen chitinous skeleton. Blood cells in ingurgitated females are also visible before and after RNA extraction (**Figure 8**).

4. Discussion

The technique of RNA extraction from a single mosquito preserving their chitinous cytoskeleton is described for the first time, and its use can contribute not only to the detection of infectious agents with RNA genome but also to the evolutionary and morphological studies of Diptera since the RNA molecule is an important tool to understand the physiology and evolutionary relationships among organisms [32], and the physical structure of the insect is maintained [21]. Also, vectorial capability of arthropods to several infectious agents can be investigated using specific molecules, with conditional expression profiles, as biomarkers. Molecular identification

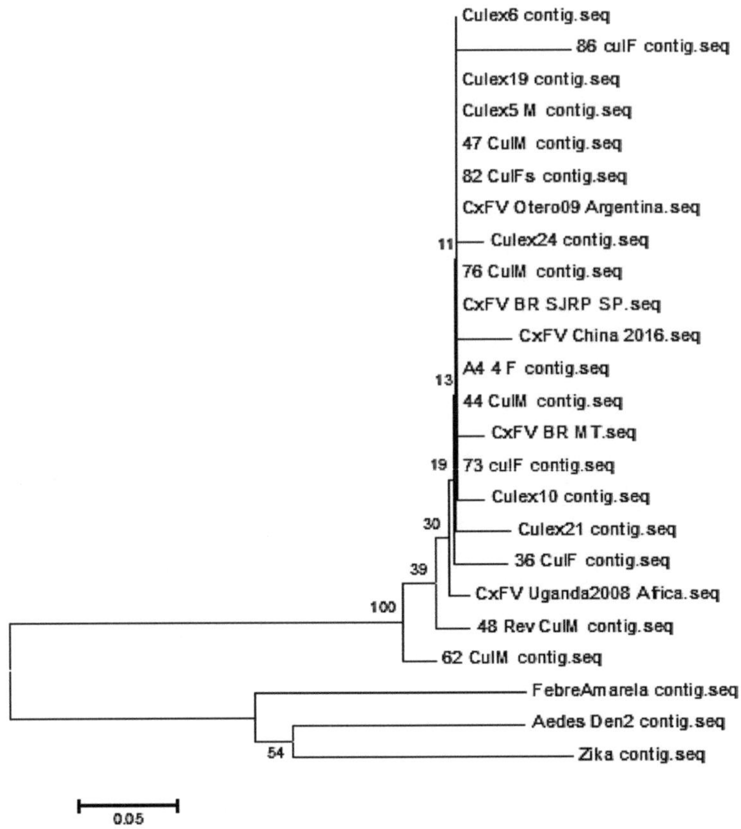

Figure 6.
Phylogenetic analysis based on partial amino acid sequence of NS5 from C. flavivirus. *The figure shows the best tree obtained after Neighbor-Joining phylogenetic analysis with the sum of branch lengths of 0.98879448. The tree was constructed after alignment of 75 amino acids of 16 translated NS5 partial sequences of* C. flavivirus *obtained from Culicidae mosquitoes from Marilia—São Paulo, YFV vaccine strain, Zika Virus, and DENV2 sequences recovered from GenBank of* C. flavivirus *isolated from China in Shanghai (MG602497), Argentina (KU726615), Africa in Uganda (GQ165808), the Brazilian states of Mato Grosso (KY349933) and São Paulo, and the city of São José do Rio Preto (KT726939).*

of the arthropod specimen can be performed by RT/PCR on RNA using oligonucleotides complementary to barcode genes. Also, if DNA is necessary, after proteinase K solution treatment, an aliquot of the arthropod nucleic acid solution can be used for DNA extraction.

Genome of the most important medical arboviruses is composed of RNA, and research works on the detection of these viruses in hematophagous mosquitoes are accomplished on pools of 20–50 specimens, which are macerated and destroyed [33–36]. In this work, a good quality of RNA was obtained from a single dipteran specimen, which was confirmed by electrophoresis in agarose gels (**Figure 1**) and by a specific amplification of a 464 bp fragment of the 28S fraction of diptera rRNA, after DNase I treatment (**Figure 2**). The RNA obtained from a single insect was appropriately to detect DENV-2 in frozen *in vitro* infected *Ae. aegypti* stored for approximately 15 years (**Figure 3**). Probably, the extraction of nucleic acid without maceration of mosquito cells circumvents liberation of high amounts of proteases, which when associated with slow tissue proteinase K digestion preserves the quality of the RNA. These results point toward the possibility to use the presented methodology to investigate undisclosed arthropod vectors through analysis of specific pathogen molecules expressing in the arthropod host. Moreover, since hematophagous dipterans are broadly disseminated, it can also be used as sentinels

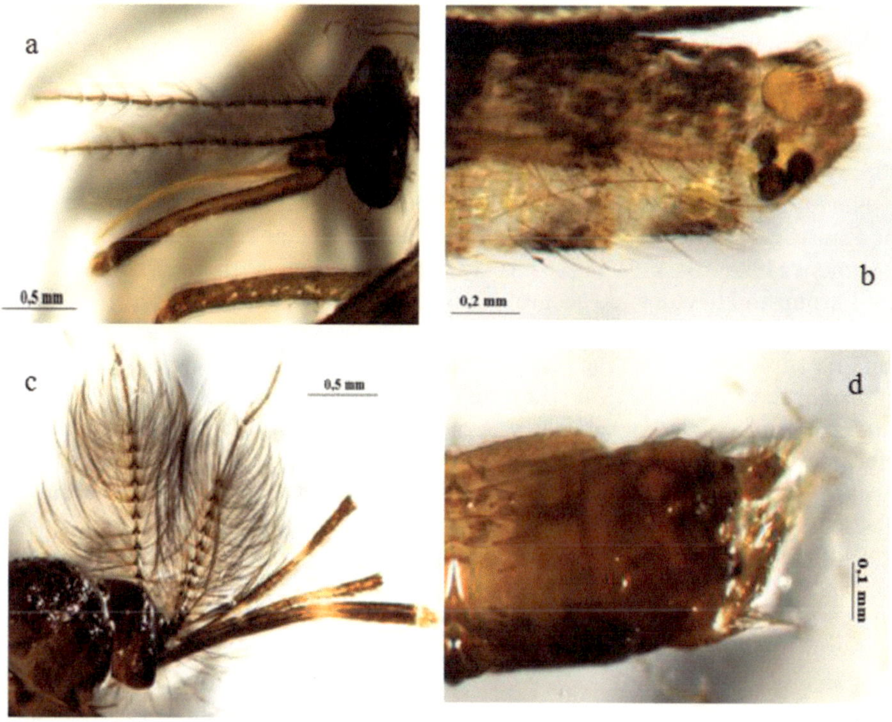

Figure 7.
Morphology of sexual dimorphic structures of Diptera from Culicidae mosquitoes infected with C. flavivirus *after RNA extraction. Head (a) and posterior segment of the abdomen (b) of a female; head (c) and posterior segment of the abdomen (d) of a male.*

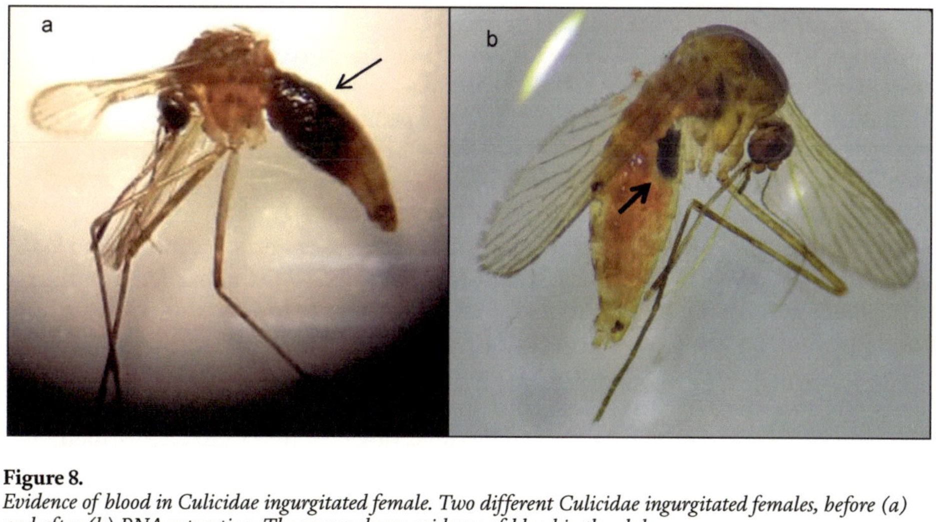

Figure 8.
Evidence of blood in Culicidae ingurgitated female. Two different Culicidae ingurgitated females, before (a) and after (b) RNA extraction. The arrow shows evidence of blood in the abdomen.

of infectious agent presenting RNA genome, contributing directly to epidemiological surveillance of arboviruses.

Different geographical regions present divergences in arthropod infectious diseases vectors diversity and distribution. In Brazil, the main urban vector for YFV is *Ae. aegypti*, whereas in the wild, it is the *Haemagogus janthinomys* [18, 37]. Moreover, a Brazilian study carried out in the Recife city of Pernambuco State revealed the transmission of ZIKV not only by *Culex quinquefasciatus* and but also by *Aedes* mosquitoes, as traditionally accepted [38]. The single insect RNA extraction method facilitates the identification of arboviruses and also the blood source ingurgitated by a dipteran through molecular techniques, since each individual insect feeds on few vertebrates [35] (**Figure 8**). Furthermore, even after nucleic acid extraction, the taxonomic position of the dipteran can be reevaluated (**Figure 7**).

Flavivirus diagnosis of 100 culicids collected in the city of Marilia, from São Paulo Brazilian State, based on NS5, revealed the occurrence of 19 positive specimens (19%) to CxFV. These viruses are part of the insect-specific flavivirus (ISF) group and have a wide geographic distribution, encompassing tropical and temperate regions, in various insect groups [39]. There is evidence that ISF infection may suppress or raise the rate of *in vitro* and/or *in vivo* replication of medical important flaviviruses [40]. A study conducted with Palm Creek virus (PCV), another ISF, originally found in Northern Australia, demonstrated that previously infected insect cells were suppressed for WNV and Murray Valley Encephalitis Virus replication, two important human arboviruses [41]. Virus replication suppression by ISF is also associated with mosquito strains [42], as demonstrated for WNV infection in two different lineages of *C. quinquefasciatus*. The mosquitoes isolated in Honduras presented increased WNV transmission rate when infected with CxFV. The ISF Nhumirim virus (NHUV), first isolated in the Pantanal region of Brazil, was evaluated in the growth and replication rates of ZIKV in insect cells [43]. They found that both in the previously inoculated cells and in cells coinoculated with NHUV, growth, and replication rates of ZIKV were significantly reduced. Also, in this work, the rates of ZIKV infection in *Ae. aegypti* infected with NHUV were significantly reduced, but the transmission rate was maintained. According to Romo (2018), ISFs can be used as models to understand the mechanisms involved in virus interference infection process, which may be used to reduce or suppress infections of important human pathogens in arthropod virus vectors. The methodology described in this work enables investigations of interactions among medical important flavivirus and ISFs at natural mosquito's population level through the use of field collected specimens.

It is believed that *Culex flaviviruses* may be specific to the culicid species and also to the region from which it is obtained [44]. In order to investigate the specificity of CxFV from Marilia, a phylogenetic reconstruction analysis was performed using homologous partial NS5 sequences of CxFV isolates from China, Africa, Argentina, and two Brazilian isolates (one in Mato Grosso and the other in São José of Rio Preto, São Paulo). The nucleotide and amino acid sequences corresponding to the *Flavivirus* partial NS5 protein varied little among then (about 0–3%). Two Neighbor-Joining-based phylogenetic trees constructed with partial NS5 nucleotide (**Figure 5**) and amino acid (**Figure 6**) homologous sequences showed the clustering of flaviviruses in two main branches, one formed by human pathogens (DENV, YFV, and ZIKV), and the other formed by the CxFV. The first branch is formed by taxa that share the same capacity to infect mammalian vertebrate cells, including humans, and present the *Ae. aegypti* as the main vector [45, 46]. The second branch is formed by organisms that differ in origin and time of collection. However, in the tree obtained with the nucleotide sequences, it is possible to observe a clade formed by all the records obtained from Marília, except for the specimen identified by number 48, which was closest to the CxFV of China. This result was different when the tree was constructed with amino acid sequences, where there was no geographical clustering of CxFV. Perhaps, the molecular marker employed in this work is not appropriate to investigate *CxFV* geographical specificity, and more studies are needed to explore the association of their genetic variability with geographical distribution and/or with *Culex* species and strains.

5. Conclusions

The single dipteran RNA extraction technique described in this work permits the use of hematophagous insects as sentinels to detect arboviruses, preserving the chitinous skeleton of the insect and guaranteeing the subsequent morphological studies. The possibility to obtain RNA from a single dipteran also makes possible the investigation of infectious agent's vector capability and the identification of the ingurgitated blood meal source, enabling the description of arthropod alimentary habit and an indication of which vertebrates may be implicated in a virus life cycle. The method also opens the possibility for constant arbovirus surveillance, which can be used to prevent and control epidemics that affect millions of people each year. The presence of CxFV in *C. flavivirus* vectors may interfere with replication, transmission, and infection rates of arboviruses of medical importance, and the method described facilitates natural population studies.

Acknowledgements

Aedes aegypti infected and noninfected with DENV-2 was kindly donated by Dr. Margareth de Lara Capurro Guimarães from the Parasitology Department of the Instituto de Ciências Biomédicas da Universidade de São Paulo. All authors are grateful to the Master Daubian Santos who contributed to morphological analysis of dipterans.

This work was supported by the Fundação de Amparo a Pesquisa do Estado de São Paulo (FAPESP) [grant number 2016/14514-4 and scholarships to Leticia Abrantes Andrade, fellow number 2018/05133-2 and Luana Prado Rolim de Oliveira, fellow number 2019/11384-0]; the Pró-reitoria de Extensão da Universidade Federal do ABC (PROEC-UFABC) [grant number PJ010-2017]; Coordenação de Aperfeiçoamento de Pessoal de Nível Superior (CAPES); and Universidade Federal do ABC (UFABC).

Conflict of interest

The authors declare no conflict of interest.

Author details

Juliana Sá Teles de Oliveira Molina[1], Andreia Moreira dos Santos Carmo[2], Gabriel Lopes Pereira[1], Leticia Abrantes de Andrade[1], Felipe Trovalim Jordão[1], Rodrigo Buzinaro Suzuki[1,3,4], Luana Prado Rolim de Oliveira[1], Aline Diniz Cabral[1] and Márcia Aparecida Sperança[1*]

1 Centro de Ciências Naturais e Humanas, Universidade Federal do ABC, São Paulo, Brazil

2 Secretaria do Estado da Saúde do Estado de São Paulo, Centro de Laboratório Regional VIII, Instituto Adolfo Lutz, São Paulo, Brazil

3 Departmet of Parasitology, Marilia Medical School, São Paulo, Brazil

4 School of Medicine, University of Marilia, São Paulo, Brazil

*Address all correspondence to: marcia.speranca@ufabc.edu.br

References

[1] Coffey LL, Forrester N, Tsetsarkin K, Vasilakis N, Weaver SC. Factors shaping the adaptive landscape for arboviruses: implications for the emergence of disease. Future Microbiology. 2013;**8**(2):155-176

[2] Gubler DJ. The global emergence/resurgence of arboviral diseases as public health problems. Archives of Medical Research. 2002;**33**(4):330-342

[3] Weaver SC. Vector biology in viral pathogenesis. In: Nathanson N, editor. Viral Pathogenesis. New York: Lippincott-Raven; 1997. pp. 329-352

[4] Salimi H, Cain MD, Klein RS. Encephalitic Arboviruses: Emergence, Clinical Presentation, and Neuropathogenesis. Neurotherapeutics. 2016;**13**(3):514-534

[5] Meltzer E. Arboviruses and viral hemorrhagic fevers (VHF). Infectious Disease Clinics of North America. 2012;**26**(2):479-496

[6] Gould E, Pettersson J, Higgs S, Charrel R, de Lamballerie X. Emerging arboviruses: Why today? One Health. 2017;**4**:1-13

[7] Figueiredo LT. Emergent arboviruses in Brazil. Revista da Sociedade Brasileira de Medicina Tropical. 2007;**40**(2):224-229

[8] Kraemer MUG, Reiner RC Jr, Brady OJ, Messina JP, Gilbert M, Pigott DM, et al. Past and future spread of the arbovirus vectors Aedes aegypti and Aedes albopictus. Nature Microbiology. 2019;**4**(5):854-863

[9] Leta S, Beyene TJ, De Clercq EM, Amenu K, Kraemer MUG, Revie CW. Global risk mapping for major diseases transmitted by Aedes aegypti and Aedes albopictus. International Journal of Infectious Diseases. 2018;**67**:25-35

[10] Neumayr A, Munoz J, Schunk M, Bottieau E, Cramer J, Calleri G, et al. Sentinel surveillance of imported dengue via travellers to Europe 2012 to 2014: TropNet data from the DengueTools Research Initiative. Euro Surveillance: Bulletin Europeen Sur les Maladies Transmissibles = European Communicable Disease Bulletin. 2017;**22**(1):1-9

[11] Kraemer MU, Sinka ME, Duda KA, Mylne AQ, Shearer FM, Barker CM, et al. The global distribution of the arbovirus vectors Aedes aegypti and Ae. albopictus. eLife. 2015;**4**:e08347

[12] Javelle E, Florescu SA, Asgeirsson H, Jmor S, Eperon G, Leshem E, et al. Increased risk of chikungunya infection in travellers to Thailand during ongoing outbreak in tourist areas: Cases imported to Europe and the Middle East, early 2019. Euro Surveillance: Bulletin Europeen Sur les Maladies Transmissibles = European Communicable Disease Bulletin. 2019;**24**(10):1-5

[13] Bhatt S, Gething PW, Brady OJ, Messina JP, Farlow AW, Moyes CL, et al. The global distribution and burden of dengue. Nature. 2013;**496**(7446):504-507

[14] Brady OJ, Gething PW, Bhatt S, Messina JP, Brownstein JS, Hoen AG, et al. Refining the global spatial limits of dengue virus transmission by evidence-based consensus. PLoS Neglected Tropical Diseases. 2012;**6**(8):e1760

[15] WHO. Dengue and Severe Dengue. Global: WHO; 2019

[16] Brasil MS. Guia de Vigilância em Saúde. In: Serviços CGdDdEe, vol. único, 2 edn. Brazil: Secretaria de Vigilância em Saúde; 2017

[17] Brasil MS. Boletim Epidemiológico. In: Epidemiológica DdV, vol. 48. Brazil: Secretaria de Vigilância em Saúde; 2018

[18] Mayer SV, Tesh RB, Vasilakis N. The emergence of arthropod-borne viral diseases: A global prospective on dengue, chikungunya and zika fevers. Acta Tropica. 2017;**166**:155-163

[19] Javelle E, Al Balushi A, Jespersen S, Al Abri S, Gautret P, Petersen E. Should travellers be offered vaccination against the dengue virus? Travel Medicine and Infectious Disease. 2019;**27**:2-4

[20] Teixeira Mda G, Barreto ML, Costa Mda C, Ferreira LD, Vasconcelos PF, Cairncross S. Dynamics of dengue virus circulation: A silent epidemic in a complex urban area. Tropical Medicine & International Health. 2002;**7**(9):757-762

[21] Santos D, Ribeiro GC, Cabral AD, Speranca MA. A non-destructive enzymatic method to extract DNA from arthropod specimens: Implications for morphological and molecular studies. PLoS One. 2018;**13**(2):e0192200

[22] Tautz D, Hancock JM, Webb DA, Tautz C, Dover GA. Complete sequences of the rRNA genes of Drosophila melanogaster. Molecular Biology and Evolution. 1988;**5**(4):366-376

[23] Lanciotti RS, Calisher CH, Gubler DJ, Chang GJ, Vorndam AV. Rapid detection and typing of dengue viruses from clinical samples by using reverse transcriptase-polymerase chain reaction. Journal of Clinical Microbiology. 1992;**30**(3):545-551

[24] Scaramozzino N, Crance JM, Jouan A, DeBriel DA, Stoll F, Garin D. Comparison of flavivirus universal primer pairs and development of a rapid, highly sensitive heminested reverse transcription-PCR assay for detection of flaviviruses targeted to a conserved region of the NS5 gene sequences. Journal of Clinical Microbiology. 2001;**39**(5):1922-1927

[25] Mount DW. Using the Basic Local Alignment Search Tool (BLAST). Cold Spring Harbor Protocols. 2007. DOI: 10.1101/pdb.top17

[26] Saitou N, Nei M. The neighbor-joining method: A new method for reconstructing phylogenetic trees. Molecular Biology and Evolution. 1987;**4**(4):406-425

[27] Felsenstein J. Confidence limits on phylogenies: An approach using the bootstrap. Evolution. 1985;**39**(4):783-791

[28] Tamura K, Nei M. Estimation of the number of nucleotide substitutions in the control region of mitochondrial DNA in humans and chimpanzees. Molecular Biology and Evolution. 1993;**10**(3):512-526

[29] Zuckerkandl E, Pauling L. Molecules as documents of evolutionary history. Journal of Theoretical Biology. 1965;**8**(2):357-366

[30] Tamura K, Dudley J, Nei M, Kumar S. MEGA4: Molecular Evolutionary Genetics Analysis (MEGA) software version 4.0. Molecular Biology and Evolution. 2007;**24**(8):1596-1599

[31] Higgins DG, Thompson JD, Gibson TJ. Using CLUSTAL for multiple sequence alignments. Methods in Enzymology. 1996;**266**:383-402

[32] Madigan MT, Martinko JM, Bender KS, Buckley DH, Stahl DA. Microbiologia de Brock - 14ª Edição: Artmed Editora. Brazil: Rio Grande do Sul; 2016

[33] Serra OP, Cardoso BF, Ribeiro AL, Santos FA, Slhessarenko RD. Mayaro virus and dengue virus 1 and 4 natural infection in culicids from Cuiaba, state of Mato Grosso, Brazil. Memórias do Instituto Oswaldo Cruz. 2016;**111**(1):20-29

[34] Ridgeway JA, Timm AE. Comparison of RNA isolation methods from insect larvae. Journal of Insect

Science. 2014;**14**(268):1-5. https://doi.org/10.1093/jisesa/ieu130

[35] Roiz D, Vazquez A, Rosa R, Munoz J, Arnoldi D, Rosso F, et al. Blood meal analysis, flavivirus screening, and influence of meteorological variables on the dynamics of potential mosquito vectors of West Nile virus in northern Italy. Journal of Vector Ecology. 2012;**37**(1):20-28

[36] Machado DC, Mondini A, dos Santos SV, Yonamine PT, Chiaravalloti Neto F, Zanotto PM, et al. First identification of Culex flavivirus (Flaviviridae) in Brazil. Intervirology. 2012;**55**(6):475-483

[37] Brasil MS. Febre Amarela: Ministtério da Saúde atualiza casos no país. In: Epidemiológica DdV. 2018

[38] Guedes DR, Paiva MH, Donato MM, Barbosa PP, Krokovsky L, Rocha S, et al. Zika virus replication in the mosquito Culex quinquefasciatus in Brazil. Emerging Microbes & Infections. 2017;**6**(8):e69

[39] Kim DY, Guzman H, Bueno R Jr, Dennett JA, Auguste AJ, Carrington CV, et al. Characterization of Culex flavivirus (Flaviviridae) strains isolated from mosquitoes in the United States and Trinidad. Virology. 2009;**386**(1):154-159

[40] Blitvich BJ, Firth AE. Insect-specific flaviviruses: a systematic review of their discovery, host range, mode of transmission, superinfection exclusion potential and genomic organization. Viruses. 2015;7(4):1927-1959

[41] Hobson-Peters J, Yam AW, Lu JW, Setoh YX, May FJ, Kurucz N, et al. A new insect-specific flavivirus from northern Australia suppresses replication of West Nile virus and Murray Valley encephalitis virus in co-infected mosquito cells. PLoS One. 2013;**8**(2):e56534

[42] Kent RJ, Crabtree MB, Miller BR. Transmission of West Nile virus by Culex quinquefasciatus say infected with Culex Flavivirus Izabal. PLoS Neglected Tropical Diseases. 2010;**4**(5):e671

[43] Romo H, Kenney JL, Blitvich BJ, Brault AC. Restriction of Zika virus infection and transmission in Aedes aegypti mediated by an insect-specific flavivirus. Emerging Microbes & Infections. 2018;**7**(1):181

[44] Bittar C, Machado DC, Vedovello D, Ullmann LS, Rahal P, Araujo Junior JP, et al. Genome sequencing and genetic characterization of Culex Flavirirus (CxFV) provides new information about its genotypes. Virology Journal. 2016;**13**(1):158

[45] Baleotti FG, Moreli ML, Figueiredo LT. Brazilian Flavivirus phylogeny based on NS5. Memórias do Instituto Oswaldo Cruz. 2003;**98**(3):379-382

[46] Moureau G, Cook S, Lemey P, Nougairede A, Forrester NL, Khasnatinov M, et al. New insights into flavivirus evolution, taxonomy and biogeographic history, extended by analysis of canonical and alternative coding sequences. PLoS One. 2015;**10**(2):e0117849